Cardiology

First and second edition authors

Anjana Siva

Mark Noble

Mohamed K Al-Obaidi

Third edition authors

Ajay Jain

Matthew Ginks

Fourth edition authors

Antonia Churchhouse

Julian Ormerod

5th Edition
CRASH COURSE

SERIES EDITORS

Philip Xiu
MA, MB BChir, MRCP
GP Registrar
Yorkshire Deanery
Leeds, UK

Shreelata Datta
MD, MRCOG, LLM, BSc (Hons), MBBS
Honorary Senior Lecturer
Imperial College London
Consultant Obstetrician and Gynaecologist
King's College Hospital
London, UK

FACULTY ADVISOR

David Newby
BA, BSc (Hons), PhD, BM, DM, DSc, MRCP, FRSE, FMedSci, FESC, FACC
British Heart Foundation John Wheatley Chair of Cardiology
University of Edinburgh
Edinburgh, UK

Cardiology

Thomas Foster
MBChB, BMedSci (Hons)
Junior Doctor
Edinburgh, UK

Jasmine Shen
MBChB
Junior Doctor
Edinburgh, UK

For additional online content visit StudentConsult.com

ELSEVIER

ELSEVIER

Content Strategist: Jeremy Bowes
Content Development Specialist: Alexandra Mortimer
Project Manager: Andrew Riley
Design: Christian Bilbow
Illustration Manager: Karen Giacomucci
Illustrator: MPS North America LLC
Marketing Manager: Deborah Watkins

First edition 1999
Second edition 2004
Third edition 2008
Fourth edition 2013
Updated fourth edition 2015
Fifth edition 2019

The right of Thomas Foster and Jasmine Shen to be identified as author of this work has been asserted by them in accordance with the Copyright, Designs and Patents Act 1988.

Notices
Practitioners and researchers must always rely on their own experience and knowledge in evaluating and using any information, methods, compounds or experiments described herein. Because of rapid advances in the medical sciences, in particular, independent verification of diagnoses and drug dosages should be made. To the fullest extent of the law, no responsibility is assumed by Elsevier, authors, editors or contributors for any injury and/or damage to persons or property as a matter of products liability, negligence or otherwise, or from any use or operation of any methods, products, instructions, or ideas contained in the material herein.

ISBN: 978-0-7020-7357-1
eISBN: 978-0-7020-7358-8

your source for books,
journals and multimedia
in the health sciences
www.elsevierhealth.com

  Working together to grow libraries in developing countries

www.elsevier.com • www.bookaid.org

The publisher's policy is to use **paper manufactured from sustainable forests**

Printed in China
Last digit is the print number: 9 8 7 6 5 4 3 2 1

Series Editors' foreword

The *Crash Course* series was conceived by Dr Dan Horton-Szar who as series editor presided over it for more than 15 years – from publication of the first edition in 1997, until publication of the fourth edition in 2011. His inspiration, knowledge and wisdom lives on in the pages of this book. As the new series editors, we are delighted to be able to continue developing each book for the twenty-first century undergraduate curriculum.

The flame of medicine never stands still, and keeping this all-new fifth series relevant for today's students is an ongoing process. Each title within this new fifth edition has been re-written to integrate basic medical science and clinical practice, after extensive deliberation and debate. We aim to build on the success of the previous titles by keeping the series up-to-date with current guidelines for best practice, and recent developments in medical research and pharmacology.

We always listen to feedback from our readers, through focus groups and student reviews of the *Crash Course* titles. For the fifth editions we have reviewed and re-written our self-assessment material to reflect today's 'single-best answer' and 'extended matching question' formats. The artwork and layout of the titles has also been largely re-worked and are now in colour, to make it easier on the eye during long sessions of revision. The new on-line materials supplement the learning process.

Despite fully revising the books with each edition, we hold fast to the principles on which we first developed the series. *Crash Course* will always bring you all the information you need to revise in compact, manageable volumes that still maintain the balance between clarity and conciseness, and provide sufficient depth for those aiming at distinction. The authors are junior doctors who have recent experience of the exams you are now facing, and the accuracy of the material is checked by a team of faculty editors from across the UK.

We wish you all the best for your future careers!

Philip Xiu and Shreelata Datta

Prefaces

Authors

Cardiology is a popular and competitive specialty that combines history taking and clinical examination with a wide range of investigations and interventions. As cardiovascular disease is the leading cause of death in developed countries a sound understanding of cardiology is vital.

The specialty is constantly evolving with advances in diagnostic tests and novel treatment options. This is reflected in this fully revised fifth Edition, which incorporates both underlying science and its clinical application, combining the material of the *Cardiology* and *Cardiovascular System* textbooks of the fourth edition. As recent graduates we are aware that assessments are changing and as a result have developed an up to date self-assessment section, including Short Answer Questions, Extended Matching Questions, OSCE cases and online-only Clinical Cases.

With this book, our intention is to give quick clear summaries to save you time during a busy rotation or during exam revision. We aim to provide additional details and tips to add to your insight into clinical practice, gain extra points in exams and become a competent junior doctor. We hope that this book also gives you an opportunity to further your interest and enjoyment of cardiology.

We wish you all the best with your studies and future careers!

Jasmine Shen and Thomas Foster

Faculty Advisor

The excellent *Crash Course* series summarizes the key learning points for the 'information overloaded' undergraduate medical student. The series format enhances learning through concise text, comprehension check boxes, and hints and tips boxes. The key salient points are presented in a user friendly and easy to read manner that enables the rapid assimilation of core knowledge.

The fourth edition of *Crash Course: Cardiovascular System* has been integrated with the *Crash Course: Cardiology,* to provide a comprehensive single text bringing together all the knowledge you need for cardiology and cardiovascular medicine. The book incorporates all the essential basic knowledge that provides an invaluable foundation for application to clinical practice. The book takes the reader through first principles to inform the basis and presentation of cardiovascular disease, ultimately leading to the investigation and management of common cardiovascular disorders. This logical sequential progression enhances learning and understanding of the cardiovascular system in clinical medicine.

This book is a 'must' for the time pressed student who needs to use their revision time efficiently and effectively in the modern era of systems-based medical education.

David Newby

Acknowledgements

We would firstly like to thank Professor David Newby for all his help and advice. We also want to acknowledge the whole team at Elsevier and all our clinical teachers over the past few years. Lastly, we would like to thank our families and friends for all their support.

Jasmine Shen and Thomas Foster

Series Editors' acknowledgements

We would like to thank the support of our colleagues who have helped in the preparation of this edition, namely the junior doctor contributors who helped write the manuscript as well as the faculty editors who check the veracity of the information.

We are extremely grateful for the support of our publisher, Elsevier, whose staffs' insight and persistence has maintained the quality that Dr Horton-Szar has set-out since the first edition. Jeremy Bowes, our commissioning editor, has been a constant support. Alex Mortimer and Barbara Simmons our development editors has managed the day-to-day work on this edition with extreme patience and unflaggable determination to meet the ever looming deadlines, and we are ever grateful for Kim Benson's contribution to the online editions and additional online supplementary materials.

Philip Xiu and Shreelata Datta

Contents

Contents

Cardiac anatomy, physiology and development

1

WHY DO WE NEED A CARDIOVASCULAR SYSTEM?

The cardiovascular system serves to provide rapid transport of nutrients to the tissues in the body and allow rapid removal of waste products. In smaller, less complex organisms than the human body there is no such system because their needs can be met by simple diffusion. Evolution of the cardiovascular system provided a means of aiding the diffusion process, allowing the development of larger organisms. The cardiovascular system allows nutrients:

- To diffuse into the system at their source (e.g., oxygen from the alveoli).
- To travel long distances quickly.
- To diffuse into tissues where they are needed (e.g., oxygen to working muscle).

This is an active process requiring a pump: the heart. The functions of the cardiovascular system rely on a transport medium: blood. Blood is made up of cells (mainly red and white blood cells) and plasma (water, proteins, electrolytes, etc.).

Functions of the cardiovascular system

The main functions of the cardiovascular system are:

1. Rapid transport of nutrients (oxygen, amino acids, glucose, fatty acids, water, etc.).
2. Removal of waste products of metabolism (carbon dioxide, urea, creatinine, etc.).
3. Hormonal control, by transporting hormones to their target organs and by secreting its own hormones (e.g., atrial natriuretic peptide).
4. Temperature regulation, by controlling heat distribution between the body core and the skin.
5. Reproduction, by producing penis erection and providing nutrition to the foetus via a complex system of placental blood flow.
6. Host defence, by transporting immune cells, antigens and other mediators (e.g., antibodies).

ANATOMY OF THE HEART AND GREAT VESSELS

Overview of the heart and circulation

The heart consists of two muscular pumps (the left and right ventricles). Each pump has its own reservoir (the left and right atria). The two pumps each serve a different circulation.

The right ventricle is the pump for the pulmonary circulation. It receives blood from the right atrium, which is then pumped through the pulmonary artery into the lungs. Here it is oxygenated and gives up carbon dioxide; it then returns via the pulmonary veins into the left atrium of the heart, and then enters the left ventricle.

The left ventricle is the pump for the systemic circulation. Blood is pumped from the left ventricle via the aorta to the rest of the body. In the tissues of the body, nutrients and waste products are exchanged. Blood returns to the right atrium via the superior and inferior vena cavae.

The two circulations operate simultaneously and are arranged in series. Unidirectional flow is ensured by valves in the heart, pressure differences in the arterial tree and valves in the veins (Fig. 1.1).

CLINICAL NOTE

As the heart consists of two separate pumps, failure of an individual pump is possible, e.g., right heart failure as a result of severe lung disease (cor pulmonale).

The circulatory system is made up of arteries, veins, capillaries and lymphatic vessels:

1. Arteries transport blood from the heart to the tissues.
2. Capillaries are where diffusion of nutrients and waste products takes place.
3. Veins return blood from the tissues to the heart. (The hepatic portal vein is an exception. This transports blood from the intestines to the liver.)
4. Lymphatic vessels return to the blood any excess water and nutrients that have diffused out of the capillaries.

HINTS AND TIPS

Arteries carry oxygenated blood and veins carry deoxygenated blood. The two exceptions to this rule are the umbilical vessels (supplying the foetus) and pulmonary vessels where this is reversed.

The volume of blood ejected from one ventricle during 1 minute is called the cardiac output. The cardiac output of each ventricle is equal overall, but there may be occasional

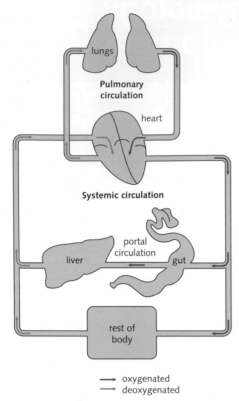

Fig. 1.1 Systemic and pulmonary circulations.

beat-by-beat variation. The entire cardiac output of the right ventricle passes through the lungs and into the left side of the heart. The cardiac output of the left ventricle passes into the aorta, and it is distributed to various organs and tissues according to their metabolic requirements or particular functions (e.g., the kidney receives 20% of cardiac output so that its excretory function can be maintained). This distribution can be changed to meet changes in demand (e.g., during exercise, the flow to the skeletal muscle is increased considerably).

Blood is driven along the vessels by pressure. This pressure, which is produced by the ejection of blood from the ventricles, is highest in the aorta (about 120 mmHg above atmospheric pressure) and lowest in the great veins (almost atmospheric). It is this pressure difference that moves blood through the arterial tree, through the capillaries, and into the veins.

The mediastinum

This is the space between the two pleural cavities. It contains all the structures of the chest except the lungs and pleura. The mediastinum extends from the superior thoracic aperture to the diaphragm and from the sternum to the vertebrae and is divided into superior and inferior parts by the plane passing from the sternal angle to the T4/T5 intervertebral disc. The inferior mediastinum is then

further subdivided into anterior, middle and posterior parts (Fig. 1.2). The contents of each part are shown in Table 1.1. The structures in the mediastinum are surrounded by loose connective tissue, nerves, blood vessels, and lymph vessels. It can accommodate movement and volume changes.

The heart is in the middle mediastinum, and it has the following relations:

1. Superiorly, the great vessels and bronchi.
2. Inferiorly, the diaphragm.
3. Laterally, the pleurae and lungs.
4. Anteriorly, the thymus.
5. Posteriorly, the oesophagus.

The structures visible on a normal chest X-ray are shown in Fig. 1.3.

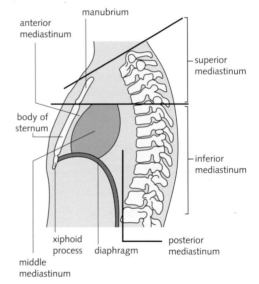

Fig. 1.2 Lateral view of the mediastinum.

Table 1.1 Contents of the mediastinum

Mediastinal compartment	Contents
Superior	Great vessels Thymus Trachea Oesophagus
Anterior	Internal thoracic arteries Thymus
Middle	Heart and pericardium Origins of the great vessels
Posterior	Descending aorta Oesophagus Sympathetic chain

Fig. 1.3 Normal posteroanterior (PA) chest X-ray. *1*, Arch of aorta/aortic knuckle; *2*, clavicle; *3*, left atrial appendage; *4*, left dome of diaphragm; *5*, left lung; *6*, left hilum; *7*, left ventricular border; *8*, pulmonary trunk; *9*, right atrial border; *10*, right dome of diaphragm; *11*, right lung; *12*, right hilum; *13*, spine of vertebrae; *14*, trachea. (Courtesy Professor Dame M. Turner-Warwick, Dr. M. Hodson, Professor B. Corrin and Dr. I. Kerr.)

Pericardium

This is the fibroserous sac that surrounds the heart. It consists of two layers, between which there is a small amount of pericardial fluid. The pericardium is fused with the central tendon of the diaphragm at its base, the sternum by the sternopericardial ligament anteriorly and with the tunica adventitia of the great vessels.

CLINICAL NOTE

When fluid accumulates within the pericardial sac this is called a pericardial effusion. If it builds up quickly and begins to affect cardiac function this is called cardiac tamponade. (Both are described in Chapter 17.)

External structure of the heart

The heart lies obliquely about two-thirds to the left and one-third to the right of the median plane (Figs 1.4–1.6). It has the following surfaces:

1. The base of the heart is located posteriorly and formed mainly by the left atrium.
2. The apex of the heart is formed by the left ventricle and is posterior to the fifth intercostal space.

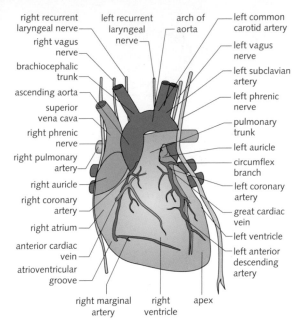

Fig. 1.4 Sternocostal external view of the heart.

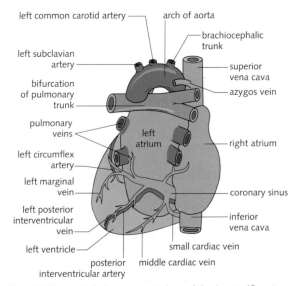

Fig. 1.5 Posteroinferior external view of the heart. (Courtesy of Professor Dame M. Turner-Warwick, Dr. M. Hodson, Professor B. Corrin and Dr. I. Kerr.)

3. The sternocostal surface of the heart is formed mainly by the right ventricle.
4. The diaphragmatic surface is formed mainly by the left ventricle and part of the right ventricle.
5. The pulmonary surface is mainly formed by the left ventricle.

The heart borders of the anterior surface are as follows:

1. Right: right atrium.
2. Left: left ventricle and left auricle.
3. Inferior: right ventricle mainly and part of left ventricle.
4. Superior: right and left auricles.

Fig. 1.6 Surface markings of the heart (*a*, aortic valve; *m*, mitral valve; *p*, pulmonary valve; *t*, tricuspid valve). These are anatomical relations – see Fig. 5.5 for auscultatory areas.

Internal structure of the heart

The internal structure of the heart is shown in Fig. 1.7. The right atrium contains the orifices of the superior and inferior venae cavae and coronary sinus. The right ventricle is separated from the right atrium by the tricuspid (three cusps) valve. The right ventricle is separated from its outflow tract (the pulmonary trunk) by the pulmonary valve. This has three semilunar valve cusps.

The left atrium has the orifices of four pulmonary veins in its posterior wall and is separated from the left ventricle by the mitral (sometimes referred to as bicuspid, i.e., two cusps) valve. The left ventricle is separated from its outflow tract (the aorta) by the aortic valve, which also has three semilunar valve cusps.

Coronary arteries

The coronary arteries are shown in Figs 1.8 and 1.9. The left coronary artery arises just distal to the left anterior cusp of the aortic valve. The right coronary artery arises from the right anterior aortic sinus just above the right anterior cusp of the aortic valve. The coronary arteries are the first branches of the aorta; the heart supplies itself with a blood supply before any other organ.

Coronary veins

The coronary veins drain mainly into the coronary sinus, which drains directly into the right atrium (Figs 1.10 and 1.11). There are some small veins that drain directly into the heart chambers. Generally, these drain into the right side of the heart.

Great vessels

'Great vessels' is the term used to denote the large arteries and veins that are directly related to the heart. The great arteries include the pulmonary trunk and the aorta (and sometimes its three main branches: the brachiocephalic, the left common carotid, and the left subclavian). The great veins include the pulmonary veins and the superior and inferior venae cavae. The great vessels and their thoracic branches are illustrated in Figs 1.12–1.14.

Tissue layers of the heart and pericardium

Figure 1.15 shows the tissue layers of the heart and pericardium.

Pericardium

The pericardium consists of an outer fibrous pericardial sac, enclosing the whole heart, and an inner double layer of flat mesothelial cells, called the serous pericardium. The two layers of the serous pericardium are:

1. The parietal pericardium, which is attached to the fibrous sac.
2. The visceral pericardium, which forms part of the epicardium and which covers the heart's outer surface.

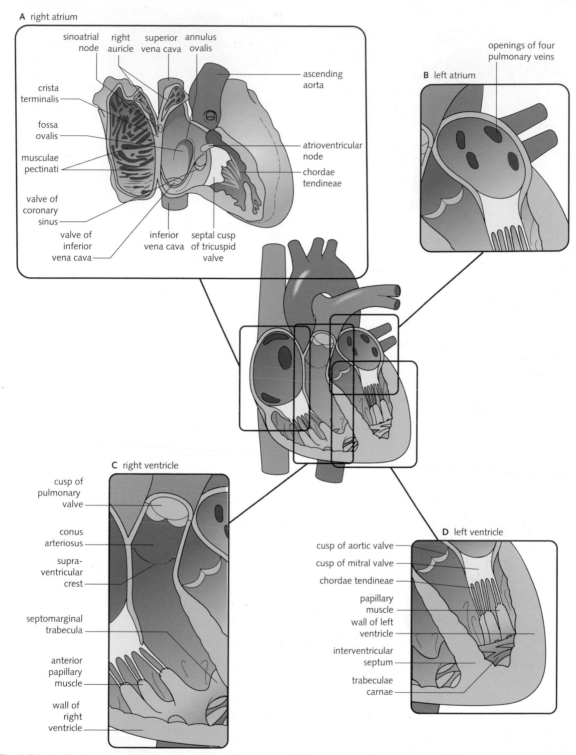

A right atrium

sinoatrial node
right auricle
superior vena cava
annulus ovalis

openings of four pulmonary veins

B left atrium

ascending aorta

crista terminalis

fossa ovalis

musculae pectinati

atrioventricular node

chordae tendineae

valve of coronary sinus

valve of inferior vena cava

inferior vena cava

septal cusp of tricuspid valve

C right ventricle

cusp of pulmonary valve

conus arteriosus

supra-ventricular crest

septomarginal trabecula

anterior papillary muscle

wall of right ventricle

D left ventricle

cusp of aortic valve

cusp of mitral valve

chordae tendineae

papillary muscle

wall of left ventricle

interventricular septum

trabeculae carnae

Fig. 1.7 Internal structure of the four chambers of the heart. (A) Right atrium. (B) Left atrium. (C) Right ventricle. (D) Left ventricle.

Fig. 1.10 Anterior view of the heart showing coronary veins.

Fig. 1.8 Anterior surface of the heart showing coronary arteries. The left coronary artery has two terminal branches: the anterior interventricular branch (also called the left anterior descending artery, or 'widow's artery') and the circumflex branch. The anterior interventricular branch supplies both ventricles and the interventricular septum. The circumflex branch supplies the left atrium and the inferior part of the left ventricle. The right coronary artery supplies the sinoatrial node via the right atrial branch.

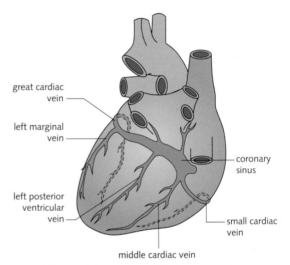

Fig. 1.11 Posteroinferior view of the heart showing coronary veins.

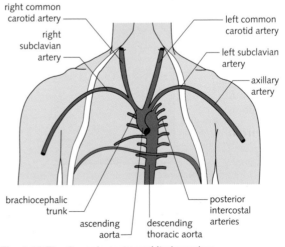

Fig. 1.9 Posteroinferior surface of the heart showing coronary arteries. The right coronary artery gives off a right marginal branch and a large posterior interventricular branch. Near the apex, the posterior interventricular branch may anastomose with the anterior interventricular branch of the left coronary artery. The right coronary artery mainly supplies the right atrium, right ventricle, and interventricular septum. It may also supply part of the left atrium and left ventricle. The nodal branch supplies the atrioventricular node.

Fig. 1.12 The thoracic aorta and its branches.

Fig. 1.13 Veins of the thorax.

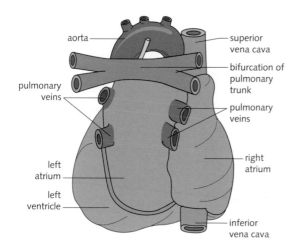

Fig. 1.14 Posterior view of the pulmonary vessels.

The serous pericardium produces approximately 50 mL of pericardial fluid, which sits in the pericardial cavity formed by the parietal and visceral layers. The primary function of this fluid is to provide lubrication so that the heart can move within the pericardium during the cardiac cycle.

Heart

The heart itself contains three layers:

- Epicardium.
- Myocardium.
- Endocardium.

Epicardium

The epicardium is a thin layer of connective tissue that contains adipose tissue, nerves and the coronary arteries and veins.

Myocardium

The myocardium is the thickest layer of the heart, and it is made up of cardiac muscle cells. The myocardium is thickest in the left ventricle and thinnest in the atria.

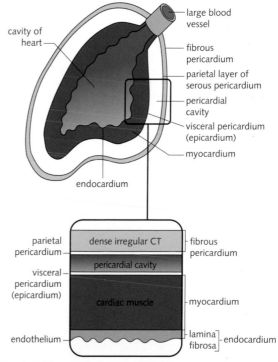

Fig. 1.15 Tissue layers of the heart and pericardium (*CT*, connective tissue).

All the muscle layers attach to the fibrocollagenous heart skeleton, which provides a stable base for contraction. The atrial myocardium secretes atrial natriuretic peptide (ANP) when stretched, promoting salt and water excretion. The ventricular myocardium secretes brain natriuretic peptide (BNP) when stretched, which seems rather a misnomer. BNP is sometimes used to monitor left ventricular dysfunction in heart failure.

Endocardium

The endocardium has three layers: an outermost connective tissue layer (which contains nerves, veins and Purkinje fibres) a middle layer of connective tissue and an endothelium of flat endothelial cells.

Heart valves

The heart valves are avascular (i.e., they have no blood supply) (Fig. 1.16). This is important if bacteria invade the valves because there is little immune reaction and infective endocarditis may result. Their avascular nature also means that they can be replaced with a porcine (pig) or bovine (cow) tissue valve without generating a rejection-like immune response.

Cardiac myocytes

There are three types of myocytes – work myocytes, nodal cells and conduction fibres:

1. Work myocytes are the main contractile cells.
2. Nodal cells make up the SA node and AV node, and generate cardiac electrical impulses.
3. Conduction (Purkinje) fibres have a greater diameter than work myocytes (70–80 μm) and allow fast conduction of action potentials around the heart.

Ultrastructure of the typical cardiomyocyte

The typical cardiac myocyte (Fig. 1.17) has the following features:

1. Length of 50–100 μm (shorter than skeletal muscle fibres).
2. Diameter of 10–20 μm.

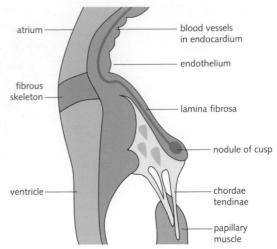

Fig. 1.16 Structure of a heart valve.

3. Single, central nucleus.
4. Branched structure.
5. Attached to neighbouring cells via intercalated disks at the branch points. These cell junctions consist of desmosomes (which hold the cells together via proteoglycan bridges) and gap junctions (which allow electrical conductivity).
6. Many mitochondria arranged in rows between the intracellular myofibrils.

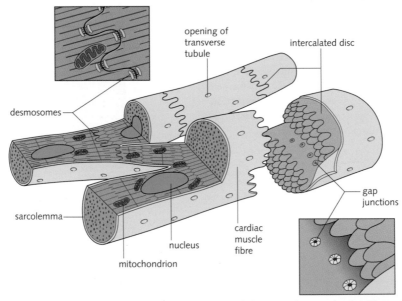

Fig. 1.17 Cardiac myocyte arrangement. Myocytes are branched, and they attach to each other through desmosomes to form muscle fibres. Gap junctions enable rapid electrical conductivity between cells. There is an extensive sarcoplasmic reticulum, which is the internal Ca²⁺ store. The contractile elements within each cell produce characteristic bands and lines. In between each myofibril unit there are rows of mitochondria. Accompanying blood vessels and connective tissue lie alongside each muscle fibre. (Redrawn with permission from Tortora, G.J., Grabowski, S.R., 2000. Principles of anatomy and physiology, ninth ed. John Wiley & Sons, New York.)

7. T (transverse) tubules organized in diads with cisternae of sarcoplasmic reticulum (Fig. 1.18), which enable rapid electrical conduction deep into the cell, activating the whole contractile apparatus.
8. Extensive sarcoplasmic reticulum, which stores Ca^{2+} ions necessary for electrical activity and contraction.

Each myocyte contains many myofibril-like units (similar to the myofibrils of skeletal muscle) (see Fig. 1.18). These units are made up of sarcomeres attached end-to-end and collected into a bundle. A sarcomere is the basic contrac-

tile unit. It is composed of two bands, the A band and the I band, between two Z lines.

1. The A (anisotropic) band is made up of thick myosin filaments and some interdigitating actin filaments.
2. The I (isotropic) band is made up of thin actin filaments that do not overlap with myosin filaments. Troponin and tropomyosin are also contained in the thin filaments.
3. The Z line is a dark-staining structure containing α-actinin protein that provides attachment for the thin filaments.

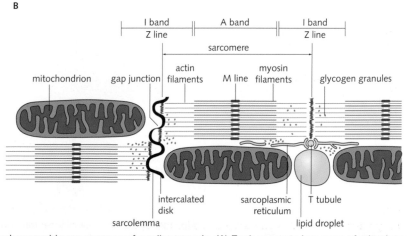

Fig. 1.18 Electron micrographic appearance of cardiac muscle. (A) Each myocyte has rows of mitochondria in between myofibril-like units. There is also an extensive sarcoplasmic reticulum and T tubule system. (B) Close-up of a myofibril-like unit shows the following bands: A band, myosin with some actin; I band, actin; Z line, attachment point for actin; M line links myosin fibres. (Reproduced with permission from [A] Williams, P.L. (Ed.), 1989. Gray's anatomy, thirty-seventh ed. Churchill Livingstone, Edinburgh; [B] Davies, A., Blakeley, A.G.H., Kidd, C., 2001. Human physiology. Churchill Livingstone, Edinburgh.)

DEVELOPMENT OF THE HEART AND GREAT VESSELS

The heart develops in the cardiogenic region of the mesoderm from week 3. This region is at the cranial end of the embryonic disc. Angioblastic cords (aggregates of endothelial cell precursors) develop and here they coalesce to form two lateral endocardial tubes. During week 4, these tubes fuse together to form the primitive heart tube and the heart begins to pump (Fig. 1.19).

From weeks 5 to 8, the primitive heart tube folds and remodels to form the four-chambered heart. Initially, the primitive heart tube develops a series of expansions separated by shallow sulci (infoldings) (Fig. 1.20).

The primitive atrium will give rise to parts of both future atria. The primitive ventricle will make up most of the left ventricle. The bulbus cordis will form the right ventricle. The truncus arteriosus will form the ascending aorta and the pulmonary trunk.

Venous blood initially enters the sinus horns of the sinus venosus from the cardinal veins (a branch of the umbilical vein). Within the next few weeks, the whole systemic venous return is shifted to the right sinus horn through the newly formed superior and inferior venae cavae. The left sinus horn becomes the coronary sinus, which drains the myocardium.

HINTS AND TIPS

Embryology terms can be understood by considering what process the term describes. For example, the septum primum is the first septum to form (*primus* means first in Latin), and septum secundum is the second septum to form.

In weeks 5–6, the septum primum and the septum secundum grow to separate the right and left atria (Fig.1.21). These septa are incomplete and leave two openings (foramina or ostia) that allow blood to move between the atria. The septum primum grows downwards from the superior posterior wall. The foramen (ostium primum) it creates narrows as the septum grows.

While the septum primum is growing, the thicker septum secundum also starts to form. This septum secundum does not meet the septum intermedium, leaving an opening called the foramen ovale near the floor of the right atrium.

Blood now has to shunt from the right to the left atrium through the two staggered openings in the septum, the foramen ovale and the ostium secundum (Fig. 1.22). At

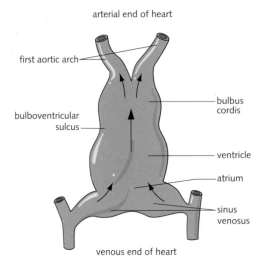

Fig. 1.19 Primitive heart tube at 21 days.

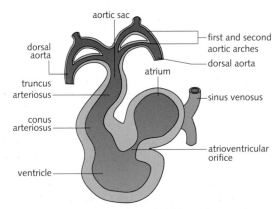

Fig. 1.20 Primitive heart tube as it folds and expands.

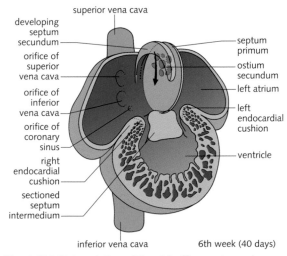

Fig. 1.21 Initial septation of the atria. The septum primum forms at day 33, and eventually leaves a hole (the ostium secundum). The septum secundum develops later, at day 40, and is deficient at the foramen ovale. (Redrawn with permission from Larsen, W.J., 1997. Human embryology, second ed. Churchill Livingstone, Edinburgh.)

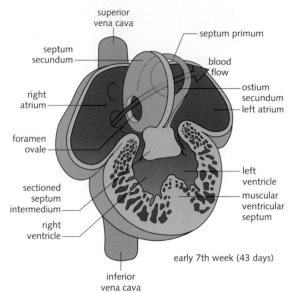

superior
vena cava

septum primum

septum
secundum

blood
flow

right
atrium

ostium
secundum

left atrium

foramen
ovale

left
ventricle

sectioned
septum
intermedium

muscular
ventricular
septum

right
ventricle

early 7th week (43 days)

inferior
vena cava

Fig. 1.22 Completed septation of the atria. The septum primum is deficient superiorly at the ostium secundum. The septum secundum is deficient inferiorly at the foramen ovale. Blood shunts from the right atrium through these two holes in the septa to the left atrium. In this way, blood bypasses the lungs in the foetal circulation. As these two openings are staggered, fusion of the septum primum and secundum will abolish any shunt between the atria. (Redrawn with permission from Larsen, W.J., 1997. Human embryology, second ed. Churchill Livingstone, Edinburgh.)

birth, the two septa are fused together to abolish any foramen between the two atria.

During weeks 5–6, the atrioventricular (tricuspid and mitral) valves develop. The heart undergoes some changes that bring the atria and ventricles into their correct positions and align the outflow tracks with the ventricles.

The inferior part of the bulboventricular sulcus grows into the muscular ventricular septum. Growth stops in week 7 to wait for the left outflow track to develop, leaving an interventricular foramen.

In weeks 7–8, the truncus arteriosus (the common outflow tract of the heart) is divided in two by a spiral process of central septation, which results in the formation of the aorta and pulmonary trunk. This septum is called the truncoconal septum. This septum also grows into the ventricles, and it forms the membranous ventricular septum, which joins the muscular ventricular septum. This completes the septation of the ventricles. Swellings develop at the inferior end of the truncus arteriosus, and these give rise to the arterial (pulmonary and aortic) valves.

Development of the vasculature

The vasculature develops from the angioblastic cords of mesoderm. The aortic ends of the primitive heart tube become the aortic arches and dorsal aortae. The aortic arches develop into the great arteries of the neck and thorax, and the dorsal aortae develop branches which supply the rest of the body. The paired dorsal aortae connect to the umbilical arteries, which carry blood to the placenta.

The umbilical veins carry oxygenated and nutrient-rich blood from the placenta to the foetus. The venous system (from the foetus, yolk sac and umbilical veins) drains into the sinus horns, and subsequently into the venae cavae and right atrium.

The ductus venosus shunts a portion of blood from the umbilical vein directly into the inferior vena cava during gestation. This is vital as it allows oxygenated blood to enter the right atrium of the heart, to be pumped around the foetus.

The lungs are not functional during gestation, negating the need for a large pulmonary circulation. The pulmonary circulation is largely bypassed by two mechanisms. The foramen ovale enables most of the oxygenated blood in the right atrium to pass into the left atrium and reach the systemic circulation. The ductus arteriosus develops from the sixth aortic arch, and connects the pulmonary arteries to the descending aorta. This allows oxygenated blood not shunted through the foramen ovale to enter the systemic circulation directly. The duct is kept open during foetal life by circulating prostaglandins, and this stimulation may be continued artificially early in the neonatal period.

Circulatory adaptations at birth

A series of changes convert the single system of blood flow around the foetus into dual systems at birth (Figs 1.23 and 1.24). Blood flow in the umbilical vessels drastically declines in the first few minutes after birth because of:

- Compression of the cord.
- Vasoconstriction in response to cold, mechanical stimuli and circulating foetal catecholamines as a result of the stress of descending through the birth canal.

At birth, the pulmonary vascular resistance falls rapidly because:

- The thorax of the foetus is compressed on descent, emptying the amniotic fluid from the lungs.
- The mechanical effort of ventilation opens the constricted alveolar vessels.
- Raising PO_2 and lowering PCO_2 cause vasodilatation of the pulmonary vessels.

This produces an increase in the pulmonary blood flow.

The sudden cessation of umbilical blood flow and the opening of the pulmonary system cause a change in the pressure balance in the atria. There is a pressure drop in the right atrium and a pressure rise in the left atrium (caused by an increased pulmonary venous return to the left atrium). This changes the pressure gradient across the atrial septum and forces the flexible septum primum against the rigid septum secundum, closing the foramen ovale. These two septa fuse together after about 3 months.

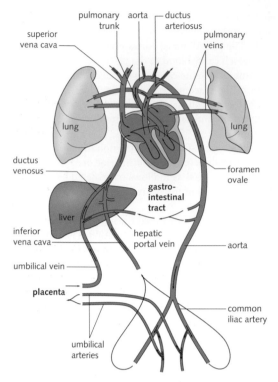

Fig. 1.23 Foetal circulation in utero.

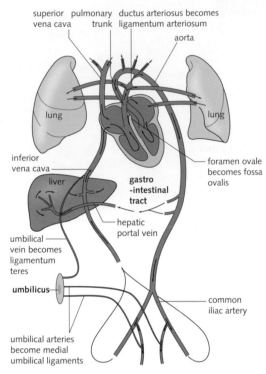

Fig. 1.24 Neonatal circulation after birth. Note the closure of the foetal shunts (foramen ovale, ductus arteriosus, and ductus venosus) and umbilical vessels.

The ductus arteriosus closes 1–8 days after birth. It is thought that as the pulmonary vascular resistance falls, the pressure drop in the pulmonary trunk causes blood to flow from the aorta into the pulmonary trunk through the ductus arteriosus. This blood is oxygenated and the increase in PO_2 causes the smooth muscle in the wall of the ductus to constrict due to decreased prostaglandin production, obstructing the flow in the ductus arteriosus. Eventually, the intima of the ductus arteriosus thickens – complete obliteration of the ductus results in the formation of the ligamentum arteriosum, which attaches the pulmonary trunk to the aorta.

The ductus venosus closes soon after birth and becomes a remnant known as the ligamentum venosus. The mechanism is unclear, but it is thought to involve prostaglandin inhibition. The closure is not vital to life as the umbilical vein no longer carries any blood.

● Chapter Summary

- The cardiovascular system is vital to the survival of all other tissues in the human body.
- The right ventricle pumps blood to the pulmonary circulation, and the left ventricle pumps blood to the rest of the body.
- Knowledge of the coronary arterial anatomy is important when considering which region of the myocardium is affected in ischaemic heart disease, and allows prediction of clinical sequelae.
- Appreciation of the development of the foetal circulation and its changes after birth are essential to understanding congenital heart abnormalities and their effects.

CARDIAC ELECTROPHYSIOLOGY

Unlike skeletal muscle, the heart possesses intrinsic electrical activity and does not require nervous input to initiate contraction. This activity originates at the sinoatrial (SA) node, a cluster of specialized myocytes that depolarize spontaneously, sometimes referred to as the heart's pacemaker. Cardiomyocytes can be broadly divided into two categories in terms of their electrophysiological behaviour and function, and the appearance of their action potentials:

- Fast depolarizing cells, such as atrial and ventricular myocardial cells, and cells of the His–Purkinje system. These are often referred to as work myocytes.
- Slow depolarizing cells, such as those forming the SA node and atrioventricular (AV) node. These are often referred to as pacemaker cells or nodal cells.

The conduction system

In order for the heart to function effectively, the electrical impulse/action potential generated by the SA node must propagate through the heart in a coordinated manner. This is facilitated by a specialized conduction system (Fig. 2.1) and the presence of low resistance gap junctions, which allow direct spread of depolarization between cells. The SA node is located in the posterior wall of the right atrium at the junction with the superior vena cava. From the SA

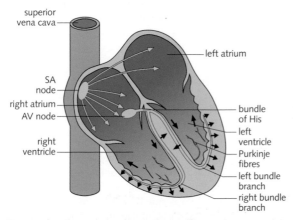

Fig. 2.1 Cardiac conduction pathway. The action potential is initiated in the sinoatrial (*SA*) node and spreads throughout the atria. It travels through the atrioventricular (AV) node and then to the bundle of His. From here it travels down the left and right bundle branches and into Purkinje fibres. The action potential is then spread throughout the ventricles.

node, the impulse passes through the atrial myocardium to the AV node, where conduction is delayed by approximately 100 ms to allow completion of atrial contraction before ventricular depolarization.

The AV node, located at the top of the interventricular septum, is the only point where current can pass through the fibrous skeleton from the atria to the ventricles (in a healthy heart). The AV node is also able to act as a back-up pacemaker in situations when the SA node ceases to function or communication between the SA node and AV node is interrupted. The impulse then enters the bundle of His, which splits into right and left bundle branches. The left bundle branch is sub-divided into anterior and posterior hemifascicles. These bundles give off fine fibres composed of specialized cardiomyocytes (called Purkinje fibres) that penetrate into the ventricular myocardium.

HINTS AND TIPS

Remember that the cells comprising the conduction systems are specialized cardiac muscle cells, NOT nerves.

Resting membrane potential

The electrical potential across a plasma membrane is determined by two main factors:

- Distribution of ions across the membrane.
- Selective permeability of the cell membrane.

In cardiomyocytes, potassium (K^+) ions are the major determinant of resting membrane potential because large numbers of K^+ channels are open constitutively. These 'leak' K^+ channels mean that permeability to K^+ is high and there is a constant efflux of K^+, referred to as the 'outward background current'. The resting membrane is only slightly permeable to sodium (Na^+), and because both the electrical and chemical gradients favour inward movement of Na^+ ions, there is a very small inward Na^+ current, which is often referred to as the 'inward background current'. The intracellular and extracellular concentrations of these ions (Fig. 2.2) are maintained by the activity of the Na^+/K^+ATPase on the sarcolemmal membrane (muscle cell membrane).

Cardiac action potential

An action potential is a transient depolarization of the cell membrane. Action potentials are initiated when the membrane is depolarized (i.e., becomes less negative) to

Fig. 2.2 Ion distribution and movement across the resting plasma membrane. Intracellular and extracellular concentrations of sodium [Na$^+$] and potassium [K$^+$] are shown. These concentrations are maintained by the action of the Na$^+$/K$^+$ATPase.

Fig. 2.3 Fast cell action potential. The phases of the action potential (0–4) are shown. Changes in membrane ion conductance throughout the action potential are shown below (*ARP*, absolute refractory period; *RRP*, relative refractory period).

a threshold potential, which can occur spontaneously (in nodal cells), but is usually stimulated by transmission from adjacent myocytes through gap junctions.

Fast cell action potential

Action potentials in fast depolarizing cells (Fig. 2.3) occur in five phases (0–4, described hereafter) and are initiated by an action potential in an adjacent cell.

Phases of the fast cell action potential:

- Phase 0: rapid depolarization (upstroke). When the membrane is depolarized to its threshold potential, fast voltage-gated Na$^+$ channels open, allowing rapid influx of Na$^+$ down its electrochemical gradient, causing further depolarization.
- Phase 1: initial repolarization. As the membrane potential approaches neutral, voltage-gated Na$^+$ channels become inactivated, terminating the rapid inward Na$^+$ current. The persistent outward background K$^+$ current causes a slight repolarization. Phase 1 is most prominent in the Purkinje fibres.
- Phase 2: plateau. This phase is mediated by opening of L-type calcium (Ca^{2+}) channels. These are voltage-gated channels that are activated slowly. The slow inward Ca^{2+} current is balanced by K$^+$ efflux and thus membrane potential remains relatively steady. Towards the end of phase 2, Ca^{2+} channels close, the steady potential is maintained by an inward current brought about by action of the Na$^+$/Ca^{2+} exchanger. The plateau phase prolongs the cardiac action potential to 150–300 ms and is a key difference between the cardiac and neuronal action potentials. This prolongation is critical in allowing contraction to occur.

- Phase 3: repolarization. Additional K$^+$ channels open, increasing K$^+$ efflux. This brings about membrane repolarization to its resting potential. A delay or defect in the opening of these K$^+$ channels caused by a genetic defect delays repolarization and manifests as a long QT syndrome.
- Phase 4: resting potential. When repolarization is complete, the membrane potential is restored to its resting value and the cycle repeats.

Slow cell action potential

Nodal cells do not have a stable resting membrane potential. There is a relatively lower density of constitutively open leak K$^+$ channels on these cells compared to fast depolarizing cells/work myocytes. This membrane potential decays (de-polarizes) slowly until it reaches a threshold potential and an action potential is triggered spontaneously (Fig. 2.4). This decaying potential is a result of a gradual reduction in the K$^+$ permeability, reducing K$^+$ efflux, along with a gradual increase in Na$^+$ and Ca^{2+} influx through slow channels. This unstable pacemaker potential (phase 4) means that an action potential may occur spontaneously if the cell is not stimulated by depolarization transmitted from adjacent cells.

Nodal cells do not express functional fast voltage-gated Na$^+$ channels and the upstroke of the action potential

Fig. 2.4 Slow cell action potential. The phases of the action potential (0–4) and changes in membrane ion conductance are shown (*ARP*, absolute refractory period; *RRP*, relative refractory period).

(phase 0) is produced by a slow inward Ca^{2+} current through L-type Ca^{2+} channels. As a result, the upstroke of the action potential is much slower than that of the fast cells. After the upstroke, K^+ channels open and outward K^+ current brings about repolarization (phase 3). There is no plateau phase in the action potential of nodal cells.

The 'funny current'

The funny current (I_f for short) is an electric current that is highly prevalent in spontaneously depolarizing areas of the heart (such as the nodal cells). It is so-named due to unusual features when compared to other ion channels in the heart (including mixed permeability to sodium and potassium ions, unusual kinetics and activation). The I_f current is activated when the membrane potential is hyperpolarized (during diastole), supplying inward current and depolarization of the action potential. As a result, this current is important for bringing about spontaneous activity of these nodal cells and therefore also the underlying heart rate. Ivabradine (an anti-anginal) acts to inhibit this current, thereby preventing the I_f current's contribution to depolarization of the nodal cells' action potentials and slowing the heart rate as a result.

Refractory period

During an action potential, cardiac cells are refractory to excitation, i.e., another action potential cannot be generated. There are two different refractory periods:

- Absolute refractory period, during which another action potential cannot be elicited, no matter how great the stimulus.
- Relative refractory period, during which an action potential can be initiated only if the stimulus is strong.

The two are shown in Figs 2.3 and 2.4. The *absolute refractory period* begins at the onset of phase 0 and lasts until midway through phase 3. This refractory period prevents a new action potential being initiated during the previous one, allowing adequate time for ventricular filling before the next contraction. The absolute refractory period in ventricular myocytes is approximately 250 ms in a healthy heart, thus the maximum rate the heart can beat in a coordinated manner is 240 beats per minute (bpm).

During phase 3, some of the fast voltage-gated Na^+ channels are reset and primed to be activated again; however, only a small number are primed so a large stimulus is required. This is the *relative refractory period*, which in work myocytes, lasts until resting membrane potential is reached and can persist into phase 4 in nodal cells.

Control of heart rate

In nodal cells, the rate at which spontaneous depolarization occurs depends on the slope of the pacemaker potential. Both the SA and AV nodes are innervated by sympathetic and parasympathetic fibres, which exert opposing chronotropic stimuli (effects on heart rate) by altering the slope of the pacemaker potential. In a denervated heart, the SA node spontaneously depolarizes at a rate of approximately 100 bpm and the AV node at between 30 and 50 bpm. Under normal circumstances the SA node is the dominant pacemaker and determines heart rate. If the SA node ceases to function, or conduction from the SA node to the AV node is interrupted, the AV node becomes the dominant pacemaker.

Sympathetic fibres release noradrenaline/norepinephrine, which acts on β_1 receptors, increasing the permeability of the nodal cell plasma membrane to Na^+ and Ca^{2+}, increasing the slope of the pacemaker potential. This causes an increased firing rate of the SA node, increasing heart rate and decreases the conduction delay at the AV node.

Parasympathetic fibres release acetylcholine, which acts on muscarinic M2 receptors, increasing the permeability to K^+ and decreasing the Na^+ and Ca^{2+} permeability. This decreases the slope of the pacemaker potential, decreasing heart rate. In addition, increased parasympathetic activity causes a slight hyperpolarization at the end of each action potential, further slowing heart rate.

Under resting conditions, the parasympathetic nervous system (PNS) exerts a constant influence on the SA node via the vagus nerve, resulting in a resting heart rate of approximately 70 bpm. If this parasympathetic influence is blocked (with atropine, for example), then the resting heart rate will increase. The effects of autonomic innervation on the action potential in the SA and AV nodes are shown in Fig. 2.5.

A

sympathetic → NA → β₁ receptor → ↑pNa⁺ + ↑pCa²⁺

B

parasympathetic → Ach → M2 receptor → ↑pK⁺

Fig. 2.5 Autonomic influences on the nodal action potential. (A) Sympathetic stimulation increases the slope of the pacemaker potential by acting on β₁ adrenoceptors and increasing Na⁺ and Ca²⁺ permeability. (B) Parasympathetic stimulation decreases the slope of the pacemaker potential and hyperpolarizes the plasma membrane by acting on M2 receptors and increasing K⁺ permeability. *Dotted lines* represent baseline trace, *solid lines* represent potential after given alteration in autonomic activity (*NA*, noradrenaline/norepinephrine; *ACh*, acetylcholine).

HINTS AND TIPS

Pacemaker rate is also affected by temperature. This is why heart rate increases when a person has a fever. It is estimated that heart rate increases by 10 bpm for every °C increase in temperature.

Excitation contraction coupling

Excitation contraction coupling (Fig. 2.6) is the process that couples an action potential with contraction in cardiac muscle, a process underpinned by an increase in cytosolic calcium concentration ($[Ca^{2+}]$). During the plateau phase of the cardiac action potential (phase 2), calcium enters the cytosol through the L-type Ca^{2+} channels. This stimulates further Ca^{2+} release from the sarcoplasmic reticulum (SR),

a process termed 'Ca^{2+} induced Ca^{2+} release'. Once in the cytosol, Ca^{2+} ions bind troponin C, altering the position of tropomyosin and exposing the myosin heads so they can bind actin filaments, allowing contraction to take place. Greater increases in cytosolic $[Ca^{2+}]$ increase contraction strength. Therefore the amount of Ca^{2+} entry determines the contractility of the myocyte. Contractility is defined as the force generated by cardiac muscle for a given fibre length.

Following myocyte contraction, rapid reduction of the cytosolic $[Ca^{2+}]$ is crucial to allow relaxation and ventricular filling during diastole (Fig. 2.7). The Ca^{2+}ATPase on the SR is activated by increased cytosolic $[Ca^{2+}]$ and pumps approximately 80%–90% of the Ca^{2+} back into the SR. The remainder is removed from the cell by the Na^+/Ca^{2+} exchanger on the plasma membrane, which utilizes the Na^+ gradient created by the activity of the Na^+/K^+ATPase to remove Ca^{2+} from the cell.

Fig. 2.6 Excitation and its effect on the myocyte.

Fig. 2.7 Ion exchanges that take place during relaxation (*ATP*, adenosine triphosphate; *SR*, sarcoplasmic reticulum).

THE CARDIAC CYCLE

The cardiac cycle is the sequence of pressure and volume changes that take place during cardiac activity (Fig. 2.8 and Table 2.1). At a resting heart rate of approximately 75 bpm, the cardiac cycle lasts 0.80 s. This is divided into diastole and systole, which last approximately 0.53 s and 0.27 s respectively. When considering the cardiac cycle, it is useful to remember that:

- Blood flows down a pressure gradient.
- The position of a valve is dependent on the pressure gradient across it.

The ventricular cycle

The ventricular cycle consists of four phases. The duration and order of each of these phases is shown in Table 2.1.
1. Ventricular filling (diastole). The atria and ventricles are initially relaxed, with passive filling occurring due to central venous pressure (CVP) and pulmonary venous pressure. Filling distends the ventricle, causing pressure to rise. Passive ventricular filling stops when ventricular pressure reaches pulmonary venous pressure. Contraction of the atria further increases the filling of the ventricles. This accounts for about 15%–20% of ventricular filling at rest but is more important during exercise as the time for passive ventricular filling is reduced. The volume of blood in the ventricle at the end of diastole is termed the end-diastolic volume (EDV).

CLINICAL NOTE

The 'atrial kick' is absent in people with atrial fibrillation due to ineffective atrial contraction. This has little effect on cardiac output at rest.

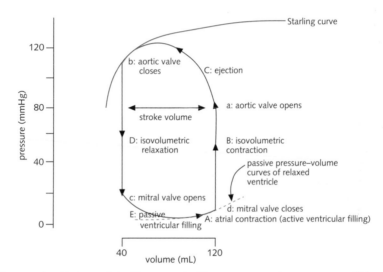

Fig. 2.8 Pressure–volume cycle of left ventricle. The most significant pressure changes occur within the ventricles during the isovolumetric stages.

Table 2.1 Summary table of the stages of the cardiac cycle

	Diastole	Systole		Diastole
Stage	Ventricular filling	Isovolumetric contraction	Ejection	Isovolumetric relaxation
Atrioventricular (AV) valves	Open	Closed	Closed	Closed
Arterial valves	Closed	Closed	Open	Closed
Ventricular pressure	Falls then slowly rises	Rapid rise	Rises then slowly falls	Rapid fall
Ventricular volume	Increases	Constant	Decreases	Constant

Note: changes at fixed volume are referred to as isovolumetric and precede the later contraction or dilation of the ventricles.

2. Isovolumetric contraction (systole). Ventricular contraction increases ventricular pressure. As ventricular pressure rises above atrial pressure, the atrioventricular valves close early in systole. This creates a closed chamber as all valves are closed. Ventricular contraction continues, causing a rapid rise in ventricular pressure. No blood is ejected from the ventricles because aortic/pulmonary pressure is greater than that in the ventricles, keeping the aortic and pulmonary valves closed.

3. Ejection (systole). As contraction continues, ventricular pressure rises, opening the aortic and pulmonary valves. This causes ejection of blood from the ventricles and a rapid rise in arterial pressure. The momentum of blood prevents immediate valve closure, even when ventricular pressure falls below arterial pressure. Eventually, the arterial valves close, creating a brief fluctuation in arterial pressure called the dicrotic notch. The ventricle does not empty completely, with an end-systolic volume (ESV) of about 40%–50%, which can be used to increase stroke volume (SV) when necessary. The ejection fraction (proportion of blood ejected during systole) is usually 50%–60%.

4. Isovolumetric relaxation (diastole). Both sets of valves are closed as the ventricles relax. When ventricular pressure falls below atrial pressure, the atrioventricular valves open and the cycle repeats.

HINTS AND TIPS

Venous return = Right heart input & output = Pulmonary blood flow = Left heart input & output = Systemic blood flow. This is because they are all in series. This idea that 'what goes in must come out' is called the Fick principle.

The atrial cycle

The pressure changes in the atria during the cardiac cycle are different from those in the ventricles. The right atrium directly communicates with the internal jugular veins (IJVs) and the absence of valves between the two means that changes in right atrial pressure are reflected by changes in the jugular venous pressure (JVP). The JVP waveform is assessed when examining the cardiovascular system and is shown in Fig. 2.9. The JVP waveform has five components:

- The A wave – atrial contraction.
- The C wave – closure of tricuspid valve.
- X descent – atrial relaxation.
- V wave – atrial filling during systole.
- Y descent – passive ventricular filling during diastole.

Fig. 2.9 The normal jugular venous pressure (JVP) waveform (*a*, a wave; *c*, c wave; *v*, v wave; *x*, x descent; *y*, y descent).

Heart sounds

Normal heart sounds (Fig. 2.10):

- First (S_1): produced by closure of the mitral and tricuspid valves.
- Second (S_2): produced by closure of the aortic and pulmonary valves.

Added heart sounds (see Fig. 2.10):

- Third (S_3): may be heard in early diastole and is due to rapid ventricular filling. A third heart sound is common in young people and athletes. It may be present in people with heart failure.
- Fourth (S_4): occurs just before the first heart sound and is due to forceful atrial contraction against a stiff ventricle. This is always abnormal and can occur in the presence of ventricular hypertrophy.

HINTS AND TIPS

To get an idea of the timing of the third and fourth heart sounds, consider the cadence of the words Kentucky (mirrors the third heart sound) and Tennessee (mirrors the fourth heart sound).

During inspiration, physiological splitting of the second heart sound can occur (Fig. 2.11). Inspiration decreases intrathoracic pressure, increasing venous return (VR) and right ventricular preload. Simultaneously, the lungs expand, decreasing return to the left atrium and decreasing left ventricular preload. As a result, right ventricular systole lasts longer than left ventricular systole and the pulmonary valve closes after the aortic valve, causing a 'split' S_2.

Fig. 2.10 Normal heart sounds (S_1, first heart sound; S_2, second heart sound) and the added third and fourth heart sounds (S_3, third heart sound; S_4, fourth heart sound).

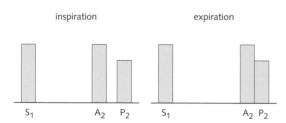

inspiration   expiration

S_1 A_2 P_2 S_1 A_2 P_2

Fig. 2.11 Splitting of the second heart sound. S_2 may show physiological splitting into A_2 and P_2. This is usually more pronounced on inspiration. (A_2, aortic component; P_2, pulmonary component).

Figure 2.12 brings together the atrial cycle, ventricular cycle and heart sounds, showing their temporal relation to each other.

Murmurs

Murmurs result from turbulent blood flow. They are most often due to valvular disease, although a benign 'flow' murmur may be present in young people or people in high cardiac output (CO) states such as pregnancy or anaemia. Murmurs may also be present in certain congenital heart defects. See Chapter 10 for more detail.

CONTROL OF CARDIAC OUTPUT

Definitions and concepts

Cardiac output (CO) is the amount of blood ejected from the heart in 1 minute. CO = heart rate (HR) × stroke volume (SV). In a normal adult, it ranges from 4 to 7 L/min at rest, but is increased during exercise (up to 20 L/min) and decreased during sleep. Before considering how CO is regulated, it is important to understand a number of definitions:

- Stroke volume (SV): the volume of blood ejected in one ventricular contraction.
- End-diastolic volume (EDV): the volume of blood in the ventricle just before contraction.
- End-diastolic pressure (EDP): the pressure of blood in the ventricle just before contraction.
- End-systolic volume (ESV): the volume of blood left in the ventricle after contraction.
- Central venous pressure (CVP): the pressure of blood in the great veins as they enter the right atrium.
- Venous return (VR): the volume of blood returning to the right heart in 1 minute. In a healthy heart, VR = CO.
- Mean arterial pressure (MAP): the average blood pressure during a single cardiac cycle.
- Total peripheral resistance (TPR): the resistance to the flow of blood in the whole system (MAP/CO).
- Systemic vascular resistance (SVR): the resistance to blood flow offered by all of the systemic vasculature (this excludes the pulmonary vasculature). It is calculated as (MAP − CVP)/CO.

- Ejection fraction: the proportion of EDV that is ejected during systole.

SV, and therefore CO, is influenced by three factors:

- Preload.
- Afterload.
- Contractility.

Preload

Preload is defined as the degree of ventricular myocyte stretch at the end of diastole and is determined by the EDV. The greater the EDV, the greater the preload and vice versa. EDV is influenced by:

- Venous return.
- Heart rate.
- Atrial contraction (reduced if ineffectual, as in atrial fibrillation).

Afterload

Afterload is defined as the force or stress on myocytes during systole. It is determined by resistance to outflow from the ventricle. For the left ventricle, aortic pressure is the main determinant and for the right ventricle, pulmonary artery pressure is the main determinant.

Contractility

Contractility is the force of contraction for a given fibre length and is determined by the degree of calcium influx during the plateau phase (phase 2) of the cardiac action potential. Factors that influence contractility are termed inotropic factors and can have a positive or negative effect.

Examples of positive inotropes include:

- Catecholamine (e.g., noradrenaline/norepinephrine).
- β-Agonists (e.g., dobutamine).
- Phosphodiesterase inhibitors (e.g., milrinone).
- Ca^{2+} sensitizers (e.g., levosimendan).
- Cardiac glycosides (e.g., digoxin).

Examples of negative inotropes include:

- β-Blockers (e.g., propranolol): inhibit the action of catecholamines on β_1 receptors.
- Ca^{2+} channel blockers (e.g., verapamil): block the L-type Ca^{2+} channels on ventricular myocytes, reducing Ca^{2+} influx.
- Hypoxia.

COMMON PITFALLS

Although sympathetic stimulation causes an increase in contractility, parasympathetic stimulation does NOT decrease contractility because parasympathetic innervation to the ventricular myocardium is sparse.

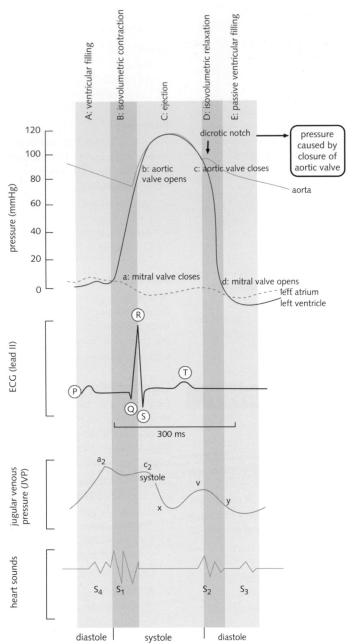

Fig. 2.12 Displayed at the top of the diagram are the pressures in the left atrium, left ventricle and aorta during the cardiac cycle. (A) Pressure in the left ventricle increases slightly as blood enters the ventricle during left atrial contraction. (B) The most rapid increase in pressure occurs during isovolumetric contraction. The increase in pressure caused by ventricular contraction closes the mitral valve (a). (C) When left ventricular pressure just exceeds aortic pressure the aortic valve opens (b) leading to ejection. Pressure rises to a peak and then falls, leading to aortic valve closure (c). (D) Isovolumetric relaxation then occurs and eventually left ventricular pressure is just below left atrial pressure, leading to the opening of the mitral valve (d). (E) This allows passive filling of the ventricles. Below this the normal electrocardiogram is displayed as it relates to the cardiac cycle. The jugular venous pressure (*JVP*) (shown below) reflects right atrial pressure due to the close proximity of the central veins to the right atrium. Finally, the heart sounds are displayed (S_1, closure of the mitral and tricuspid valves 'lubb'; S_2, closure of the aortic and pulmonary valves 'dupp').

Starling's law of the heart

Starling's law of the heart (also called the Frank-Starling law) states that the energy released during contraction depends upon the initial fibre length, within physiological limits (Fig. 2.13). The greater the heart is stretched by filling (preload), then the greater the energy released by contraction. This is due to stretch-dependent sensitivity of myocardial contractile proteins to calcium ions, which influences numbers of actin–myosin cross-bridges formed. It is important to distinguish this from contractility (see earlier).

Although initial stretch of the ventricular myocardium is produced by the EDV, EDP is easier to measure, and the relationship between the two is almost linear (providing myocardial compliance is normal). In the right ventricle, EDP is closely related to the CVP. EDP plotted against SV produces the Starling curve (Fig. 2.14). Excessively high filling pressures cause excessive myocyte stretch and the relationship is no longer valid, such that when a certain EDP is exceeded, any further increase will decrease SV.

Starling's law is the principle that matches right and left ventricular SVs and understanding it is central to understanding how CO is controlled.

Change in preload

Increased preload will increase CO. Within a few beats, the increased stretch of right ventricular myocardium and increased right ventricular SV will increase pulmonary pressures and thus increase filling of the left ventricle. This increases left ventricular SV. A decrease in preload will in the same way decrease CO.

Fig. 2.13 Sarcomere length compared with tension. Increasing the initial sarcomere length increases tension, up to the maximum stretch possible for an individual myocyte.

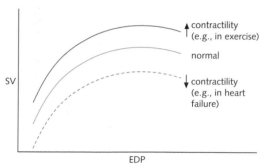

Fig. 2.14 Stroke volume (*SV*) compared with end-diastolic pressure (*EDP*). This produces the Starling curve, which shows that an increase in EDP (and therefore end-diastolic volume (EDV) as they have an almost linear relationship) causes an increased SV. There is, however, a limit at which the curve turns downwards and the relationship is no longer valid. The mechanism for this downturn is complex, and it mainly reflects excessive stretching of the ventricular myocytes. Changes in contractility are characterized by upward (positively inotropic) and downward (negatively inotropic) displacement of the Starling curve.

Change in afterload

An increase in afterload will reduce left ventricle SV, therefore increasing ESV. This will result in a greater EDV during the next cycle. The increased preload increases the force of the next contraction to restore SV despite increased afterload.

Figure 2.15 shows the pressure–volume loop for the left ventricle and how this is affected by changes in EDV and contractility.

These pressure–volume loops are important in understanding the importance of:

- Adequate, but not excessive filling of the ventricles (e.g., in heart failure, high EDV may be pathological).
- Keeping peripheral resistance as low as possible to maximize CO (reducing afterload).
- Maintaining a sufficient level of contractility to maintain life when the previous determinants have been optimized.

These factors are particularly important when considering the treatment of patients with heart failure.

HINTS AND TIPS

Remember that cardiac output is limited by venous return – without integrated regulation of the cardiovascular system, increased heart rate will be compensated for by reduced stroke volume.

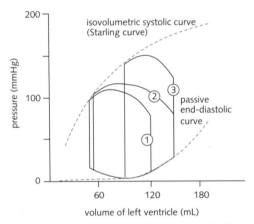

Fig. 2.15 Pressure–volume loops (*1*, normal state; *2*, increased end-diastolic volume (EDV) leads to increased stroke volume (SV) if arterial pressure is constant; *3*, increased EDV and increased mean arterial pressure (MAP) result in a decreased SV). The end-systolic points of the loops produce the Starling curve so long as contractility remains constant.

HAEMODYNAMICS AND VASCULAR FUNCTION

Blood flow and velocity

In normal arteries and veins, blood flow is described as laminar (Fig. 2.16), in which blood flows in a number of parallel planes, with those in the centre flowing faster than those towards the vessel wall. This occurs due to increased shear forces between outermost layers of blood and the vessel wall, resulting in slower flow.

Turbulent flow occurs in the ventricles and 'single-file' flow occurs in capillaries where the diameter of the vessel is the same (or often less than) that of red and white blood cells.

Disruption of laminar flow can occur at areas of stenosis or branching. This promotes atherosclerotic change.

HINTS AND TIPS

Alteration in normal blood flow (such as turbulence, stasis, etc.) is one of the three main contributing factors for thrombus formation, as described by Virchow's triad. The other two factors are endothelial injury/dysfunction and hypercoagulability.

The velocity of blood flow within the vessels is inversely related to the total cross-sectional area (Fig. 2.17). The branching nature of the circulatory system means that the total cross-sectional area of the capillaries is much greater than that of the large arteries or veins. This substantially reduces velocity in the capillaries, allowing diffusion to take place.

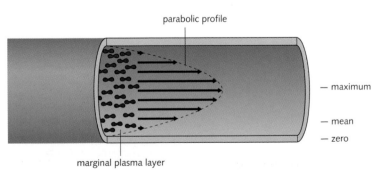

Fig. 2.16 Laminar flow. The dashed line indicates the parabolic profile of the different speeds across the vessel. Cells tend to accumulate in the centre of the flow, leaving a marginal plasma layer with fewer red cells at the periphery.

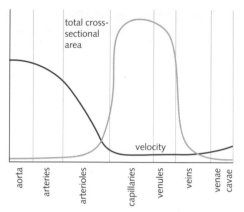

Fig. 2.17 Total cross-sectional area and mean velocity within the different anatomical classifications of vessels. Velocity in the arterial side actually varies during the cardiac cycle – the mean velocity is shown.

Vascular resistance

Total resistance in the vasculature (Fig. 2.18) is greatest in the arterioles, through a combination of their length and reduced radius without a significant change in total cross-sectional area. Total resistance is dependent upon the arteriolar radius, which is tightly controlled.

Capillary resistance is less than arteriolar resistance because capillaries are shorter (0.5 mm), large numbers of capillaries occur in parallel and they have single-file flow rather than laminar flow. Remember, however, that due to its smaller radius, a given length of capillary will have greater resistance than the same length of arteriole.

Blood viscosity

Viscosity is the measure of the internal friction within a moving fluid. According to Poiseuille's law, resistance is proportional to viscosity and so, blood viscosity plays a role in determining resistance, and therefore flow. The main de-

terminant of viscosity is the haematocrit (the percentage of red cells in the blood volume).

A normal haematocrit (generally 40%–50%) is the optimal level for oxygen delivery. An elevated haematocrit (polycythaemia) increases the carriage of oxygen, but increases viscosity, impeding flow and increasing cardiac work. Polycythaemia may occur with:

- Chronic hypoxia (e.g., severe respiratory disease).
- High altitude living – as a physiological adaptation.
- Myeloproliferative disease (e.g., polycythaemia rubra vera).
- Severe dehydration – haemoconcentration due to reduction in circulating volume without loss of red blood cells.
- Right to left shunting (e.g., Eisenmenger syndrome or cyanotic congenital heart disease).

Plasma viscosity is also determined by the level of plasma proteins (mainly albumins and globulins) and is increased in conditions such as myeloma, in which there is increased production of immunoglobulin. In addition to increasing plasma viscosity, this increase in plasma proteins promotes aggregation of red blood cells, further increasing viscosity. Vessel diameter and the rate of flow also influence red blood cell aggregation and as a result, the viscosity of blood is different throughout the vascular system.

Arteries

The pulse waveform

The waveform of arterial pressure during the cardiac cycle is shown in Fig. 2.19:

- During the early part of ventricular ejection, the rate of blood flowing into the aorta is greater than the rate of blood flowing off into the peripheral circulation. This increases the volume of blood in the aorta and thus the pressure. The peak pressure reached is known as the systolic blood pressure (SBP).
- As ejection declines and during diastole, flow from the aorta into the peripheral vessels is greater than flow into the aorta and the pressure drops. The pressure at

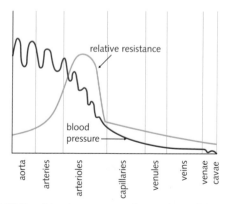

Fig. 2.18 How blood pressure and vascular resistance change across the vascular system. Pressure in the arterial side and in the great veins varies with the cardiac cycle.

Fig. 2.19 Pulse waveform. The dicrotic notch is caused by closure of the aortic valve.

the end of diastole (which is the lowest in the cycle) is termed diastolic blood pressure (DBP).

- Closure of the aortic valve causes a small backflow of blood in to the ventricles and a visible dip in the pressure readings – this is referred to as the 'dicrotic notch'.

During systole, when aortic pressure increases, the walls of these elastic arteries are stretched and store some of the energy generated by ventricular contraction. They then recoil during diastole to maintain pressure and convert the intermittent flow from the left ventricle into the aorta into more continuous flow into the peripheral vasculature, maintaining perfusion pressure.

Factors that alter the rate of ventricular ejection or outflow from the aorta to the peripheral circulation will alter the shape of the pulse waveform. Aortic stenosis decreases the rate of ejection and causes what is described as a 'slow rising' pulse, whereas aortic regurgitation, in which blood flows back into the heart through the aortic valve, causes a 'collapsing' pulse. These are shown in Fig. 2.20.

Arterial blood pressure

Arterial blood pressure is determined in the elastic arteries, such as the aorta and its major branches, and, in the presence of steady venous pressures, determines the perfusion pressure for the body's tissues. Arterial blood pressure is expressed as the SBP/DBP.

Normal blood pressure

Normal blood pressure for a healthy adult male at rest is 120/80 mmHg. However, this value can vary due to many factors:

- Ageing increases SBP due to decreased arterial compliance.
- During sleep, blood pressure falls because of decreased metabolic demands.
- Anger, sexual excitement and stress increase blood pressure, as a result of sympathetically mediated responses.
- In the young, mean arterial pressure falls by a small amount during inspiration because of a transient fall in SV.
- In pregnancy, blood pressure falls gradually in the first trimester, reaching a minimum in the second trimester and then rises to normal in the third trimester.

Mean arterial pressure (MAP)

This is the average blood pressure over a single cardiac cycle and not the average of the systolic (SBP) and diastolic pressures (DBP). Mean arterial blood pressure is equal to CO multiplied by TPR. It can be estimated using the equation:

$$MAP = DBP + 1/3(SBP - DBP)$$

Pulse pressure

This is the difference between systolic and diastolic blood pressure. Pulse pressure can be altered under different circumstances:

- Ageing: the aortic wall becomes less elastic with age. This causes greater increases in pressure during ventricular ejection, resulting in a higher SBP. DBP, on the other hand, is reduced due to lack of elastic recoil meaning that pressure drops at a greater rate during diastole. This increases pulse pressure.
- Haemorrhage: when blood volume is reduced, SV is reduced due to decreased preload, decreasing SBP. To maintain MAP (and perfusion pressure), TPR is increased, raising DBP and decreasing pulse pressure.
- Aortic valve disease (see Fig. 2.20). Pulse pressure is decreased in aortic stenosis and increased in aortic regurgitation.

Arterioles

Arterioles are the site of greatest resistance to blood flow in the circulatory system. The abundant smooth muscle in the wall of these vessels allows tight control of lumen diameter. Control over arteriolar diameter has a number of important functions:

- Coordinated constriction or dilatation of a large proportion of arterioles will alter the TPR and thus arterial blood pressure.
- Constriction or dilatation of arterioles in single organs allows the distribution of the CO to different organs to be regulated.
- Constriction or dilatation of arterioles influences the hydrostatic forces in the capillaries and as a result has an effect on fluid filtration. Constriction of arterioles increases resistance and causes a greater pressure drop, reducing the pressure in the distal vessels.

Fig. 2.20 Normal, slow-rising and collapsing pulse waveforms.

Control of vascular smooth muscle tone

Tight control over the arteriolar vascular smooth muscle tone is achieved via numerous mechanisms. These mechanisms can be broadly divided into local and systemic influences. Vasoconstriction is an active process brought about by the contraction of vascular smooth muscle. Vasodilatation occurs when vascular smooth muscle relaxes.

Local factors are numerous and include:

- Intrinsic tone of vascular smooth muscle – higher internal pressures cause increased myogenic constriction.
- Endothelium-derived dilator factors (e.g., nitric oxide).
- Endothelium-derived constrictor factors (e.g., endothelin 1, thromboxane A_2).
- Metabolic factors – locally produced products of metabolism cause relaxation of smooth muscle and thus vasodilatation. This increases blood flow to tissues with high metabolic requirements.
- Various other factors – such as histamine, bradykinin, leukotrienes.

Local influences serve only the needs of the local tissues without taking into account the requirements of the whole body, including maintenance of blood pressure. Consider a situation in which all the tissues in the body had increased requirements, and local factors brought about vasodilatation in all the tissues simultaneously. This would cause a massive decrease in blood pressure. To maintain blood pressure, there are a number of systemic influences on vascular tone that are superimposed on those local factors:

- Sympathetic nervous system (SNS) activity – a basal level of sympathetic vasoconstriction is partly responsible for vessel tone at rest. Increased activation of these nerves causes contraction of smooth muscle and vasoconstriction. Conversely, vasodilatation can be brought about by decrease in sympathetic nerve activity. Catecholamines (adrenaline/epinephrine and noradrenaline/norepinephrine) are released from the adrenal medulla secondary to exercise, hypotension, or 'fight-or-flight' situations. Catecholamines bind to β_1 receptors in the myocardium, increasing heart rate and contractility and bind to α_1 receptors on vascular smooth muscle causing vasoconstriction. Adrenaline/epinephrine has high affinity for β_2 receptors in skeletal muscle and increases blood flow for use in 'fight-or-flight' responses.
- PNS activity – parasympathetic vasodilator nerves innervate blood vessels in the genitalia, skin, salivary glands, pancreas and gastrointestinal mucosa. Their effect on blood pressure is small, but they are important for initiating an erection and for 'rest and digest' responses.
- Antidiuretic hormone (ADH) – released from the posterior pituitary following a rise in plasma osmolarity (or to a lesser extent with hypotension). ADH promotes water retention in renal tubules and can cause vasoconstriction in most tissues (but vasodilatation in coronary and cerebral vessels).
- Natriuretic peptides – in response to increased cardiac filling pressures, specialized myocytes in the atria secrete atrial natriuretic peptide (ANP) and brain natriuretic peptide (BNP). These peptides increase excretion of salt and water in renal tubules and have a mild vasodilatory effect.
- Renin-angiotensin system – described in detail hereafter.

The renin-angiotensin system

Renin is an enzyme produced by the juxtaglomerular cells of the kidney. It converts circulating angiotensinogen to angiotensin I (Fig. 2.21). Renin production is increased by:

- A fall in blood pressure in glomerular afferent arterioles.
- Increased sympathetic activity to the renal arterioles, by binding of adrenaline/epinephrine to β_1 receptors in the kidney.
- Decreased sodium in the macula densa of the adjacent distal tubule.

Angiotensin-converting enzyme (ACE) converts angiotensin I to the peptide angiotensin II, predominantly on the endothelium of the pulmonary vascular bed. Angiotensin II is the active component of this renin-angiotensin-aldosterone system (RAAS) and has the following actions:

- Increases aldosterone secretion from the adrenal cortex, leading to salt and water reabsorption in the distal renal tubules.
- Causes vasoconstriction by acting on vascular smooth muscle, augmenting release of noradrenaline/norepinephrine and increasing SNS action.
- Stimulates release of ADH from the posterior pituitary.

Capillaries

In most tissues, tone of the vascular smooth muscle in the supplying arteriole determines perfusion of the supplied capillaries. Vascular smooth muscle in capillaries has sparse innervation and tone is predominantly controlled by local factors. Changes in terminal arteriolar diameter and capillary perfusion pressure have an impact on fluid filtration.

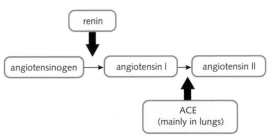

Fig. 2.21 Formation of angiotensin II. Angiotensinogen is secreted by the liver, acted on by renin (secreted by the kidney) and finally converted to the active angiotensin II by angiotensin-converting enzyme (ACE).

Capillary diameter is often smaller than red blood cell diameter (3–6 μm compared with 8–10 μm), but because the red blood cells can deform, they are still able to pass through the microvasculature.

HINTS AND TIPS

Raynaud's phenomenon is a condition whereby exposure of the extremities (fingers, toes, nose) causes excessive cutaneous vasoconstriction that impairs perfusion of the extremities resulting in ischaemia.

Veins and venules

Venules and veins are thin-walled, distensible vessels that return blood from the capillaries to the right atrium.

Veins have valves that prevent backflow of blood and without them, VR would be limited. Valve failure can result in varicosities. Venous vessels have other important functions and influences:

- Venous pressure is one of the determinants of fluid filtration by altering the capillary hydrostatic pressure.
- Due to their high compliance, venous vessels can function as a reservoir for blood, the volume of which can be controlled by numerous factors.
- The venous vessels determine the filling pressures of the heart and thus the EDV and SV according to Starling's law.

Skeletal muscle pump

Rhythmic exercise, especially of the leg muscles, produces a pumping effect, increasing movement of venous blood into the central veins, maintaining venous return. By pumping blood out of the active muscle, this muscle pump lowers venous pressure in that muscle, increasing perfusion pressure and increasing blood flow through active muscles. Incompetent valves make the skeletal muscle pump ineffective.

INTEGRATED CONTROL OF THE CARDIOVASCULAR SYSTEM AND CARDIOVASCULAR REFLEXES

Arterial baroreceptors and the baroreflex

The baroreceptor reflex is vital for minute-to-minute control of arterial blood pressure. Arterial baroreceptors are stretch receptors located in the wall of the carotid sinuses and the aortic arch. They continuously generate impulses, with frequency dependent on the degree of vessel wall stretch. Increased stretch (due to increased pressure), also known as increased baroreceptor loading, increases firing rate. The impulses generated by the baroreceptors are carried to the nucleus tractus solitarius (NTS) in the medulla by the glossopharyngeal and vagus nerves (from the carotid sinus and aortic arch respectively). In the NTS, these afferent impulses interact with other central pathways regulating autonomic nervous system activity.

When blood pressure decreases, the baroreceptors are unloaded (stretch is reduced) and the firing rate to the medulla decreases. The effect is to decrease parasympathetic (PNS) and increase sympathetic (SNS) drive. This causes the following effects (Fig 2.22):

- Increased heart rate and contractility, increasing CO (SNS and PNS).
- Peripheral vasoconstriction, increasing TPR (SNS).
- Venoconstriction, decreasing venous pooling and increasing VR and preload (SNS).
- Catecholamine secretion (SNS).
- Increased renin secretion and activation of the renin-angiotensin system, causing vasoconstriction and increasing circulating volume (SNS).

These actions increase CO and TPR, restoring blood pressure to normal. The baroreflex is rapid and very important in acute hypotension or haemorrhage. Increased loading of the baroreceptors has the opposite effect, decreasing CO and TPR.

Baroreceptor-mediated vasoconstriction primarily affects vascular beds in skeletal muscle and the gastrointestinal tract. Cutaneous circulation is important if the temperature is neutral. Cerebral and coronary circulations are largely unaffected by these changes in sympathetic activity.

The level of blood pressure that the baroreceptors take as 'normal' (the set point) can be reset by central or peripheral processes:

- Central resetting: in exercise or during fight-or-flight situations, the rise in blood pressure that occurs does not cause bradycardia because central influences reset the baroreflex set point and allow the blood pressure to increase.
- Peripheral resetting: chronic hyper- or hypotension leads to the set point being reset to this new pressure, allowing the baroreflex to operate in its optimal range. Because of this, the baroreflex is of little use for long-term control of blood pressure.

Arterial baroreceptors' sensitivity to changes in blood pressure is decreased by reduced compliance of arterial walls – this occurs with ageing and in chronic hypertension.

Central pathways

The cardiovascular system is influenced by complex interactions between the medulla, hypothalamus and cortex.

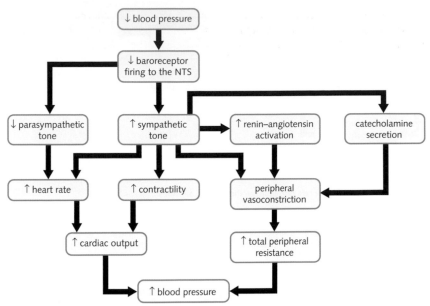

Fig. 2.22 The baroreceptor reflex. The responses to unloading of arterial baroreceptors to restore blood pressure to the set point (*NTS*, nucleus tractus solitarius).

Medulla

It is thought that there are complex signals between the hypothalamus, cortex and cerebellum, as well as signals within the vasomotor centre of the medulla:

- The rostral ventrolateral medulla is responsible for sympathetic outflow.
- The nucleus ambiguus is responsible for parasympathetic (vagal) outflow.

Together, these two areas mediate the neural control of vascular tone and heart rate. Information from baroreceptors and other cardiovascular receptors is received at the NTS in the medulla. The afferent inputs are integrated and relayed to other areas in the brain.

Hypothalamus

The hypothalamus contains four areas of interest:

- Depressor area – receives input from the NTS and can produce the baroreflex.
- Defence area – responsible for the alerting (fight-or-flight) response.
- Temperature-regulating area – controls cutaneous vascular tone and sweating.
- ADH-secreting area – produces antidiuretic hormone (vasopressin).

Cardiorespiratory interactions

During inspiration, reduced intrathoracic pressure increases venous return. This increases SV by Starling's law. In addition to this mechanical interaction, there are also neurally mediated cardiorespiratory interactions.

Sinus arrhythmia

Sinus arrhythmia describes the physiological phenomenon of increased heart rate during inspiration. It is more profound in younger people. The mechanisms that underlie sinus arrhythmia are detailed in Fig. 2.23.

These mechanisms also explain the increase in heart rate that occurs in any situation where respiratory rate is increased. Examples include systemic hypoxia, exercise and stress.

Arterial chemoreceptors

Peripheral chemoreceptors are located in the carotid and aortic bodies. They are involved in the regulation of pH and oxygen/carbon dioxide levels in arterial blood. Their fibres travel with afferent baroreceptor fibres in the glossopharyngeal and vagus nerves. Their activity is increased by increased carbon dioxide, decreased oxygen and reduced pH in arterial blood.

Increased stimulation of these chemoreceptors results in increased parasympathetic drive to the heart, decreasing the heart rate and increasing sympathetic drive to the arterioles, causing vasoconstriction. This reflex is in place to reduce oxygen requirements; however, it is only apparent if the respiratory rate is not able to increase, for example during artificial ventilation or in a fetus in the womb.

HINTS AND TIPS

This chemoreceptor reflex explains why a decrease in heart rate in the fetus suggests hypoxia.

B

Sinus arrhythmia (change of heart rate due to inspiration and expiration)

Every QRS complex has a preceding P wave. There is a normal PR interval, but the heart rate increases during inspiration. This is seen by the decreased R–R interval. This is normal, especially in children and healthy adults.

Fig. 2.23 Sinus arrhythmia. (A) Neural pathways underpinning sinus arrhythmia and the increase in heart rate in response to an increased respiratory rate or increased tidal volume. (B) ECG trace of sinus arrhythmia (*NTS*, nucleus tractus solitarius).

Under normal circumstances, when respiratory rate can increase, increased stimulation of the chemoreceptors increases outflow from the inspiratory centre, increasing respiratory rate and tidal volume. This causes an increase in heart rate, and the greater degree of pulmonary stretch receptor stimulation that accompanies increased tidal volume further augments this response. Under normal circumstances, hypoxaemia will cause a tachycardia. Remember that hypoxaemia will also cause vasodilatation in certain vascular beds, such as skeletal muscle and the brain, via the local effects of reduced partial pressure of oxygen in the blood.

Other cardiopulmonary receptors

There are many cardiopulmonary receptors in the heart, great veins and pulmonary arteries with afferents to the NTS including:

- Atrial stretch receptors – these are located where the great veins join the atria and are stimulated by atrial stretch, which is increased when blood volume increases. Stimulation produces a reflex tachycardia (the Bainbridge reflex) by increasing sympathetic drive to the SA node. It also decreases secretion of ADH to reduce circulating volume.
- Unmyelinated mechanoreceptor fibres – these are present in both atria and in the left ventricle. Large degrees of distension in the chambers stimulate these receptors causing a reflex bradycardia and peripheral vasodilatation.
- Chemosensitive fibres – these are stimulated by bradykinin and other substances released by ischaemic myocardium. It is thought that the pain of angina and myocardial infarction is mediated by these fibres. Stimulation increases respiratory rate, reduces heart rate and peripherally vasodilates.

Coordinated cardiovascular responses

Orthostasis

Orthostasis means maintenance of an upright posture. When moving from a supine position to standing, gravity causes venous pooling in vessels below the heart, thereby increasing venous pressures and distending veins. This reduces apparent circulation volume and venous return. Cardiac filling is reduced and SV and CO fall. Arterial blood pressure drops, but only transiently as the baroreceptor reflex corrects it almost immediately.

CLINICAL NOTE

Failure of the mechanisms that maintain orthostatic BP control leads to postural hypotension. This is defined as a decrease in SBP of >20 mmHg or a decrease in DBP of >10 mmHg on standing. This may result in symptoms of light-headedness or even collapse.

Valsalva manoeuvre

The Valsalva manoeuvre is a forced expiration against a closed glottis. This commonly occurs when coughing, defecating, or lifting heavy weights. It causes increased intrathoracic pressure, which brings about a response that proceeds in four phases (Fig. 2.24):

1. Increased intrathoracic pressure increases blood flow from the pulmonary circulation into the left atrium. This increases left ventricular EDV and SV.

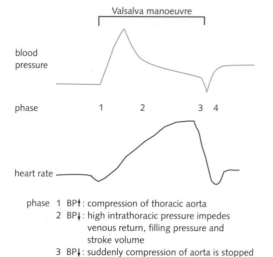

phase 1 BP↑: compression of thoracic aorta
2 BP↓: high intrathoracic pressure impedes venous return, filling pressure and stroke volume
3 BP↓: suddenly compression of aorta is stopped
4 BP↑: ↑venous return, ↑stroke volume, reflex bradycardia

Fig. 2.24 Response to the Valsalva manoeuvre (*BP*, blood pressure).

There is also compression of the aorta, increasing blood pressure.

2. High intrathoracic pressure impedes venous return, decreasing SV and therefore also blood pressure. During this period, there is a baroreceptor-mediated increase in heart rate.
3. When the manoeuvre is released, compression on the aorta is stopped and left ventricular filling pressures are reduced temporarily as the pulmonary vessels re-expand. This causes a drop in blood pressure.
4. VR is restored, increasing cardiac filling pressures and SV. This increases BP, resulting in a baroreceptor reflex-mediated bradycardia and subsequent fall in BP to normal levels.

This manoeuvre is a useful test of baroreceptor competence. If the pressure fall in phase 2 continues and there is no bradycardia in phase 4, then the baroreflex is interrupted, and the person will be at risk of postural hypotension.

Diving reflex

The diving reflex occurs when cold water stimulates the sensory receptors of the trigeminal nerve and receptors in the nasopharynx and oropharynx. The body is expecting a period of submersion and responds to conserve the limited oxygen supply available and to preferentially divert it to the heart and brain. The reflex results in three changes:

- Apnoea – while apnoeic, changing concentrations of oxygen and carbon dioxide in the blood stimulate chemoreceptors, increasing vagal drive and decreasing heart rate.
- Bradycardia – intense vagal inhibition decreases the slope of the pacemaker action potential and decreases oxygen consumption.

- Peripheral vasoconstriction – in the splanchnic, renal and skeletal muscle vascular beds. The strong, sympathetically mediated vasoconstriction increases TPR, allowing blood pressure to be maintained despite profound bradycardia.

HINTS AND TIPS

This reflex can be exploited clinically as a method to terminate supraventricular arrhythmias. Placing an icepack on the face or submersing the face in cold water elicits this response and slows heart rate.

The alerting/defence response

This is also known as the fight-or-flight response. This is the body's response to a stressful stimulus:

- Increased sympathetic outflow (increased adrenaline/epinephrine binding to myocardial β_1 receptors) and decreased parasympathetic outflow to the heart. This increases heart rate and contractility, increasing CO.
- Increased sympathetic outflow to the gastrointestinal tract, kidneys and skin causes vasoconstriction (due to increased adrenaline/epinephrine acting on α_1 receptors).
- Increased sympathetic outflow to skeletal muscle reduces arteriolar tone causing vasodilatation (due to increased adrenaline/epinephrine acting on β_2 receptors).

The net result is increased heart rate and blood pressure, and increased skeletal muscle blood flow. During this response, the baroreceptor reflex is inhibited so hypertension is not corrected. Changes in autonomic activity also cause pupillary dilatation and piloerection. The intensity of the stimulus affects the intensity of the response and the responses of two different people to the same stimulus may be very different.

Syncope (fainting)

Syncope is a sudden, transient loss of consciousness as a result of cerebral hypoperfusion. It may be initiated by standing, hypovolaemia, arrhythmia, or psychological stress. There is often a pre-syncope period of tachycardia, cutaneous vasoconstriction, hyperventilation and sweating (due to the alerting response). Hyperventilation causes reduction in the concentration of carbon dioxide in the blood and can cause paraesthesia in the fingers and around the mouth.

A vasovagal episode proceeds as follows:

1. A sudden large increase in vagal outflow causes bradycardia.
2. Profound peripheral vasodilatation occurs due to decreased sympathetic drive.

3. This causes a fall in blood pressure, reducing cerebral blood flow.
4. If it occurs at all, loss of consciousness results within seconds.

> **HINTS AND TIPS**
>
> Fits, faints and funny turns are common presentations of cardiovascular disease. It is important to consider a number of pathologies in the nervous, cardiovascular and respiratory systems before reaching the diagnosis of a psychological cause.

A person who has fainted falls to the floor. This raises the intrathoracic blood volume and the cardiac filling pressures. Coupled with the baroreflex, this increases CO and arterial pressure and restores cerebral perfusion. Consciousness is restored rapidly. Raising the person's legs will cause a further increase in VR and thus CO.

> **COMMON PITFALLS**
>
> You should never hold a person who has fainted upright as this prevents the beneficial effects of increasing intrathoracic blood volume and may maintain cerebral hypoperfusion.

Shock and haemorrhage

Haemorrhage

Haemorrhage describes loss of blood from the vascular compartment. The body has a number of responses in place to initially compensate for the reduction in circulating volume and eventually to replace that volume. Acute haemorrhage can be classified according to the amount of blood lost or the percentage of total blood volume lost. Table 2.2 shows this classification and the changes in physiological parameters that occur at each stage.

In the absence of compensatory cardiovascular changes, haemorrhage will reduce circulating volume and reduce blood pressure. The reduction in blood pressure would be dependent on the amount of blood lost as that would determine the degree to which ventricular filling (preload) was reduced. In reality, however, changes do take place and these can be divided into three sets based on the timeframe in which they occur (Fig. 2.25).

The primary aims in the treatment of haemorrhage are, firstly, to stop the bleeding and, secondly, to replace circulating volume with intravenous fluids as appropriate. It is important to remember that replacement does not have to be with blood; the key is to restore circulating volume to ensure CO is sufficient to maintain organ perfusion.

Table 2.2 Changes in vital signs in response to acute haemorrhage

Parameter	Severity of circulatory shock			
	Class I	Class II	Class III	Class IV
Blood loss (%)	0–15	15–30	30–40	>40
Blood loss (mL)	0–750	750–1500	1500–2000	>2000
Pulse rate	↔	↑	↑	↑↑
Respiratory rate	↔	↑	↑↑	↑↑
Capillary refill time	↔	↔	↑	↑↑
Blood pressure	↔	↔	Narrowing of pulse pressure	↓

Note that higher classes of shock indicate increased severity.

Shock

Shock is an acute failure of the cardiovascular system to adequately perfuse the tissues, which may result in cellular injury and organ dysfunction. There are four broad categories:

- Hypovolaemic shock – due to a fall in circulating volume. This may be caused by internal or external losses, e.g., vomiting, diarrhoea, haemorrhage.
- Distributive shock – the result of abnormal distribution of blood flow, e.g., septic shock, anaphylaxis, neurogenic shock.
- Cardiogenic shock – when the heart is unable to maintain CO. This usually has an acute precipitant, e.g., myocardial infarction, arrhythmia.
- Obstructive shock – when there is direct obstruction to blood entering or leaving the great vessels, e.g., tamponade, massive pulmonary embolism.

Most types of shock (apart from septic shock) cause a characteristic clinical picture as the result of compensatory changes that occur in response to a decrease in CO and blood pressure:

1. Pale, cold, clammy skin caused by cutaneous vasoconstriction in an effort to maintain adequate blood flow to vital organs.
2. Sweating caused by sympathetic stimulation.
3. Rapid, weak pulse caused by compensatory tachycardia and decreased SV.
4. Reduced pulse pressure due to reduced SV (reduced SBP) and increased TPR (increased DBP).
5. Rapid, shallow breathing as a result of chemoreceptor stimulation by from metabolic acidosis caused by anaerobic cellular respiration (in the presence of inadequate oxygen delivery).
6. Reduced urine output due to renal hypoperfusion and reduced glomerular filtration.

Septic shock is the most common type of circulatory shock. Sepsis is caused by toxins (e.g., endotoxin) released from certain bacteria. This initiates a profound systemic

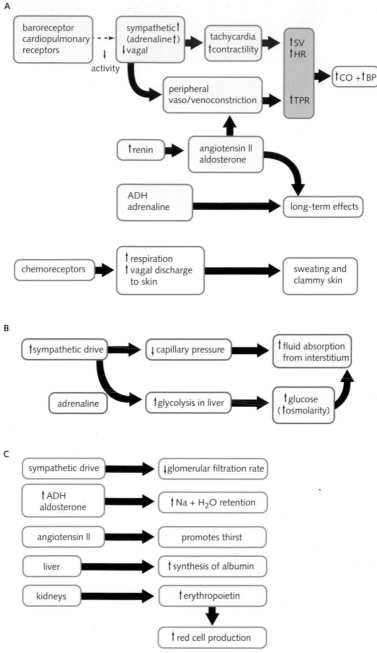

Fig. 2.25 (A) Immediate response to haemorrhage (over seconds to minutes). (B) Intermediate response to haemorrhage (over minutes to hours). (C) Long-term response to haemorrhage (over hours to days) (*ADH*, antidiuretic hormone; *BP*, blood pressure; *CO*, cardiac output; *HR*, heart rate; *SV*, stroke volume; *TPR*, total peripheral resistance).

inflammatory response, with production of cytokines and inflammatory mediators. Widespread vasodilatation and increased capillary permeability reduces TPR. Fluid moves from the vascular compartment into the interstitium. Reduced circulating volume in combination with the decrease in TPR significantly decreases blood pressure. Although the baroreceptor reflex causes a tachycardia and increases myocardial contractility, increasing CO, the peripheral vasoconstriction is ineffective. The patient will have a tachycardia, but warm skin and a low blood pressure due to the widespread vasodilatation. Treatment is with fluid replacement, antibiotics and, if severe, cardiovascular support with noradrenaline/norepinephrine may be required.

● Chapter Summary

- The electrical activity in the heart originates in the SA node and propagates through the atria and then to the ventricles via the AV node. The AV node can function as a back-up pacemaker.
- Nodal cells spontaneously depolarize and initiate an action potential without outside stimulus. Work myocytes are stimulated by adjacent cells depolarizing.
- CO is a product of SV and heart rate. It is determined by preload, afterload and cardiac contractility.
- Complex changes in cardiac volumes and pressures occur throughout the cardiac cycle.
- Blood flows in a laminar fashion in the blood vessels; disruption of this can result in atherosclerosis.
- There are a number of important local and systemic influences that provide closely regulated control of blood pressure, vascular resistance and organ perfusion.
- The body has a number of mechanisms in place to ensure homeostasis when the requirements placed upon the cardiovascular system are altered (e.g., by hypotension or haemorrhage, exercise, etc.).

THE ELECTROCARDIOGRAM (ECG)

The electrocardiogram (ECG) is a recording of the electrical activity of the heart, obtained by measuring the changes in electrical potential difference across the body surface. It is usually the first investigation used to diagnose arrhythmias and the underlying cause of chest pain.

As a wave of depolarization spreads through the myocardium there will be, at any one moment, areas of myocardium that have been excited and areas that have not yet been excited. As a result, there is a difference in potential between them: one area is negatively charged (excited), the other is positively charged (not excited), with respect to the charge in the extracellular space. These areas can be thought of as two electrical poles that comprise the cardiac dipole. This dipole depends on both the size of the charge (which depends on the amount of muscle excited) and the direction the wave of depolarization is travelling in. In the absence of electrical activity in the heart and skeletal muscle, the electrical potential across the surface of the body is uniformly positive. The cardiac dipole (electrical activity in the heart) alters the electrical potential across the body, and by placing electrodes in certain positions, the cardiac dipole and other changes in potential can be measured in different directions. This provides the basis for electrocardiography.

Figure 3.1 depicts how a wave of depolarization affects the potential difference between two electrodes, and thus how this is translated onto an ECG trace. Remember that as the dipole has both charge (amplitude) and direction, the shape of the ECG varies depending upon the position of the recording electrode. As current travels towards the positive electrode, there is an upward deflection of the ECG waveform. As the current travels towards the negative electrode (or away from the positive one), there is a downward deflection of the ECG waveform. If current is moving perpendicular to the recording pair of electrodes, there is a biphasic waveform.

The 12-lead ECG

Conventionally, the ECG is recorded using 12 'leads' (Fig. 3.2). Note that the term 'lead' is used to denote the direction in which the potential is measured and not a physical electrode – only nine electrodes are used to produce the 12 leads. The additional three lead traces show the potential difference between specific pairs of electrodes. These leads allow us to view the direction and magnitude of electrical activity in both the frontal and transverse planes and in any direction in these planes.

Fig. 3.1 The influence of the direction of depolarization on the ECG trace. Repolarization produces a deflection in the opposite direction.

Limb leads

The limb leads view the heart in the frontal plane.

Unipolar limb leads measure any positive potential difference directed towards their solitary positive electrode from an estimate of zero potential. They include aVL, aVR and aVF. The zero potential is estimated by averaging the input from the three limb leads.

The bipolar leads make up Einthoven's triangle around the heart (see Fig. 3.2). They record the differences in potential between pairs of limb leads:

- Lead I: right arm (aVR) to left arm (aVL); left arm positive.
- Lead II: right arm (aVR) to left leg (aVF); left leg positive.
- Lead III: left arm (aVL) to left leg (aVF); left leg positive.

ECG traces from each of the limb leads are shown in Fig. 3.3.

Chest leads

The chest leads (V1 to V6) are unipolar leads that measure any potential changes in the horizontal (or transverse plane), and they are arranged around the left side of the chest (as described in Fig. 3.2).

HINTS AND TIPS

Rarely, electrodes may be placed on the posterior chest wall (usually to confirm a posterior myocardial infarction). Posterior leads V7 to V9 are placed in the same horizontal plane as V6. V7 is placed in the left posterior axillary line, V8 at the tip of the left scapula and V9 in the left paraspinal region.

Fig. 3.2 Placement of ECG electrodes. The electrodes on the right arm *(RA)*, left arm *(LA)* and left leg *(LL)* give the electrocardiogram trace for the frontal leads (i.e., I, II, III, aVL, aVR and aVF). Einthoven's triangle around the heart is shown. Anterior chest lead placement is shown in the frontal and transverse planes. V1 is placed in the fourth intercostal space on the right sternal edge and V2 on the left sternal edge. V4 is placed in the fifth intercostal space in the mid-clavicular line, V5 in the anterior axillary line, and V6 in the mid-axillary line. V3 is placed between V2 and V4 *(LV,* left ventricle; *RV,* right ventricle).

Fig. 3.3 Lead directions in the anterior plane. (Redrawn with permission from Epstein, O., et al., 1997. Clinical examination, second ed. Mosby International, New York.)

The ECG trace

The components that make up an ECG tracing (Fig. 3.4) are:

- P wave – due to atrial depolarization.
- PR interval – from onset of the P wave to the onset of the QRS complex (approximately 120–200 ms). This represents the time taken for depolarization to propagate through the atria and the impulse to conduct through the atrioventricular node to the bundle of His.

Fig. 3.4 Components of the ECG trace.

Fig. 3.5 Definitions of the ECG waves. (A) If the wave following the P wave is negative, it is a Q wave. (B) If a positive deflection follows the P wave, it is called an R wave, whether it is preceded by a Q wave or not. (C) Any following negative deflection is known as an S wave, whether there has been a preceding Q wave or not.

- QRS complex – due to ventricular depolarization and is usually less than 100 ms in duration; greater than 120 ms is considered to be prolonged. The definitions of each wave within the QRS complex are depicted in Fig. 3.5.
- ST segment – coincides with the plateau phase of the ventricular action potential and ventricular contraction. It is usually isoelectric (flat) as the ventricles are depolarized throughout. Abnormalities of the ST segment can indicate ischaemia or infarction.
- T wave – due to ventricular repolarization.
- QT interval – from the onset of the Q wave to the end of the T wave (approximately 400 ms). This represents electrical depolarization and repolarization of the ventricles.
- U wave – sometimes seen as a small deflection following the T wave (and usually in the same direction). The source of the U wave is unclear – they are seen most classically in hypokalaemia but are also seen in a number of other conditions (including hypocalcaemia, hypomagnesaemia and hypothermia). It is thought they may represent delayed repolarization of Purkinje fibres.

Q waves

Small, non-significant Q waves are often seen in the left-sided leads due to the depolarization of the septum from left to right. Significant (pathological) Q waves:

- Are more than 0.04 s (one small square) in duration and more than 25% of the following R wave in depth.
- Occur after transmural myocardial infarction (MI) where the myocardium on one side of the heart dies. This myocardium has no electrical activity and therefore the leads facing it are able to pick up the electrical activity from the opposite side of the heart (effectively like looking through an electrical hole in the heart). The myocardium depolarizes from the inside out; therefore the opposite side of the heart depolarizes away from these leads, resulting in a negative deflection or Q wave.
- May also occur in patients with hypertrophic cardiomyopathy due to depolarization of the thickened septum. This may lead to an erroneous diagnosis of previous MI.

R wave progression

The wave of depolarization in the ventricles starts in the septum and then spreads into the left and right ventricles (Fig. 3.6). Because the left ventricle is usually larger than the right, the average depolarization heads towards the left ventricle. This means that V1 and V2 will have a predominant S wave (i.e., negative deflection) and a small R wave, whereas V5 and V6 will have a predominant R wave (i.e., positive deflection) with a small S wave. The interventricular septum lies where there are equal positive and negative deflections (i.e., R and S waves) and is usually at V3 or V4. This steady increase in the size of the R wave is sometimes termed R wave progression. If this is normal, then there is said to be 'good' R wave progression.

ECG abnormalities in non-cardiac disease

Non-cardiac disease may have a number of impacts upon the ECG trace, for example:

- Hypokalaemia – prolonged QT interval, small T, U wave.
- Hyperkalaemia: tall T, wide QRS, absent P.
- Hypercalcaemia: short QT interval.

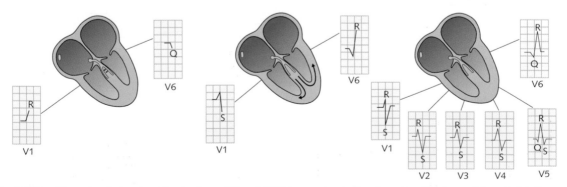

Fig. 3.6 The different anterior chest leads show different QRS traces due to the changing directions of the electrical activity. Lead V4 is usually over the interventricular septum and therefore usually shows equal R and S waves. Note the changing relative heights of Q, R and S waves between leads. The changing height of the R wave from V1 to V6 is known as 'R wave progression'.

- Hypocalcaemia: long QT interval.
- Hypothermia: bradycardia, J waves/Osborn waves (positive deflections at the junction between QRS complex and ST segment), baseline artefact due to shivering, risk of arrhythmia as patient is warmed up.
- Digoxin – downsloping ST segment ('reverse tick' shape), T wave inversion.
- Digoxin toxicity – atrioventricular block, atrial tachycardia, ventricular arrhythmias.

Some of these abnormalities are seen in Fig 3.7.

Assessment of cardiac axis

The average direction of the wave of depolarization is the electrical axis of the heart, usually referred to as the cardiac axis (Fig. 3.8). This usually lies closest to lead II but is within normal limits if between −30 and +90 degrees. Any deviation from this range is referred to as right or left axis deviation. Right axis deviation can be caused by right ventricular hypertrophy and left axis deviation by left ventricular hypertrophy. When interpreting an ECG, it must be established whether the axis is normal or not.

When the depolarization wave in the ventricles is moving towards a lead, then the R wave will be larger than the S wave in that lead. When the ventricular depolarization wave is moving away from a lead, then the S wave will be larger than the R wave in that lead. If the S wave and R wave are equal, then the depolarization is moving (on average) at right angles to that lead. The simplest way to assess the cardiac axis is to look at leads I and II. If the overall deflection in leads I and II is positive, then the axis is normal. If lead

Causes of left axis deviation	Left bundle branch block, left anterior hemiblock, left ventricular hypertrophy, ostium primum atrial septal defect
Causes of right axis deviation	Right bundle branch block, cor pulmonale, right ventricular hypertrophy, ostium secundum atrial septal defect

Fig. 3.8 (A) Cardiac axis (*IA*, indeterminate axis; *LAD*, left axis deviation; *RAD*, right axis deviation). (B) Causes of left and right axis deviation.

I is positive and II negative, it is left axis deviation. If lead I is negative and II is positive, then it is right axis deviation. If both are negative, check you have the leads on correctly!

Fig. 3.7 (A) U waves. (B) J waves. (C) Not all ST depression is due to ischaemia.

Do not get confused between the orientation of the heart and the cardiac axis. The cardiac axis is an electrical entity and is the angle at which the maximum amplitude ECG R wave is generated.

The vector method for calculating cardiac axis

The cardiac axis can be calculated more accurately by considering the net deflection (in terms of numbers of small squares) from the isoelectric line in leads I and aVF. The net deflection values can then be plotted as vectors (Fig. 3.9) to accurately calculate the cardiac axis.

Note that positive displacement in aVF is plotted down the y-axis. If the net deflection in a lead is negative, it should be plotted in the opposite direction to that lead (i.e., 180 degrees for a negative displacement in lead I and 270 degrees for a negative displacement in aVF).

Assessment of rate and rhythm

The standard paper speed is 25 mm/s, which means that in 1 second the paper has moved by five large squares (i.e., 0.2 s per large square and 0.04 s per small square). The rate can be measured in a variety of ways:

- Divide 300 by the number of large squares between QRS complexes. That will give you a rate in beats per minute (bpm).

Fig. 3.9 Calculation of the cardiac axis. The net positive displacement of the QRS in leads I and aVF is (A) measured and (B) plotted on a graph. The angle subtended by a line between this point and 0 degrees is equal to the mean QRS axis.

- Count the number of beats in the rhythm strip (which represents 10 seconds of electrical activity on a standard trace) and multiply this number by 6.

Assessing rhythm is usually achieved by looking at lead II (often used to form the rhythm strip), but looking at V1 is also helpful, as P waves cannot always be seen in lead II. Note whether the distance between the R wave peaks is consistent. If it is not, try and establish whether it is regularly irregular or irregularly irregular. See Chapter 15 for more detail.

ECG machines will often attempt to interpret the ECG trace. Do not accept this without question as it is often wrong!

Ambulatory ECG monitoring

A standard 12-lead ECG gives a 10-second snapshot of the heart's rhythm. In some cases, a longer recording may be beneficial. Ambulatory ECG monitoring allows continuous monitoring of cardiac electrical activity, normally over a period of 24 hours or longer. The patient wears an ambulatory ECG device (sometimes called a Holter monitor) for the monitoring period. See Chapter 8 and Chapter 15 for more details.

PRESENTING AN ECG

When reading or presenting an ECG it is helpful to have a systematic approach to ensure no abnormalities are missed. The following is an example of such an approach, but with experience you may develop your own system:

- Name, age and sex of the patient.
- Date and time the ECG was taken.
- Rate.
- Rhythm.
- Axis.

Next, note any abnormalities and in which lead they occur:

- P waves – width and height.
- PR interval.
- QRS complex – width and height.
- QT interval.
- ST segment – any elevation or depression?
- T waves – negative/positive and height.

If there are abnormalities, look to see whether they are global or territorial. Remember the territories:

- Anterior – V3–V4.
- Septal – V1–V2.
- Inferior – II, III and aVF.
- Lateral – I, aVL, V5–V6.
- Posterior – V7–V9 (may see reciprocal changes in V1–V2).

CLINICAL NOTE

Abnormalities may be present across more than one territory. For example, an anterolateral ST elevation myocardial infarction may be seen as ST elevation in leads V3–6, I and aVL.

● Chapter Summary

- A standard 12-lead ECG has 6 limb leads and 6 chest leads. There are, however, only 9 physical electrodes.
- P waves represent atrial depolarization. QRS complexes represent ventricular depolarization. T waves represent ventricular repolarization.
- Not all ECG abnormalities are the result of cardiac disease.
- When reading an ECG, ensure a methodical approach is used to avoid missing abnormalities.

Other common investigations

EXERCISE ECG

Indications for exercise testing

Current National Institute for Health and Care Excellence (NICE) guidelines recommend that exercise ECG testing should not be used routinely to diagnose or exclude stable angina in people without known coronary artery disease. The assessment of ischaemic heart disease was one of the main uses of this investigation previously; however, it can still be helpful to aid diagnosis in some cases, and it can provide prognostic information.

Other indications include:

1. To detect exercise-induced arrhythmias – the increased catecholamine levels and metabolic acidosis caused by exercise potentiate arrhythmias in those patients vulnerable to this. This gives an indication of prognosis and whether treatment is required or not.
2. Driver and Vehicle Licensing Agency (DVLA) requirements, e.g., for holders of an Heavy Goods Vehicle (HGV) licence.
3. Risk assessment in hypertrophic cardiomyopathy.
4. Cautious use in patients with aortic stenosis and unclear symptoms.
5. Preoperative non-cardiac surgery assessment.

Methods of exercise

The aim of the exercise test is to stress the cardiovascular system; hence, it is referred to as an exercise stress test (EST) or exercise tolerance test (ETT). All exercise protocols have a warm-up period, a period of exercise with increasing grades of intensity and a cool-down period.

The best method is treadmill exercise. Other methods, such as bicycle testing, are often less effective because many patients are not used to the cycling action, and therefore leg fatigue may set in before cardiovascular fatigue, resulting in early termination of the test. However, bicycle testing has the advantage that the workload can be controlled and recorded in watts.

The Bruce protocol is often used in conjunction with treadmill testing. This involves 3-minute stages starting with a speed of 1.7 mph and a slope of 10 degrees. Subsequent stages are at incrementally higher speeds and steeper gradients. The final stage (stage 6) is at a rate of 5.5 mph and a gradient of 20 degrees.

The modified Bruce protocol is sometimes used for patients likely to have poor exercise tolerance. An additional two stages are added to the beginning of the standard Bruce protocol. Again, they are 3 minutes in duration and at a speed of 1.7 mph, but the gradient starts at 0 degrees and increases to 5 degrees in the first and second stages, respectively.

Patient preparation

The following should be completed before testing:

1. All patients should have been seen and examined by a physician to ensure there are no contraindications to testing (see later).
2. The test and its indications and risks should have been fully explained to the patient.

Certain patients may be advised to stop medication before the test. The operator should be aware of patients still taking their medication (especially drugs affecting the heart rate, such as β-blockers) because these affect the response to exercise. Other medicines, such as digoxin, can give rise to ST segment abnormalities and false positive results.

Variables measured

The following variables are measured before, during and after exercise. Measurements are stopped once all variables have returned to their pre-exercise levels.

12-lead electrocardiogram

The patient is fitted with the standard 12-lead ECG equipment. Poor electrode contact is avoided by shaving hair.

Blood pressure

Normal response to exercise involves an increase in blood pressure. An inadequate response or a fall in blood pressure with exercise indicates the likelihood of the following disorders:

1. Coronary artery disease – the most common cause.
2. Cardiomyopathy.
3. Left-ventricular outflow tract obstruction, such as aortic stenosis.
4. Anti-hypertensive medication.

Heart rate response

Heart rate normally increases with exercise. If the increase is inadequate, ischaemic heart disease or sinus node disease must be suspected (also ingestion of β-blockers and calcium channel antagonists).

An excessive increase in heart rate indicates reduced cardiac reserve secondary to left-ventricular failure (LVF) or anaemia.

Test end-points

The following denote successful completion of the exercise test:

1. Attainment of maximal heart rate (maximal heart rate is 220 minus age in years; however attainment of 85% of maximal heart rate is satisfactory).
2. Completion of all stages of the test with no untoward symptoms and without attaining maximum heart rate.

Appropriate premature termination of the exercise test is indicated if any of the following occur:

1. The patient requests to stop due to excessive dyspnoea or fatigue – the most common cause.
2. Chest pain.
3. Dizziness or faintness.
4. Any form of arrhythmia.
5. Failure of blood pressure to increase with exercise (or fall in blood pressure).
6. An excessive increase in blood pressure (e.g., systolic 220 mmHg).
7. Failure of heart rate to increase.
8. ST segment depression or elevation greater than 1 mm.

Positive exercise test

The following are indications of a positive exercise test:

1. ST segment depression (horizontal or downsloping) of more than 1 mm in two or more contiguous leads. (Upsloping ST segments are normal with exercise) (Fig. 4.1).
2. ST segment elevation.
3. Characteristic angina.
4. Ventricular arrhythmias.
5. Exertional hypotension.

Causes of ST segment depression are listed in Table 4.1.

COMMON PITFALLS

Exercise testing has variable sensitivity (40%–60%) and specificity (80%–90%) for detecting coronary artery disease, and both values are lower in women. Therefore it cannot be used to rule in or rule out coronary artery disease definitively. This is even more problematic in low-risk populations where positive results are more likely to be a false-positive than true. Problems arise when clinicians do not fully understand how to use and interpret the test. Beware a negative exercise test with good history of angina; other investigations will be more helpful.

Fig. 4.1 Computer-averaged exercise ECG report showing ST depression after exercise *(right-hand trace)* compared with resting ECG *(left-hand trace)* in each of the ECG leads. There is a good tachycardia in response to exercise and the blood pressure rises to 166/84 mmHg. The ST depression is in the lateral leads V3–V6 and the inferior leads II, III and aVF ETT, exercise tolerance test.

Table 4.1 Causes of segment depression

Source	Pathology
Cardiac	Ischaemia, AS, LVH, intraventricular conduction defect (e.g., LBBB)
Non-cardiac	Hypokalaemia, digoxin, hypertension

AS, aortic stenosis; *LBBB*, left bundle branch block; *LVH*, left-ventricular hypertrophy.

Contraindications to exercise testing

This list includes conditions in which additional stress on the heart may be hazardous:

1. Severe aortic stenosis – gradient >40 mmHg with normal left-ventricular function.
2. Severe hypertrophic cardiomyopathy – except in specific cases to assess for surgical treatment.
3. Uncontrolled cardiac failure.
4. Unstable angina or acute myocardial infarction (MI).
5. Myocarditis or pericarditis.
6. Second- or third-degree atrioventricular block.
7. History of sustained ventricular arrhythmias.
8. Severely uncontrolled hypertension.

Despite adhering to these rules, exercise testing does have a mortality rate of approximately 0.5–1/10 000.

In all cases, there should be trained staff and full cardiopulmonary resuscitation facilities available.

COMMUNICATION

You need to have a working knowledge of the common cardiac investigations so that you can explain to patients what is involved and how the findings may guide further treatment.

ECHOCARDIOGRAPHY

Echocardiography (echo) is the use of ultrasound to investigate the structure and function of the heart. The frequency of the ultrasound waves used is between 1 and 10 MHz. This is above the upper limit of audible sound (20 kHz).

The ultrasound waves are generated by a piezoelectric element within the transducer. Certain structures (e.g., blood) transmit waves much more than others (e.g., muscle or bone), and wave reflection varies with different tissue interfaces. The transducer picks up the reflected waves and, by knowing the time taken for the sound to return and the speed of the waves through the medium, the distance of the reflecting object from the transducer can be calculated.

By rapidly generating waves and detecting reflected waves, a picture of the heart can be built up.

M mode echocardiography

The transducer is stationary and records only a single line through the heart producing an image on a moving page. The activity along the beam is seen changing with time. This mode of echocardiography allows rapid motion to be visualized and accurate timing of cardiac events. It is useful for:

1. Visualizing the movement of the mitral and aortic valve leaflets.
2. Assessing left-ventricular dimensions and function.
3. Assessing aortic root size.
4. Assessing left atrial size.

Two-dimensional echocardiography

The ultrasound generator moves from side to side so a sector of the heart is visualized, and the series of scan lines are brought together to form a two-dimensional (2D) image. This is the mainstay of echocardiography and provides anatomical reference for other imaging modalities.

Standard views of the heart are taken in transthoracic echocardiography (Fig. 4.2) to provide information on:

1. Valve structure and function.
2. Left-ventricular contractility.
3. Size of the chambers.
4. Congenital cardiac malformations.
5. Pericardial disease.

Although this is a non-invasive, harmless and well-tolerated investigation, this approach has certain inadequacies:

1. Ultrasound does not transmit well through air, therefore the presence of lung between the heart and chest wall impedes ultrasound travel, and only windows that avoid the lungs are useful.
2. The posterior part of the heart is furthest from the transducer and may not be viewed adequately, particularly when searching for thrombi and vegetations; therefore transoesophageal echocardiography may be required.

Doppler echocardiography

This records blood flow within the heart and great vessels by using the Doppler shift phenomenon (where the change in frequency of ultrasound reflected off moving objects (e.g., blood cells) varies according to the speed and direction of movement). Colour Doppler echocardiography assigns colours to different directions of blood flow, to enable the operator to assess both the speed and the direction of blood flow.

Doppler echocardiography is used for assessment of:

1. Valve stenosis and regurgitation.
2. Atrial and ventricular septal defects, patent ductus arteriosus and other congenital anomalies.
3. Pulmonary hypertension.

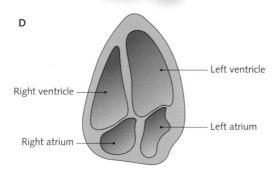

A relatively new modality called tissue Doppler imaging uses the same principles to assess the motion of the myocardium, rather than blood. This can give enhanced information about left-ventricular systolic function and, in particular, diastolic relaxation of the heart.

Other echocardiography modalities

Three-dimensional (3D) echo can produce detailed anatomical recordings, which can then be manipulated in a similar way to magnetic resonance imaging (MRI) scans. Real-time 3D echo can be used to guide intervention. Miniaturized echo probes can also be deployed through catheters to produce intracardiac echo images. These modalities may become more common in the future.

Transoesophageal echocardiography

Transoesophageal echocardiography (TOE) uses a flexible probe with a 2D transducer incorporated into the tip. Images are obtained by introducing the transducer into the distal oesophagus (Fig. 4.3). The advantage of TOE is that images are much clearer because the transducer is in close apposition to the heart. This is why TOE is the investigation of choice for assessment of:

1. Intracardiac thrombus – transthoracic echocardiography (TTE) is unreliable.
2. Prosthetic valve function – the planes used in TTE result in a great deal of artefact generated by the prosthesis.
3. Valve vegetations – usually cannot be excluded without TOE.
4. Congenital heart lesions (e.g., atrial and ventricular septal defects).

TOE imaging can be performed in multiple planes, whereas TTE is restricted to a few planes. TOE can also be used intraoperatively during cardiac surgery to provide information on valve function and left-ventricular function.

Fig. 4.2 Two-dimensional echocardiography. (A) The top illustration shows a long axis view of the heart taken from the left parasternal position with the transducer placed at the left sternal edge. Rotating the probe 90 degrees gives the parasternal short axis view. (B) Shows the mitral valve (MV), looking like the mouth of a fish. (C) Tilting the probe upwards from this point shows the three-pointed star of the aortic valve, and downwards shows the apex of the left ventricle. (D) Placing the probe over the apex of the heart gives the apical four-chamber view. Tilting the probe anteriorly to include the left-ventricular outflow tract and aortic valve gives a five-chamber view. *IVS,* interventricular septum; *LA,* left atrium; *LV,* left ventricle; *RA,* right atrium; *RV,* right ventricle.

Fig. 4.3 Transoesophageal echocardiography.

Stress echocardiography

This can be used to look for the presence of myocardial ischaemia. When myocardium is ischaemic, it contracts less strongly and efficiently. Stress echo aims to demonstrate transient reduced function in a region of myocardium supplied by a narrowed coronary artery.

The patient's heart is stressed with a drug such as dobutamine, which increases the rate and force of contraction and causes peripheral vasodilatation, so mimicking exercise. With a skilled operator, echocardiography images are obtained before, during and after dobutamine. Areas of ischaemia are seen as areas of regional wall motion abnormality, which recover at rest.

COMPUTED TOMOGRAPHY CORONARY ANGIOGRAPHY

To obtain clear, detailed images of a moving structure such as the heart is inherently challenging. The advent of rapid-acquisition of images has allowed heart motion artefact to be overcome and led to the use of computed tomography (CT) as a non-invasive alternative for imaging the coronary arteries. Modern scanners give ever-higher spatial resolution at a lower dose of radiation.

CT coronary angiography (CTCA) has recently become the first-line investigation in patients with new chest pain due to suspected coronary artery disease. Coronary artery lesions and their degree of obstruction can be assessed accurately.

HINTS AND TIPS

CTCA is useful as a 'rule-out' test. CTCA does not carry the risks of an invasive procedure, but clearly does not allow the option to intervene, and some cases may benefit from further invasive angiography for angioplasty. However, it is still not as sensitive or specific as coronary angiography, which remains the gold standard.

CT calcium scoring, which uses a single beam of electrons and multiple detectors, gives an even lower dose of radiation to calculate a risk score for future MI and cardiac death. However, it does not provide anatomical and functional information of coronary artery disease and is perhaps most useful for population risk assessments and potentially guiding the prescription of preventative therapies, such as statins.

CARDIAC MAGNETIC RESONANCE

Cardiac magnetic resonance (CMR) is increasingly common. It has a number of advantages:

1. It is non-invasive.
2. It does not expose the patient to ionizing radiation.
3. It can be gated by an ECG trace, so producing detailed still images from each stage of the cardiac cycle.

Depending on which imaging mode is used, MRI has a number of uses in the assessment of:

1. Ischaemic heart disease. Myocardial perfusion and scar (infarcted) tissue can be assessed using contrast techniques. Myocardial function before and after pharmacological stress can be assessed.
2. Cardiomyopathy. Particularly useful in the assessment of the degree of myocardial fibrosis and occasionally in rare diseases associated with deposition of proteins or lipids into the myocardium (e.g. amyloidosis or Fabry disease).
3. Congenital heart disease.
4. Valvular heart disease.
5. Myocarditis.
6. Aortic disease.

Contraindications:

1. Permanent pacemaker or implantable cardioverter defibrillator, or temporary pacing wires.
2. Intracerebral clips.
3. Metallic foreign bodies.
4. Severe claustrophobia.

CARDIAC CATHETERIZATION

This invasive investigation is the gold standard and the most frequently performed procedure for the assessment of coronary artery disease.

Technique

Access to the right side of the heart (right heart catheterization) is gained by a large vein (e.g., right antecubital fossa, femoral, or internal jugular vein).

Access to the left side of the heart is gained by a peripheral artery (e.g., right radial or femoral artery).

The vessel is punctured using a large hollow (Seldinger) needle and a wire is passed through the needle. The needle is then removed, and a sheath passed over the wire. Using a long radio-opaque guide-wire, hollow catheters can then be passed to the heart and inserted into the desired chamber or vessel, where a number of investigations may be carried out:

- The pressure in the chamber or vessel can be recorded.
- Oxygen saturation of the blood can be measured at different locations.

- Radio-opaque contrast can be injected via the catheter to provide information, depending on the location of the catheter. For example, if in the aortic root (aortography), the size and tortuosity of the aortic root can be seen by the outline of the dye within it, and aortic regurgitation can be detected.

Left heart catheterization and coronary angiography

Indications
This can be indicated for patients who have:

- Suspected coronary heart disease: positive exercise test or myocardial perfusion scan, a good history of, and multiple risk factors for, ischaemic heart disease.
- Valvular heart disease.
- Previous cardiac arrest.
- Heart failure.
- Occupational reasons – for patients who have chest pain even if non-invasive tests are negative (e.g., airline pilots).

Note that the list of indications is more complicated, but you only need to have a general idea of the common indications.

Patient preparation
The following must be completed prior to the procedure:

- A detailed history to ensure that the indications are appropriate and that the patient has no other serious diseases that may affect the decision to proceed. Any history of allergy to iodine must be noted.
- Examination to ensure that the patient is well enough.
- The procedure must be carefully explained to the patient.
- The risks must be explained.
- Informed consent is obtained.
- Peripheral pulses must all be felt for and their absence or presence noted. If the femoral approach is to be used, the groin area will need to be shaved just before the procedure.

Left ventriculography
This assesses left-ventricular cavity size and function and mitral regurgitation. Contrast is injected rapidly to fill the left ventricle. X-ray images are obtained to visualize left-ventricular contractility and the direction in which contrast is ejected from the left ventricle.

Coronary angiography
The left and right coronary ostia are located in turn and contrast is gently injected into the arteries. Several images are obtained of each artery from different angles so a detailed picture of the anatomy and patency of the arteries can be obtained. Images are recorded using X-ray video recording.

Complications of coronary angiography
The average mortality or serious complication rate of coronary angiography is 1/1000 cases. The following complications may occur:

- Haemorrhage from the arterial puncture site – this is more common from the femoral approach compared to the radial approach. Firm pressure should be applied to the site of bleeding and a clotting screen performed; rarely, operative repair is necessary.
- Formation of a pseudoaneurysm – this results from weakening of the femoral artery wall and may require surgical repair.
- Infection of the puncture site or (rarely) septicaemia may occur. Blood cultures and intravenous antibiotics may be required.
- Thrombosis of the artery used – this results in a cold white or blue foot or hand if there is no collateral supply and necessitates peripheral angiography and referral to the vascular surgeons.
- Contrast reaction – this may range from mild urticaria and pyrexia, to full-blown anaphylactic shock.
- Arrhythmias – these may occur during the angiography due to coronary arterial spasm or occlusion by the catheter. Any form of arrhythmia may occur (ventricular arrhythmias are more common).
- Pericardial tamponade – this is rare and occurs as a result of coronary artery tear or left-ventricular tear. The patient becomes acutely cyanosed and hypotensive. Pericardial aspiration is required urgently.
- Displacement of atherosclerotic fragments, which then embolize more distally, resulting in myocardial infarction, stroke, ischaemic toes, etc.
- Death.

HINTS AND TIPS

Coronary angiography is mandatory before a patient can undergo a coronary artery bypass operation. It provides detailed information on the severity and location of coronary atherosclerotic lesions, without which surgery cannot be undertaken. Older patients undergoing valve replacement surgery also have coronary angiography before surgery to exclude coexistent coronary artery disease. If this is found, coronary artery bypass may be undertaken at the same time as valve replacement.

Right heart catheterization

A catheter can be passed to measure pressures in the right atrium, right ventricle and pulmonary arteries. A balloon tip on the end can be 'wedged' into the pulmonary artery to obtain the 'wedge' pulmonary artery pressure, an approximation of left atrial filling pressure, useful in some critically ill patients. Cardiac shunts can be identified by measuring the oxygen saturations in different parts of the heart, and thermodilution techniques (where cold fluid is injected and the rate of change of temperature with time can be used to calculate blood flow) can measure cardiac output.

RADIONUCLIDE IMAGING

Myocardial perfusion imaging

This investigation uses radiolabelled agents (e.g., technetium-99m or thallium-201), which are taken up by the myocardium proportional to local myocardial blood flow. If the image early after stress demonstrates areas of reduced uptake and the later image demonstrates normal uptake in the same areas, this suggests the presence of reversible ischaemia. It is more sensitive and specific than exercise testing alone, but much more expensive.

Methods of stressing the heart

Wherever possible, exercise should be used to create actual physiological stress.

For patients who are unable to exercise due to poor mobility, peripheral vascular disease or respiratory disease, pharmacological agents may be used to mimic physiological stress. (Patients who have severe aortic stenosis or cardiac failure should in general not have stress testing.)

The commonly used agents for pharmacological stress are:

- Dipyridamole – this blocks the reabsorption of adenosine into the cells, so increasing intravascular adenosine concentrations. Adenosine is a powerful vasodilator and vasodilates normal coronary arteries, but not diseased coronary arteries. It therefore redistributes blood flow away from diseased vessels. This relative hypoperfusion of diseased areas is picked up by radionuclide myocardial imaging.
- Adenosine – a direct infusion of adenosine may be used.
- Dobutamine – this drug mimics exercise by increasing heart rate and myocardial contractility.

Note that both dipyridamole and adenosine are contraindicated in patients who have bronchospasm.

Multigated acquisition scanning

Multigated acquisition (MUGA) scanning is a radionuclide technique for evaluating cardiac function.

Technetium-99m label is applied to the patient's red blood cells. The amount of radioactivity detected within the left ventricle is proportional to its volume, and its degree of contraction will affect this. The imaging of the cardiac blood pool is synchronized to the ECG trace. Images throughout hundreds of cardiac cycles are recorded and an overall assessment of the left-ventricular ejection fraction can be made using the averaged values for end-systolic and end-diastolic volume.

This method is used less often than in the past, but it remains superior to echocardiography for the accurate assessment of ejection fraction.

Positron emission tomography

Positron emission tomography uses radionuclides, such as rubidium-82, nitrogen-13 ammonia and 18F-fluorodeoxyglucose, to provide images of the metabolic processes of the myocardium. It is expensive, but can be used to assess myocardial viability in patients when conventional techniques (radionuclide perfusion scanning and coronary angiography) have given equivocal results.

Other common investigations

● Chapter Summary

- Exercise ECG has been superseded by CT coronary angiography as a first-line test to provide evidence for suspected angina. However, when used judiciously, it can still provide useful information with regard to risk.
- Echocardiography is commonly used for the diagnosis and assessment of valvular disease and to diagnose and assess severity of heart failure. Stress echocardiography also has a role in assessing coronary artery disease.
- Cardiac catheterization is the gold standard for assessing coronary artery disease and allows for percutaneous intervention at the same time, if suitable. However, there are low rates of significant risks involved with this procedure.
- MRI does not expose the patient to ionizing radiation and can provide detailed cross-sectional images of the heart and great vessels to evaluate congenital anomalies, problems with the great vessels (e.g., in dissection) and inflammatory/infiltrative diseases of the myocardium. Contrast also allows the assessment of myocardial perfusion and infarction.
- Radionuclide imaging is decreasing in use due to improvements in other cross-sectional imaging techniques due to its cost and radiation exposure, although it can still be useful in selected cases.
- A detailed understanding of these investigations is important to select the most likely investigation to be useful and prepare the patient, to allow timely treatment for the patient and judicious use of resources.

This chapter will cover some basic principles of history and examination. These will be elaborated on in subsequent chapters.

HISTORY

Presenting complaint

As with any history, you should let the patient tell you the natural history of the complaint, but symptoms you should specifically ask about that are relevant to the cardiovascular system include:

- Chest pain.
- Shortness of breath, orthopnoea and paroxysmal nocturnal dyspnoea.
- Oedema/leg swelling.
- Palpitation.
- Syncope (fainting) or dizziness.

Past medical history

Important past medical conditions to note include:

- Ischaemic heart disease (e.g., myocardial infarction and angina) and any previous interventions, including angioplasty, coronary artery bypass graft (CABG), etc.
- Hypertension.
- Dyslipidaemia/high cholesterol.
- Diabetes mellitus.
- Any pacemakers or other implantable devices.
- Other vascular diseases (e.g., stroke/transient ischaemic attack, peripheral vascular disease).
- Rheumatic fever.
- Renal disease.

Social history

It is particularly important to ask regarding smoking history (as an atherosclerotic risk factor) and regarding alcohol intake (alcohol has a toxic effect on the myocardium).

Family history

Ask whether there is any incidence of the following diseases in close relatives:

- Myocardial infarction – A positive family history for myocardial infarction is regarded as <55 years for a male first-degree relative and <65 for a female first-degree relative.
- Stroke.

- Angina.
- Cardiomyopathy or sudden cardiac death.

CLINICAL NOTE

If the history is consistent with any form of cardiovascular disease, it is useful to make a list of risk factors for atherosclerosis that the patient does and does not have. See Chapter 12 for more information. This can help to formulate a management plan tailored specifically to that individual patient.

Review of systems

Remember to review the other systems:

- Respiratory system – cough, sputum or haemoptysis may occur in a patient with pulmonary oedema. A dry cough is a side-effect of angiotensin-converting enzyme (ACE) inhibitors.
- Gastrointestinal system – abdominal (particularly epigastric) pain or retrosternal 'heart burn' might be caused by a myocardial infarction/ischaemia. Ascites, nausea and abdominal discomfort may be the result of heart failure.
- Genitourinary system – diabetes mellitus and diuretic therapy may cause urinary frequency. Nocturia is common in heart failure.

CLINICAL EXAMINATION

Before beginning your examination, it is always important to introduce yourself to the patient, gain consent to examine them and ensure they are adequately exposed. The patient should be seated at 45 degrees, if possible, and the whole upper body exposed.

General appearance

Note from the end of the bed the general appearance of the patient. Think about whether the patient looks comfortable or if they are in pain. The patient may be obviously short of breath, pale or may be cyanosed (blue tinge to the skin). Make a note of any oxygen masks or intravenous infusions that the patient is receiving. You may also hear the clicking sound of a mechanical heart valve replacement.

Hands and arms

Both hands should be inspected on the anterior and posterior aspects. Signs that may be present in the hands are shown in Table 5.1.

Radial pulse

Palpate the radial pulse with the tips of the fingers and gently compress the radial artery against the head of the radius. The radial pulse is used to assess heart rate and rhythm. The pulse character and volume, however, are best assessed at the carotid artery. The rate should be counted for about 30 seconds and then doubled to give a rate per minute. A normal pulse is between 60 and 100 beats per minute (bpm). Anything outside this range is termed bradycardia (<60 bpm) or tachycardia (>100 bpm). The rhythm may be:

- Regular: normal rhythm; remember sinus arrhythmia is normal (an increased rate during inspiration).
- Regularly irregular: commonly caused by ectopic systolic beats or second-degree heart block.
- Irregularly irregular: usually caused by atrial fibrillation, but an ECG is required to confirm this.

Radioradial delay is delay of the left radial pulse compared with the right; this may be due to an aortic dissection or subclavian artery stenosis. Radiofemoral delay is delay of the femoral pulse compared with the radial; this may be due to coarctation of the aorta.

Checking for a collapsing pulse (see later) is also often performed at the wrist. The flats of the examiner's fingers should be placed over the radial artery and the arm raised above the patient's head. A positive result is a bounding pulse, which rapidly falls – a so-called 'water hammer' pulse. It is worthwhile checking with the patient before carrying out this manoeuvre as some patients may find this uncomfortable, for example, if they have osteoarthritis of the shoulder.

> **HINTS AND TIPS**
>
> Taking the radial pulse affords a good opportunity to observe the patient and also to measure the respiratory rate. The respiratory rate often rises when patients think it is being measured!

Brachial pulse

Palpate just above the medial aspect of the antecubital fossa and compress the brachial artery against the humerus. If you have trouble, palpate the tendon of biceps and move your fingers medial to it. People will usually assess the brachial pulse OR the carotid pulse for the pulse volume and character.

Blood pressure

A measurement of blood pressure should be taken in all patients. As well as observing whether the blood pressure is high or low, think about whether the pulse pressure is normal, increased or decreased.

Face and neck

Signs that may be found in the face are shown in Table 5.2.

Table 5.1 Examination of the hands

Area	Sign observed	Diagnostic inference
Nails	Clubbing (loss of the angle at the base of the nail) ![normal / clubbed diagram: gap present, loss of angle]	Cardiac causes include subacute bacterial endocarditis and cyanotic congenital heart disease. Numerous other non-cardiac causes including bronchial carcinoma, bronchial empyema/abscess, bronchiectasis, fibrosing alveolitis, mesothelioma, inflammatory bowel disease, cirrhosis. May be idiopathic.
	Splinter haemorrhages (small, splinter-like, linear haemorrhages under the nail).	Infective endocarditis; commonly found after trauma to the nail, especially in manual workers.
Fingers	Tobacco stains.	Smoking.
	Osler nodes (red, painful, transient swellings on pulp of fingers and toes).	Infective endocarditis. Occur due to immune complex deposition.
Palms	Janeway lesions (small, erythematous macules on the thenar and hypothenar eminences that blanch under pressure).	Infective endocarditis. Occur due to septic emboli, forming microabscesses.
Dorsum	Tendon xanthomas (yellow nodules over the extensor tendons).	Familial hypercholesterolaemia.

Table 5.2 Examination of the face*

Area	Sign observed	Diagnostic inference
Eyes	Xanthelasma (lipid deposits above or below the eye).	Hypercholesterolaemia.
	Conjunctival pallor.	Anaemia.
	Exophthalmos (protrusion of the eyeballs from their sockets).	Thyrotoxicosis.
	Corneal arcus (crescenteric opacity in the periphery of the cornea).	Common in old people; hypercholesterolaemia.
Retina	Microaneurysm (small vascular leaks caused by capillary occlusion).	Diabetes mellitus.
	Cotton-wool spots (white exudate around the macula).	Hypertension; arterial occlusion; ischaemia of the retina.
	Flame-shaped haemorrhages (haemorrhage around optic disc spreading outwards).	Hypertension.
	Papilloedema (swelling of the optic nerve head caused by raised intracranial pressure).	Malignant hypertension; chronic meningitis; brain tumour or abscess; subdural haematoma.
	Roth spots.	Infective endocarditis.
Skin	Malar flush (peripheral cyanosis on cheeks).	Mitral stenosis.
Lips and tongue	Central cyanosis.	Pulmonary–systemic shunting; lung disease; haemoglobinopathy.
Palate	High–arched.	Marfan syndrome.
Oral cavity	Poor dentition and oral hygiene.	May be more prone to infective endocarditis.

* **Generally, this is restricted to just inspection unless other systems are also being assessed.**

CLINICAL NOTE

Fingernail clubbing is an important sign of disease and should always be checked for. It progresses as follows:

1. Increased fluctuation of the nail bed only
2. Loss of the normal angle at the base of the nail
3. Increased convexity of the nail fold
4. Clubbed or 'drumstick' appearance of the fingertip

Carotid pulse

The carotid pulse should be palpated by pressing backwards at the medial border of the sternocleidomastoid and lateral to the thyroid cartilage. The two pulses should never be palpated at the same time or you will risk restricting the cerebral blood supply. The carotid pulse should be used to assess the character of the pulse (Fig. 5.1). This may be difficult, and it is important to note that there are variations of normal pulse character. The important pulses to note are:

- Slow rising pulse – the pulse rises slowly to a peak and then falls slowly. It is of small volume. This suggests aortic stenosis.

- Collapsing (water hammer) pulse – a rapid rise to the pulse and then a rapid fall. It is usually found in aortic regurgitation but may also be found in patent ductus arteriosus.
- Bisferiens pulse – two pressure peaks are seen (both in systole). This is indicative of aortic stenosis and regurgitation (mixed aortic valve disease).
- Pulsus alternans – alternating strong and weak pulses, indicative of severe left ventricular dysfunction.
- Pulsus paradoxus – a pulse that is weaker or even disappears on inspiration. Although blood pressure can decrease slightly during inspiration in a normal individual, if it drops by more than 10 mmHg it is defined as pulsus paradoxus and is abnormal. It can occur in cardiac tamponade, constrictive pericarditis or a tension pneumothorax.

Pulse volume should also be assessed. Low volume implies a decreased stroke volume. High volume (sometimes described as bounding) may be caused by high cardiac output (e.g., due to anaemia, thyrotoxicosis, sepsis, etc.).

Jugular venous pressure (JVP)

The internal jugular venous pressure reflects right atrial pressure. The reasons behind this and the components of the normal waveform are described in Chapter 2. You should observe the maximum height of the internal

Fig. 5.1 Characters of pulses. The various pulse waveforms that can result are shown here.

jugular venous pulsation and the character of the pulsation as follows (Fig. 5.2):

1. Place the patient at a 45-degree angle, with the neck supported to relax the neck muscles. You may need to turn the patient's head away from you slightly.
2. Observe the junction of the sternocleidomastoid with the clavicle and then look up along the route of the jugular veins to see if you can see visible pulsation.
3. Try palpating the pulse. If you can feel it, then the pulse is probably from the carotid artery. The venous pulse is also usually complex, with two impulses and a dominant inward wave, whereas the arterial pulse is usually a simple dominant outward wave. The JVP decreases with inspiration under normal circumstances.
4. Measure the vertical height of the pulse from the manubriosternal angle (angle of Louis). This measurement is the jugular venous pressure (in cmH_2O), which can be used to calculate right atrial pressure (by adding $5\,cmH_2O$ to the JVP measurement).

The external jugular vein is often easier to see, as it is lateral to the sternocleidomastoid and more superficial. However, it is an unreliable indicator of central venous pressure. It contains valves and moves through many fascial planes, and so it is affected by compression from structures in the neck. Some common abnormalities of the JVP waveform are described in Table 5.3.

Table 5.3 Common abnormalities in JVP

Abnormality	Diagnostic inference
Dominant a wave	Pulmonary stenosis, pulmonary hypertension, tricuspid stenosis.
Canon a wave	Complete beat block, paroxysmal nodal tachycardia, ventricular tachycardia.
Dominant v wave	Tricuspid regurgitation.
Absent x descent	Atrial fibrillation.
Exaggerated x descent	Cardiac tamponade, constrictive pericarditis.
Sharp y descent	Constrictive pericarditis, tricuspid regurgitation.
Slow y descent	Right atrial myxoma.
Normal JVP	

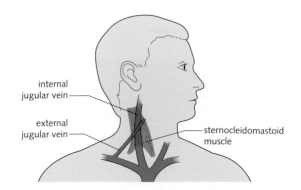

Fig. 5.2 The course of the internal and external jugular veins.

A raised jugular venous pressure (pulsation >4 cm above the manubriosternal angle with the patient positioned at 45 degrees) is usually indicative of:

- Right heart failure.
- Superior vena cava obstruction (this also abolishes any pulsations).
- Intravascular volume overload (e.g., acute nephritis, excess fluid therapy).

If the jugular venous pressure rises (rather than falls) on inspiration (Kussmaul sign) then consider:

- Constrictive pericarditis.
- Cardiac tamponade.
- Tension pneumothorax.

HINTS AND TIPS

Observing the JVP is a difficult clinical skill to master. Distinguishing the JVP from carotid pulsation is important. The JVP falls on inspiration, has a complicated waveform, fills from the top when occluded, is non-palpable and is exaggerated by the hepatojugular reflex and the Valsalva manoeuvre.

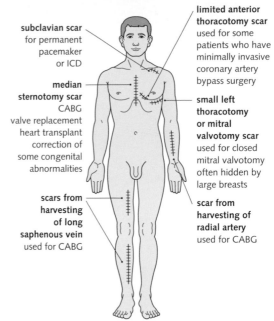

subclavian scar for permanent pacemaker or ICD

median sternotomy scar CABG valve replacement heart transplant correction of some congenital abnormalities

scars from harvesting of long saphenous vein used for CABG

limited anterior thoracotomy scar used for some patients who have minimally invasive coronary artery bypass surgery

small left thoracotomy or mitral valvotomy scar used for closed mitral valvotomy often hidden by large breasts

scar from harvesting of radial artery used for CABG

Fig. 5.3 Common scars related to cardiac surgery. Note that a larger left lateral thoracotomy is used for correction of coarctation and patent ductus arteriosus. *CABG,* Coronary artery bypass grafting; *ICD,* implantable cardioverter defibrillator.

If the JVP is not visible, you may attempt to elicit the hepatojugular reflex. This involves applying pressure over the liver, which should increase venous return, raise central venous pressure and cause the jugular venous pressure to rise and become visible. If the internal jugular venous pulsation was originally so high that it was not visible in the neck (i.e., the venous pulse was above the level of the jaw), then this manoeuvre will not elicit any change.

Central venous pressure (and therefore right atrial pressure) can be measured more accurately by the placement of a central line in the internal jugular vein. Normal central venous pressure is 0–10 cmH$_2$O.

Thorax

Inspection

Thorough inspection of the thorax should include asking the patient to lift their arms. Look for scars (Fig. 5.3), chest wall deformities, abnormal pulsations and a pacemaker/implantable cardiac defibrillator (usually just below the clavicle on the left). Important scars to be aware of include a median sternotomy, lateral thoracotomy and mitral valvotomy scar (may be hidden under the breast in a female patient).

Palpation

The apex beat should be palpated first. The apex beat is defined as the most inferior-lateral point at which the cardiac impulse can be felt and is normally located in the fifth intercostal space in the mid-clavicular line (Fig. 5.4). If the apex beat is displaced (usually inferolaterally), it generally indicates cardiac dilatation. In left ventricular hypertrophy, due to hypertension or aortic stenosis for example, the apex beat is more forceful. It is important to remember the distinction between ventricular dilatation (which causes displacement of the apex beat) and hypertrophy (which increases the force of the apex beat). The left sternal edge should be palpated with the palm of the hand for a right ventricular heave and finally, all four valve areas (see later) should be palpated with the fingertips for thrills (palpable murmurs).

HINTS AND TIPS

The apex beat may be difficult to palpate in obese patients and in patients with emphysema or pleural/pericardial effusion. If the apex beat is completely absent on the left side of the precordium, consider checking the other side: the patient may have dextrocardia! This is something that may come up in medical student exams from time to time.

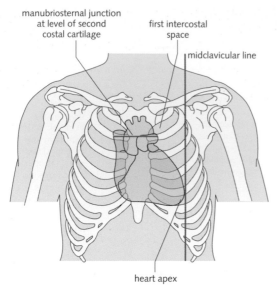

Fig. 5.4 Position of the apex beat. As a guide to identifying intercostal spaces, the second rib lies lateral to the manubriosternal angle; the second intercostal space is below this rib. The lateral position can also be described relative to the anterior axillary line and the mid-axillary line.

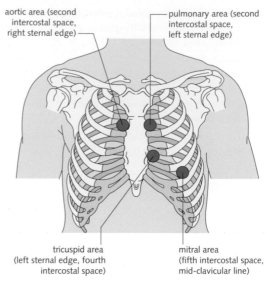

Fig. 5.5 Auscultatory areas. This shows where the valve sounds are best heard. These areas are not the surface markings of where the valves actually are.

Auscultation

The stethoscope has two ends, the bell and the diaphragm (this has a flat membrane across it like a drum). The diaphragm is better for listening to higher pitched sounds; therefore it is best for hearing:

- First and second heart sounds.
- Third and fourth heart sounds.
- Systolic murmurs.
- Aortic diastolic murmurs (aortic incompetence).

The bell of the stethoscope is best for low-pitched sounds and is best for hearing the rumbling diastolic murmur of mitral stenosis. The bell should not be placed too tightly to the skin, as it will then function as a diaphragm.

There are certain areas where auscultation should be performed (Fig. 5.5); these are the areas where murmurs from heart valves are best heard.

Heart sounds

Auscultate the heart sounds while palpating the carotid pulse, this will allow you to determine where sounds are localised within the cardiac cycle. The heart sounds (both normal and abnormal) are discussed in Chapter 2.

Patients may also have prosthetic heart valve sounds if they have previously undergone valve replacement; this is discussed in Chapter 16.

Murmurs

Murmurs are additional sounds caused by turbulent blood flow at a valve or an abnormal communication within the heart. The presence of a murmur does not always indicate disease, and the loudness does not correlate with the severity of the lesion. The common murmurs that you are likely to encounter (and how to examine for them) are discussed in Chapter 10.

Lung bases

Use the stethoscope diaphragm to auscultate the bases of the lungs to check for signs of pulmonary oedema (i.e., fine crackles) or pleural effusion (absent breath sounds).

Abdomen

If there are any signs of heart failure, it may be useful to palpate the liver. An enlarged liver can occur due to venous congestion in heart failure affecting the right ventricle. In tricuspid regurgitation, the liver may be pulsatile.

Legs

Inspect for scars that may indicate previous vein harvesting for use in coronary artery bypass grafting.

It is important to always check the ankles for pitting oedema, which is a sign of heart failure. Gently press for at least 10 seconds on the skin over a bony landmark, such as the medial malleolus, and if pitting oedema is present, an imprint of your finger will be left after you remove it. You should comment on whether it is unilateral or bilateral and how far it extends up the legs. In patients who are in bed, sacral oedema may develop, so it is often useful to check while the patient is leaning forward for you to auscultate to their lung bases.

CARDIOVASCULAR EXAMINATION SUMMARY

Examination is best practised on real patients; for a template of examination and some of the signs you might find see Table 5.4.

Table 5.4 Template for examination of the cardiovascular system

Wash your hands, introduce yourself to the patient, obtain consent and expose the patient. Position ideally supine at 45 degrees.

General inspection	General appearance, oxygen, fluids, medications, etc.
Hands	Peripheral cyanosis, fingernail inspection (clubbing, splinter haemorrhages), tar staining, tendon xanthomata, Osler nodes and Janeway lesions. Feel temperature and check capillary refill time.
Radial pulse	Rate, rhythm, volume. Examine for radioradial and radiofemoral delay and for collapsing pulse.
Blood pressure	Note pulse pressure. Consider erect and supine measurements.
Face	Central cyanosis, conjunctival pallor, corneal arcus, xanthelasma, malar flush. Consider retinal examination for Roth spots (rarely carried out).
Neck	JVP (height and waveform), carotid pulse (character and volume).
Inspection of precordium	Scars, deformity, visible pulsation/heave.
Palpation of precordium	Apex beat position and character, left parasternal heave, thrills (palpable murmurs).
Auscultation of precordium	• Mitral area, tricuspid area, pulmonary area, aortic area. • Areas of murmur radiation – axilla (e.g., mitral regurgitation), carotids (e.g., aortic stenosis). • Manoeuvres to amplify diastolic murmurs.
Back	Auscultate lung bases for crepitations. Palpate for sacral oedema.
Abdomen	Palpate liver (for hepatomegaly and/or pulsation).
Legs	Peripheral pulses and ankle oedema.

Concluding remarks: Review of observation chart (if not done initially), appropriate investigations if present.

● Chapter Summary

- As with any system, a comprehensive history is vital for diagnosis and to understand the patient's concerns.
- The main presenting complaints for cardiovascular disease include chest pain, breathlessness, peripheral oedema, palpitations, dizziness, and syncope.
- Cardiovascular disease can present with a wide range of clinical signs. It is important to be methodical to avoid missing these.
- Certain elements of the cardiovascular examination can be very difficult (e.g., JVP inspection, auscultation of murmurs); repeated practice is necessary to become competent.

Chest pain 6

Chest pain is one of the most common presenting complaints, not just in cardiology but in medicine as a whole. Of note:

- There are many causes of chest pain.
- Some causes are life-threatening and require prompt diagnosis and treatment; other causes are more benign.

DIFFERENTIAL DIAGNOSIS

The differential diagnosis of chest pain is diverse, as shown in Table 6.1. Therefore history is important to focus examination and investigation.

HINTS AND TIPS

In general practice, chest pain can often present prior to the rash of herpes zoster reactivation. It is useful to bear in mind if the patient describes unilateral burning/tingling pain from the back to the chest confined within a dermatome. Postherpetic neuralgia is also common.

Table 6.1 Differential diagnosis of chest pain (Red denotes potentially immediately life-threatening)

System	Pathology
Cardiac	Angina pectoris (myocardial ischaemia) Myocardial infarction Pericarditis Arrhythmia Prolapse of the mitral valve
Vascular	Aortic dissection Aortic aneurysm
Respiratory (most can be associated with pleuritic pain)	Pulmonary embolus Pneumothorax Pneumonia Pulmonary infarct Pulmonary neoplasm
Gastrointestinal	Oesophagitis/oesophageal spasm Oesophageal tear/rupture Peptic ulcer Biliary disease Pancreatitis
Musculoskeletal	Musculoskeletal strain Fractured rib Costochondritis (Tietze syndrome)
Neurological	Herpes zoster Nerve root compression by disc prolapse

HISTORY

If there is severe ongoing chest pain, any signs of poor perfusion or haemodynamic instability, urgent action is required. History and examination will be more focused to allow concentrated investigation and timely management.

Nature of presenting complaint

In most cases, a detailed history of the pain is vital. The mnemonic SOCRATES is helpful initially to remember the important aspects, as outlined in Table 6.2. Time of onset and duration are important in terms of ischaemic chest pain algorithms. Missing out important points, such as onset, duration and exacerbating factors, does not only lose points in exams, but can also miss the diagnosis, with possible harm to the patient, or extra investigations if the initial set were untargeted.

In clinical practice you will find your own way of taking a history smoothly. There is no need to stick to rigid structures, such as SOCRATES, once you are fluent. For example, radiation follows naturally from site of pain. Adapt your history to the patient and what he or she tells you about first. As with any system, starting with open questions identifies the patient's main concerns before narrowing the differential with closed questions.

COMMON PITFALLS

Do not use response to glyceryl trinitrate (GTN) to diagnose ischaemic chest pain. It has been shown to be unreliable. Interestingly, oesophageal spasm, or indeed any muscular spasm, can be relieved by GTN, and ongoing chest pain not relieved by GTN can signify a myocardial infarction.

Characteristics to help distinguish selected diagnoses are contrasted in Table 6.3.

For an idea of the severity of a patient's symptoms, previous and current 'exercise tolerance' clarifies the degree of deterioration. How far can he or she walk on the flat? On stairs/hills? Pain at a reproducible distance or effort is typical of angina.

Table 6.2 Evaluating the nature of chest pain (SOCRATES)

Site	Where is the pain (e.g., retrosternal, epigastric, interscapular, left or right)? Is it diffuse or localized?
Onset	What time did the pain start? What was the patient doing at the time? Did it come on gradually or suddenly?
Character	How would the patient describe the quality of the pain (e.g., crushing/heavy, tight, sharp/stabbing, burning)?
Radiation	Does the pain go anywhere else? Neck/jaw/arms? Back – from the chest to the back or vice versa? Shoulder?
Associated features	Associated symptoms (e.g., breathlessness, palpitations, nausea, sweating, change in colour observed by a relative/bystander).
Timing	Was the pain constant or intermittent? How long did it last?
Exacerbating and relieving factors	Did anything improve or worsen the pain (e.g., exertion, inspiration, food, posture, localized movement, emotion)?
Severity	Usually a numerical score (e.g., out of 10, 10 being the most severe pain ever experienced/imaginable).

Table 6.3 Classical characteristics of different types of chest pain

Characteristic	Myocardial ischaemia/ infarction	Pericarditis	Pleuritic pain	Oesophagitis/ reflux	Musculoskeletal	Aortic dissection
Quality	Crushing, heavy, dull ache, tight, bandlike	Sharp (may be dull or crushing)	Sharp	Specific to cause (e.g., burning, gnawing)	Usually sharp, although can be dull	Tearing, sharp, stabbing
Site	Central anterior chest, diffuse	Central anterior, left-sided	Anywhere in the chest, usually localized	Epigastric or retrosternal	Related to muscle involved	Retrosternal, interscapular
Radiation	Neck, jaw, arms left > right	Usually none, occasionally shoulder	Usually none	Specific to cause, occasionally throat	Related to muscle involved	Usually along the course of dissection
Exacerbating factors	Exertion, cold weather, anxiety	Recumbent position, deep inspiration	Deep inspiration, coughing, moving	Recumbent position, food, NSAIDs	Palpation of chest wall, movement by patient	Nil particular
Relieving factors	Rest (not in infarction), glyceryl trinitrate	Sitting forward, NSAIDs	Shallow breathing	Antacids	Resting affected muscles/joints	Nil particular
Associated features	Breathlessness If infarction, can be associated with nausea, sweating and shock or syncope	Fever, recent viral illness (e.g., rash, arthralgia)	Cough, haemoptysis, breathlessness, fever with pneumonia/PE, shock with large volume PE	Can be associated with nausea and sweating	Other affected joints; the patient will usually look very well	Unequal radial and femoral pulse/BP; aortic regurgitation murmur may occur, end-organ symptoms (e.g., neuro deficit)

Past medical history

This can provide clues including:

- History of ischaemic heart disease – this will increase risk of further ischaemic events. Even if the presentation is unrelated (e.g., sepsis or severe anaemia), the presence of chest pain in the context of pre-existing coronary artery disease may signify an inability to compensate and resultant myocardial ischaemia (e.g., type 2 myocardial infarction (MI)).
- History of risk factors for ischaemic heart disease (e.g., diabetes mellitus, hypertension, dyslipidaemia, other vascular disease).

- Previous arrhythmia may indicate a propensity to arrhythmia, which at extremes of heart rate may cause decompensation and myocardial ischaemia.
- Hypertension is also an important risk factor for aortic dissection.
- Pericarditis might be preceded by a prodromal viral illness.
- Recent cardiothoracic surgery may be complicated by pericarditis, mediastinitis, arrhythmia, myocardial ischaemia, pulmonary embolus and pneumonia.
- Pulmonary embolus risk is increased if there has been previous venous thromboembolism, and can be precipitated by active malignancy, a recent operation or illness or other causes of prolonged inactivity.
- Other pre-existing diseases may provide the diagnosis. Previous reflux with typical symptoms of reflux would be reassuring of the same process.
- Protracted recent vomiting could increase the risk of the rare occurrence of oesophageal tear or rupture.

Medication history, family history and social history

Other risk factors for ischaemic heart disease include a positive family history and smoking. Heavy alcohol intake and nonsteroidal antiinflammatory drug (NSAID) ingestion may predispose to gastritis and peptic ulcer disease.

> **CLINICAL NOTE**
>
> A positive family history of early ischaemic heart disease is present if there is ischaemic heart disease in first-degree male relatives <55 years old or first-degree female relatives <65 years old.

EXAMINATION

The aim of examination is to identify the severity of the condition immediately, find signs to support the underlying diagnosis and refute other differentials or place them in a sensible order and identify complications. Points to note are detailed in Fig. 6.1.

Observations, including heart rate, blood pressure, respiratory rate, oxygen saturations and temperature, are important to risk-stratify patients initially and inform the differential diagnosis.

The following points are specific to this chapter and omit differentials of examination findings that would not cause chest pain.

Inspection

- Shock (e.g., pallor, sweating, poor perfusion) – points more towards the life-threatening causes outlined in red earlier.
- Cyanosis, tachypnoea or increased work of breathing – may indicate MI leading to left ventricular failure or a respiratory cause.

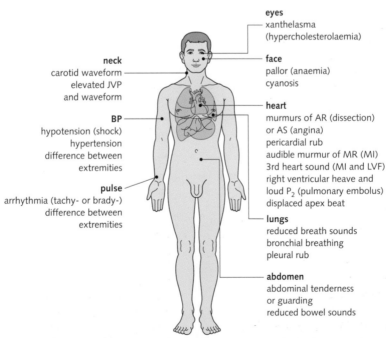

eyes
xanthelasma (hypercholesterolaemia)

neck
carotid waveform
elevated JVP and waveform

face
pallor (anaemia)
cyanosis

BP
hypotension (shock)
hypertension
difference between extremities

heart
murmurs of AR (dissection) or AS (angina)
pericardial rub
audible murmur of MR (MI)
3rd heart sound (MI and LVF)
right ventricular heave and loud P_2 (pulmonary embolus)
displaced apex beat

pulse
arrhythmia (tachy- or brady-)
difference between extremities

lungs
reduced breath sounds
bronchial breathing
pleural rub

abdomen
abdominal tenderness or guarding
reduced bowel sounds

Fig. 6.1 Points to note when examining a patient with chest pain. (*AR,* Aortic regurgitation; *AS,* aortic stenosis; *BP,* blood pressure; *LVF,* left ventricular failure; *MI,* myocardial infarction; *MR,* mitral regurgitation.)

- Vomiting – suggests MI or a gastrointestinal cause.
- Coughing – suggests a respiratory cause or, less commonly, left ventricular failure.

Cardiovascular system

- Perfusion of tissues is the best indicator of how well the cardiovascular system is functioning or compensating. This is in the form of end-organ perfusion, e.g., skin (capillary refill time and peripheral colour and warmth), brain (confusion/reduced consciousness), etc.
- Pulse and blood pressure – is there an abnormal rhythm, rate or character? A slow rising pulse may be due to severe aortic stenosis causing angina. A collapsing pulse, due to aortic regurgitation is a classic but rare complication of aortic dissection. Is there hypotension/hypertension? Uncommonly, inequalities of the pulses or blood pressure between extremities will be found and may indicate aortic dissection.
- Conjunctival pallor could suggest anaemia, which may exacerbate angina.
- Oral mucous membranes can demonstrate central cyanosis due to hypoxia or can be dry due to tachypnoea or intravascular volume depletion.
- Raised jugular venous pressure – right heart failure as a result of MI or pulmonary embolus (PE).
- Carotid pulse – useful to palpate to check if a murmur is systolic or diastolic. If there is such significant hypotension that only large central pulses are palpable, urgent action is required!
- Displaced apex beat in the context of chest pain may be a result of dilatation/aneurysm from previous MI. A nondisplaced heaving apex beat may suggest pre-existing hypertensive heart disease. A parasternal right ventricular heave may suggest a PE.
- Auscultation – pericardial rub suggests pericarditis, a pansystolic murmur may be heard in mitral regurgitation as a result of MI, a third heart sound may be found as a result of left ventricular failure, angina caused by aortic stenosis would reveal an ejection systolic murmur, an early diastolic murmur may be heard in aortic regurgitation complicating dissection.
- Bilateral crepitations may suggest left ventricular failure, and peripheral pitting oedema may be due to right ventricular or biventricular failure.
- Leg pulses may be delayed and diminished or absent in aortic dissection, and lower limb perfusion may be compromised.

> **CLINICAL NOTE**
>
> Interestingly, there is often no significant finding on examination of patients with angina. There may be signs of risk factors for angina (e.g., xanthomata/xanthelasma, tar staining/smell of tobacco, the heave of hypertensive heart disease and fingertip marks from BM testing in diabetes).

Respiratory system

- Unequal hemithorax expansion – may be present in pneumonia and pneumothorax.
- Abnormal percussion note – dullness may be present in pneumonia, hyperresonance in pneumothorax.
- Bronchial breathing and unilateral crepitations – suggestive of pneumonia.
- Pleural rub – pleural irritation (e.g., pneumonia, pulmonary infarction secondary to PE).

Gastrointestinal system

- Abdominal tenderness or guarding – looking for causes of high abdominal/lower chest pain.
- Scanty/absent bowel sounds – abdominal pathology (e.g., peritonitis due to perforated peptic ulcer is a rare cause of lower chest pain).

INVESTIGATIONS

See Table 6.4 for urgent investigations; those lower in the table would only be considered if there was clinical concern.

Blood tests

- Cardiac biomarkers – Serial high sensitivity troponins are used to diagnose or rule out MI. However, troponin may be elevated in other conditions, such as severe sepsis or major pulmonary embolism, and may reflect myocardial injury rather than infarction.
- Arterial blood gases – useful for quick results in unwell patients. Hypoxia can be seen in pulmonary oedema, PE and other respiratory causes. Hypocapnoea can be seen with tachypnoea when lung gas exchange is preserved. Lactic acidosis is concerning for tissue hypoperfusion. Other electrolyte disturbances may contribute to arrhythmia, which at extremes of rate can cause myocardial ischaemia.

Table 6.4 First-line tests to exclude a chest pain emergency

Tests	Diagnosis
ECG	Demonstrates STEMI. Lack of ST elevation may still be NSTEMI if troponin is raised, or ischaemia if it is not raised. Widespread concave ST elevation in pericarditis. May show signs of PE including right heart strain if large clot load.
Biochemical markers	Significant elevation suggests MI. Often protocols require repeat testing at 3 or 6 hours if initially mildly elevated.
CXR	Signs of LVF (see below), pneumothorax and consolidation. Widened mediastinum suggests aortic dissection.
Arterial blood gases	In unwell patients, this will quantify hypoxaemia and severity of hypoperfusion (metabolic acidosis) rather than provide direct evidence for PE, LVF or pneumonia.
CT scan	Urgently required if aortic dissection is suspected.

LVF, left ventricular failure; *NSTEMI,* non-ST elevation myocardial infarction; *PE,* pulmonary embolus; *STEMI,* ST elevation myocardial infarction

- Full blood count – significant anaemia may exacerbate angina, raised white cell count may suggest inflammation or infection.
- Renal function and electrolytes – may be abnormal due to cardiogenic shock and hypoperfusion, vomiting, diuretic therapy, etc. and will be important in decisions regarding further therapy.
- Liver function tests and amylase may be deranged in certain gastrointestinal pathologies.
- Thyroid function tests may provide an exacerbating (increased output or arrhythmic) cause of angina.
- Although lipids and glucose are less immediately important, if this is ischaemic chest pain, these will be important risk factors to tackle in ongoing management.

Electrocardiography

Relevant findings may include:

- ST elevation in contiguous leads in the same anatomical territory may indicate acute ST elevation myocardial infarction (STEMI). Very rarely it can be due to Prinzmetal angina (MI secondary to coronary vasospasm).

- New bundle branch block (BBB) in the presence of typical chest pain may indicate MI; however, this is often difficult to diagnose unless recent ECGs without BBB are instantly accessible. The results of cardiac markers may help to make the diagnosis.
- ST depression or T wave inversion in an anatomical distribution in the presence of typical chest pain suggests non-STEMI or myocardial ischaemia. (Remember ST depression may be reciprocal change in STEMI.)
- Fully developed Q waves in an anatomical territory – indicates an old MI or late presentation of STEMI.
- Nonanatomical widespread 'saddle-shaped' ST elevation is typical of pericarditis.
- Arrhythmia causing myocardial ischaemia or as a result of cardiac or pulmonary disease.
- Rarely, acute aortic dissection can cause inferior STEMI if it leads to right coronary artery dissection.

It is worth bearing in mind that there are other causes of ST elevation, including left ventricular aneurysm (deep Q waves and ST elevation in an anatomical distribution) and rarer causes, such as Brugada syndrome (ST elevation and partial right BBB in V1–2 with a 'coved' morphology) and ventricular pacing (similar to left BBB morphology with pacing spikes).

There are other causes of ST depression less pertinent to chest pain. Digoxin can cause 'reverse tick' ST depression. Hypokalaemia can cause widespread ST depression with T wave flattening/inversion and other changes. Other causes include right ventricular hypertrophy and right BBB morphology.

COMMON PITFALLS

Posterior ST elevation MIs can be easily missed if it is not appreciated that they cause anterior horizontal ST depression, along with dominant R waves (equivalent of Q waves) and importantly prominent upright T waves.

The classic changes in PE are:

- Sinus tachycardia (most commonly seen).
- Anterior T wave inversion (common).
- Atrial fibrillation.
- Tall P waves in lead II (right atrial dilatation).
- Right axis deviation and right BBB.
- S wave in lead I, Q wave in lead III and inverted T wave in lead III (the classic, and relatively uncommon, S1Q3T3 pattern).

An exercise 12-lead ECG or computed tomography (CT) coronary angiogram may be performed in intermittent stable exertional chest pain, to risk stratify suspected angina if there are no contraindications. For this and other investigations in stable chest pain, see Chapter 13.

Chest X-ray

Signs include:

- Signs of heart failure – cardiomegaly, pulmonary oedema, effusions, upper venous diversion, septal lines.
- Lung field abnormalities corresponding to respiratory causes.
- Oligaemic lung fields in PE – this is rarely seen and unreliable; CT pulmonary angiography is required if PE is suspected.
- Pericardial effusion – better assessed with echocardiography.
- Mediastinal widening in aortic dissection.

Echocardiography

This may reveal:

- Regional myocardial dysfunction – a feature of infarction or ischaemia, although less useful in the acute setting.
- Pericardial effusion – suggests pericarditis or dissection.
- Aortic dissection with false lumen.
- Aortic valve or mitral valve or septal abnormalities.
- More useful acutely to look for evidence of right heart strain in an unwell patient with suspected PE.

Computed tomography

A CT aortogram may be acutely required to diagnose aortic dissection. CT pulmonary angiography (CTPA) is a sensitive and specific test for PE if renal function allows for contrast. It is rapid and can also give detailed information about the lungs.

Increasingly, CT coronary angiograms are being performed to diagnose or exclude the presence of coronary artery disease.

Ventilation/perfusion scan

This is only sensitive for PE in selected patients and is only useful in patients with otherwise normal lungs and is rarely performed now.

Angiography, myocardial perfusion imaging or stress echocardiography

For further information about both acute and stable chest pain, see Chapter 13.

NEW ONSET CENTRAL CHEST PAIN AT REST IN AN ILL PATIENT

This is clearly a medical emergency requiring rapid diagnosis and treatment. It is necessary to rapidly distinguish between:

- MI (see Chapter 13) (high risk of hypoperfusion, arrhythmia and arrest).
- Crescendo angina (see Chapter 13) (high risk of MI).
- Arrhythmia (see Chapter 15).
- Pericarditis (see Chapter 17).
- Dissection of the thoracic aorta.
- Mediastinitis secondary to oesophageal rupture.
- PE.

Therefore urgent actions include:

- Rapid clinical assessment.
- Troponin and other bloods sent for processing and intravenous access.
- ECG.
- Chest X-ray.
- Further imaging if required.

RED FLAG

ST elevation MI usually indicates proximal occlusion of a major coronary artery. If untreated, myocardial necrosis begins within 30 minutes. Urgent restoration of coronary blood flow (reperfusion) prevents further myocardial damage and improves prognosis. Immediate treatment is detailed below. Primary percutaneous coronary intervention (PCI) is the preferred reperfusion option if available within 90 minutes, otherwise thrombolysis is still used. This is discussed further in Chapter 13.

Myocardial infarction/ischaemia

Immediate treatment for STEMI and non-STEMI (follow local acute coronary syndrome protocols):

- Targeted O_2 therapy if SpO_2 <94%; aim for 94%–98%.
- Cardiac rhythm monitoring.
- Glyceryl trinitrate.
- Intravenous opiate analgesia titrated to pain and intravenous antiemetic.
- Aspirin 300 mg orally.
- Second antiplatelet by local protocol (clopidogrel, ticagrelor, prasugrel).
- Transfer to specialist cardiac unit.
- If not transferring direct to primary PCI or considering thrombolysis, antithrombotic by local protocol (fondaparinux, low-molecular weight heparin).
- Local protocols regarding further treatment.

Dissection of the thoracic aorta

This less common, but potentially life threatening cause of chest pain is important to keep in mind during history and examination, and rapidly investigate when suspected. Risk factors include hypertension, connective tissue disorders (e.g., Marfan syndrome) and pregnancy. It is also important to remember that proximal extension of dissection can be associated with coronary artery dissection (classically inferior MI), aortic regurgitation or tamponade.

CXR may demonstrate a widened mediastinum, although its absence does not rule out aortic dissection. If aortic dissection is clinically suspected and the patient is stable enough, urgent confirmation is required using CT, magnetic resonance imaging (MRI) or transoesophageal echocardiography, if available.

Thrombolysis is contraindicated because it can cause massive haemorrhage from the aorta. Therefore it is important to decide whether the history is typical of coronary artery disease before disregarding other possible causes. Careful blood pressure control in a coronary care unit is required, with dissections involving the ascending aorta requiring immediate emergency surgery.

Further information can be found in Table 6.5 and Fig. 6.2. A sagittal MRI scan of an aortic dissection is shown in Fig. 6.3.

Table 6.5 Overview of aortic dissection

Predisposing factors	Hypertension Aortic atherosclerosis and other risk factors of atherosclerosis (male gender, increased age, smoking, etc.) Aortic aneurysm Aortitis (autoimmune diseases, syphilis) Aortic trauma or instrumentation Connective tissue disorders – Marfan syndrome, Ehlers-Danlos syndrome Aortic coarctation Bicuspid aortic valve Pregnancy Cocaine use
Pathophysiology	A false lumen is created within the aortic wall as a result of a tear in the tunica intima; blood enters and can extend the dissection. It usually occurs in the thoracic aorta due to the high luminal pressure exerted on the vessel wall.
Classification	Stanford classification: type A (DeBakey types I and II) – any dissection involving the ascending aorta; type B – does not involve the ascending aorta. DeBakey classification: type I – involving the ascending and descending aorta; type II – involving the ascending aorta only; type III – involving the descending aorta only.
Symptoms	Severe sudden onset central tearing/ripping/sharp chest pain radiating to the back. Pain can migrate when the dissection extends. Further complications if the dissection involves branches of the aorta: coronary ostia – myocardial infarction, carotid arteries – focal neurological deficit; spinal arteries – paraplegia; renal arteries – oliguria/anuria and renal failure; mesenteric arteries – abdominal pain; iliac and femoral arteries – limb ischaemia.
Signs	Shock, cyanosis, sweating. Blood pressure and pulse difference between extremities. Aortic regurgitation (if involving the aortic valve). Cardiac tamponade (if causing haemopericardium). Cardiac failure. Signs associated with involvement of other aortic branches as above, including pulse deficit or reduced perfusion in the lower limbs.
Investigation	If renal branches involved, may have renal dysfunction. If coronary ostia involved, troponin may be raised and ECG may demonstrate ST elevation. CXR – widened mediastinum. May demonstrate pericardial or cardiophrenic angle effusion if catastrophic leak; however, unlikely to see this as likely rapidly fatal. CT or MRI aortogram – the investigations of choice, will accurately demonstrate aortic false and true lumens and their extent. The false lumen often becomes larger than the true lumen. Echocardiography – may demonstrate the intimal flap and the false and true lumens. Transoesophageal echo has higher diagnostic accuracy than transthoracic. Aortic regurgitation, pericardial effusion or tamponade may also occur.

(Continued)

Table 6.5 Overview of aortic dissection—cont'd

Management	Intravenous access. Analgesia – morphine. If the patient is moribund, treatment is supportive with fluid/blood replacement and other aspects of resuscitation. If the patient is more stable, blood pressure control is essential – hypertension must be controlled urgently to avoid any further extension. This is usually achieved with intravenous infusions of labetalol ± nitroprusside. Aim for systolic BP 100–120 mmHg within 20 min. This will require invasive monitoring; transfer to a coronary care/critical care/high dependency unit. Seek early consultation with cardiothoracic and vascular surgeons. Stanford type A dissections are treated surgically by replacing the affected aortic segment with a synthetic graft. For Stanford type B dissections, medical management is the priority, with possible surgical or endovascular treatment.
Prognosis	Acute type A dissection carries with it a mortality rate of 1%–2% per hour during the first 48 hours and a 90% mortality rate at 30 days if left untreated, therefore urgent treatment is critical. Acute type A dissection has a high risk of rupture, and type B dissection has a lower risk of rupture. If rupture occurs, this is almost always rapidly fatal.

CT, computed tomography; *CXR,* chest X-ray; *ECG,* electrocardiography; *MRI,* magnetic resonance imaging.

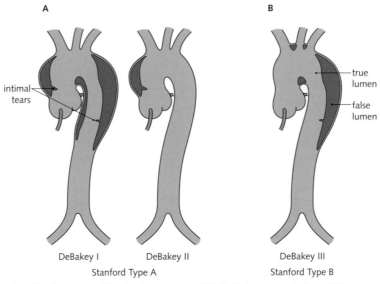

Fig. 6.2 Classification of aortic dissection: Stanford types A and B; DeBakey types I, II and III.

Mediastinitis

This is unusual but should be considered where there is a possibility of oesophageal leak, most likely after endoscopy or oesophageal surgery. Occasional oesophageal rupture occurs following protracted vomiting and is known as Boerhaave syndrome.

Pulmonary embolus

PE is common and can present as acute chest pain and breathlessness in an ill patient, or as intermittent chest pain and breathlessness in a relatively well patient. Therefore this is an important differential, especially if the chest pain is not entirely typical of angina.

Chest pain in PE is typically pleuritic, but can also be tight, and can be located anywhere in the chest. Features include:

- Dyspnoea.
- Dry cough.
- Haemoptysis.
- Hypotension/autonomic features.
- Sudden syncope or cardiac arrest.

The last two points are associated with massive PE. The ECG may show ventricular tachyarrhythmia or sinus rhythm with electromechanical dissociation, known as pulseless electrical activity. Patients may experience a sense of 'impending doom' or profound anxiety. Thrombolysis, or rarely clot-directed thrombolysis or surgery, may be attempted as lifesaving therapy in massive PE where there is haemodynamic compromise.

Fig. 6.3 Sagittal MRI scan showing extensive aortic dissection. Note how the descending aorta seems to have two lumens (double-barrelled). (Courtesy Dr A. Timmis and Dr S. Brecker.)

Table 6.6 Conditions predisposing to venous thromboembolism

Condition	Examples
Hypercoagulable states	Malignancy, oral contraceptive pill, thrombophilia such as protein C/protein S deficiency, etc.
Postoperative	Abdominal and pelvic surgery, leg and hip surgery
Venous stasis	Congestive cardiac failure, atrial fibrillation (formation of thrombus in the right ventricle can result in PE)
Immobility	Prolonged bed rest for any reason, long air journeys
Haemoconcentration	Diuretic therapy, polycythaemia
Pregnancy	Hypercoagulable state with possible immobility, venous stasis, haemoconcentration or surgery (Caesarean section)

Risk factors for PE are set out in Table 6.6.

As the mortality rate resulting from PE is approximately 10%, appropriate investigation to confirm or exclude PE should be carried out promptly if suspected.

Treatment in most cases is with anticoagulation using low-molecular-weight heparin or novel oral anticoagulants. If renal function does not allow these, intravenous heparin infusions can be used. Once PE is confirmed, longer term treatment is with warfarin or with continued novel oral anticoagulant.

● Chapter Summary

- In a patient presenting with chest pain, a clear history (if possible!) provides more information than examination to narrow the differential diagnosis and will ensure appropriate investigations are chosen. This is achieved through careful consideration of the differential diagnosis and their features.
- Examination will indicate how unwell a patient is and may provide some additional important clues.
- Information gathered directs immediate investigation. Potentially life-threatening causes to look for, or rule out early, include acute coronary syndrome, myocardial ischaemia as a consequence of arrhythmia, PE, pneumothorax, aortic dissection and oesophageal rupture.
- Urgent treatment of life-threatening causes reduces risk of death and serious complications.
- Treatment of STEMI involves some universal principles, but also involves carefully planned protocols suited to the setting (e.g., proximity to cardiology intervention units), therefore familiarize yourself with local protocols.

Shortness of breath, also known as dyspnoea, is an uncomfortable awareness of one's own breathing. It is a normal sensation on heavy exertion and considered abnormal only when it occurs at a level of physical activity not normally expected to cause any problem. This is a common presenting complaint and there are a number of possible underlying causes – the majority of these are cardiovascular or respiratory in nature.

Peripheral oedema is caused by an increase in extracellular fluid. This fluid follows gravity and therefore tends to affect the ankles initially. Ankle swelling is indicative of oedema if there is not a local acute or chronic traumatic cause. Oedema may be a feature of generalized fluid retention or obstruction of fluid drainage from the lower limbs.

DIFFERENTIAL DIAGNOSIS

There is a wide range of differential diagnoses for patients presenting with dyspnoea or breathlessness (Table 7.1).

Similarly, peripheral oedema may be the result of a number of different pathologies (Table 7.2).

In the patient presenting with dyspnoea and ankle swelling, the main diagnosis of concern is heart failure (see Chapter 14). There are many causes of cardiac failure, including:

- Ischaemic heart disease.
- Hypertension.
- Valvular disease.
- Cardiomyopathies.
- Chronic lung disease (cor pulmonale).
- Pulmonary embolism (PE).
- Primary pulmonary hypertension.

The multitude of underlying causes means that a history and examination encompassing all aspects of cardiac and respiratory disease is needed to identify the possible causes of the patient's symptoms.

HISTORY

When taking a history from a patient presenting with dyspnoea, be sure to include sufficient detail with particular emphasis on:

- Timing – is the dyspnoea acute or chronic? Continuous or intermittent?

Table 7.1 Differential diagnosis for patients presenting with dyspnoea and features of these conditions

Diagnosis	Features of breathlessness
Pulmonary oedema	Acute or chronic; exacerbated by lying flat (orthopnoea) or patient may be woken at night by episodes of severe breathlessness (paroxysmal nocturnal dyspnoea); may have cough with pink frothy sputum.
Ischaemic heart disease	Acute; exacerbated by exertion and cold weather, relieved by rest and nitrates; associated with chest pain and sweating.
Chronic obstructive pulmonary disease (COPD)	Chronic; exacerbated by respiratory infections; may be associated with cough and sputum; almost always associated with smoking.
Interstitial lung disease	Chronic; no real exacerbating/relieving factors; may have history of exposure to occupational dusts or allergens.
Pulmonary embolus	Acute; associated pleuritic chest pain and/or haemoptysis.
Pneumothorax	Acute; pleuritic chest pain.
Pneumonia	Acute; may be systemic features of infection; may be associated with cough, sputum and pleuritic chest pain.
Lung neoplasms	May be associated with history of weight loss, cough, haemoptysis and pleuritic chest pain.
Anaemia	History of blood loss, change in bowel habit, epigastric pain, peptic ulcers, recent operations, etc.
Anxiety	Associated with stress; may have associated perioral or peripheral paraesthesia.
Pregnancy	Gradual progression due to splinting of diaphragm (and sometimes anaemia).
Obesity	Gradual progression due to effort of moving and restriction of chest wall.
Trauma/musculoskeletal	Shortness of breath due to pain.

Table 7.2 Differential diagnosis for patients presenting with oedema

Diagnosis	Notes
Cardiac failure	Due to increased sodium retention secondary to activation of the renin-angiotensin-aldosterone system (RAAS).
Hypoalbuminaemia	Loss of fluid from the intravascular space due to loss of oncotic pressure within the capillaries.
Hepatic failure/cirrhosis	Due to a number of mechanisms: hypoalbuminaemia, peripheral vasodilation and activation of RAAS with sodium retention.
Renal failure	Reduction in sodium excretion, resulting in water retention.
Other	Drugs (including corticosteroids, calcium channel blockers), venous disease, obesity, lymphoedema.

- Exacerbating and relieving factors – exertion, lying flat (orthopnoea), sleep (the patient may describe paroxysmal nocturnal dyspnoea – waking up gasping for breath).
- If there is cough – ask for details of sputum production. Yellow-green sputum suggests pneumonia or exacerbation of chronic obstructive pulmonary disease (COPD); pink frothy sputum suggests left ventricular failure (LVF); haemoptysis can be a feature of PE or malignancy.
- If there is wheeze – this is suggestive of airways obstruction (i.e., asthma, COPD or neoplasm of the lung causing airway obstruction). Wheeze can also occur during LVF.
- If there is chest pain – ask for details of location, nature of pain, radiation, etc.
- If there are palpitations – ask about rate and rhythm; may suggest arrhythmia.

CLINICAL NOTE

Some patients may have breathlessness as their only symptom of ischaemic heart disease; this is sometimes called 'angina equivalent'.

If there is peripheral oedema, the patient's dyspnoea may be the result of cardiac failure and pulmonary oedema, but it is important when taking the history to remember other pathologies. A full systemic enquiry is important for this purpose, for example:

- Change in bowel habit, epigastric discomfort or dyspepsia may raise suspicion of anaemia.
- Diarrhoea, poor appetite or weight loss may raise suspicion of hypoalbuminaemia.

Past medical history

A detailed history of previous illnesses and operations will provide clues in a patient who has long-standing cardiac, respiratory, renal or liver disease.

Drug history

Important points include the following:

- Some drugs may be nephrotoxic (e.g., nonsteroidal antiinflammatory drugs, angiotensin-converting enzyme inhibitors).
- Some drugs may be hepatotoxic (e.g., methotrexate).
- Dihydropyridine calcium channel blockers (such as amlodipine) cause ankle oedema in approximately 8% of patients.

CLINICAL NOTE

Oedema commonly appears in patients treated with dihydropyridine calcium channel blockers (e.g., nifedipine, amlodipine). This is due to disturbance of oncotic and hydrostatic pressures in the tissue, not to general fluid retention. This type of oedema should not be treated with diuretics, which cause electrolyte depletion.

Social history

Important findings may include:

- Cigarette smoking – a risk factor for ischaemic heart disease.
- Alcohol abuse – not only a risk factor for hepatic cirrhosis, but also a common cause of cardiomyopathy. A detailed alcohol consumption history is therefore important.
- Intravenous drug abuse – a risk factor for hepatitis.
- Recent social stressors – may suggest a psychogenic cause for breathlessness.

CLINICAL NOTE

Causes of localized oedema in either the arms or legs include:

- Local venous thrombosis, cellulitis or trauma.
- Lymphoedema secondary to impaired lymphatic drainage – either due to obstruction (e.g., secondary to malignancy) or as the result of previous lymph node clearance.

EXAMINATION

A thorough examination is needed due to the wide range of differential diagnoses; see Fig. 7.1 for a summary.

Inspection

Note the following:

- Signs of shock (e.g., pallor, sweating) – suggest acute LVF, pneumonia or PE.
- Signs of anaemia (e.g., conjunctival pallor).
- Appearance of hands and fingers – such as clubbing or flapping tremor (carbon dioxide retention or liver flap).
- Laboured or obstructed breathing, tachypnoea or cyanosis. One or more are usually seen with resting dyspnoea.
- Cough – may suggest acute LVF, pneumonia; note the appearance of the sputum (always ask to look in the sputum pot if it is present).
- Appearance of chest – a barrel-shaped chest (hyperexpansion) is a feature of emphysema; kyphoscoliosis may impede ventilation.
- Signs of chronic liver disease, such as jaundice, spider naevi, gynaecomastia, loss of body hair, or testicular atrophy. Confusion may be indicative of encephalopathy.
- There might be evidence of ongoing dialysis, either through the presence of fistulae (usually in the forearms) or tubing attached to the abdomen in ambulatory peritoneal dialysis.
- Pyrexia – suggests infection (although note PE and myocardial infarction may be associated with a low-grade pyrexia).

Cardiovascular system

Check the following:

- Pulse and blood pressure – any abnormal rhythm, tachycardia (often seen in cardiac failure), bradycardia, hypotension, hypertension (common in both ischaemic heart disease and chronic renal disease).
- Mucous membranes – pallor suggests anaemia; cyanosis suggests hypoxia (e.g., LVF, COPD, PE, pneumonia and lung collapse).
- Carotid pulse waveform and jugular venous pressure (JVP) – JVP is elevated in fluid retention, cardiac failure and conditions causing pulmonary hypertension with associated right heart failure (e.g., PE, COPD). JVP assessment is one of the most important signs to elicit when looking for signs of heart failure. Assess it carefully.
- Palpation – lateral displacement of apex beat suggests cardiac enlargement, and a left parasternal heave suggests right ventricular hypertrophy or pulmonary hypertension.
- Heart sounds – note any audible murmurs (valvular lesions may cause LVF) or added heart sounds (third and fourth heart sounds may be heard in LVF).
- Dip the urine – this is part of every examination of the cardiovascular system. Proteinuria is a feature of nephrotic syndrome and other causes of renal impairment. Haematuria is seen in some diseases causing renal impairment.
- Peripheral oedema.

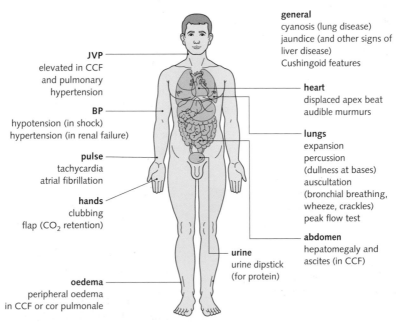

Fig. 7.1 Points to note when examining a patient presenting with dyspnoea or ankle swelling. *BP*, Blood pressure; *CCF*, congestive cardiac failure; *JVP*, jugular venous pressure.

Examination of oedema

Oedema of generalized fluid retention is pitting in nature. To demonstrate this, the area in question should be pressed firmly for at least 10 s – this will leave an indent. Be careful: ankle oedema may be tender. The severity of oedema can be gauged by the extent to which the oedema can be felt up the leg. Lymphoedema and chronic venous oedema do not 'pit'.

Respiratory system

Check the following:

- Expansion – unequal thorax expansion is a sign of pneumonia, pneumothorax or effusion.
- Vocal resonance/fremitus – when enhanced suggests consolidation; when reduced is a sign of effusion or pneumothorax.
- Abnormal dullness over hemithorax with reduced expansion – suggests pneumonia.
- Stony dullness at one or both lung bases – suggests pleural effusion.
- Hyperresonance over hemithorax with unilaterally reduced expansion – suggests pneumothorax.
- Bilateral hyperresonance with loss of cardiac dullness – suggests emphysema.
- Bronchial breathing – suggests pneumonia.
- Crepitations – coarse crepitations are heard in bronchitis, emphysema and pneumonia. Bilateral basal fine inspiratory crepitations suggest LVF. Fine mid-inspiratory crepitations may suggest pulmonary fibrosis.
- Wheeze – asthma, COPD, cardiac asthma in LVF.
- Peak flow test – always ask to perform this test as part of any respiratory examination. Explain the technique to the patient clearly and then perform three attempts and take the best out of three. Peak flow will be reduced in active asthma and COPD.

Gastrointestinal system

Examine for hepatomegaly and ascites – seen in congestive cardiac failure, isolated right-sided failure and in hepatic failure.

INVESTIGATIONS

A summary of immediate investigations for emergency causes of dyspnoea is shown in Table 7.3.

Blood tests

These include:

- Full blood count – might reveal anaemia or leucocytosis (in pneumonia).

Table 7.3 Important immediate tests to investigate for dyspnoeic emergencies

Test	Diagnosis
Chest X-ray	Acute left ventricular failure – pulmonary oedema, large heart shadow, effusions, Kerley B lines, upper lobe venous diversion.
	Acute asthma – clear overexpanded lungs.
	Pneumothorax – absence of lung markings between lung edge and chest wall, deviation of mediastinum if tension present.
	Pneumonia – consolidation (may be lobar or diffuse).
Electrocardiography	Look for evidence of myocardial infarction, ischaemia, pulmonary embolus.
Arterial blood gases	Hypoxia suggests left ventricular failure or significant lung disease (use the level of hypoxia to guide the need for oxygen therapy or artificial ventilation).
Peak flow	Reduced in airway obstruction (asthma, chronic obstructive pulmonary disease), but may also be reduced in sick patients because of weakness (it is an effort-dependent test).

- Urea and electrolytes – may be deranged due to diuretic treatment of cardiac failure, possible syndrome of inappropriate antidiuretic hormone secretion in pneumonia. This will be abnormal in primary renal disease and commonly in liver disease.
- Cardiac biomarkers – elevated if dyspnoea secondary to myocardial infarction or myocarditis. Modest elevations are also seen with ongoing heart failure.
- Liver function tests – this is abnormal in liver disease but note that hepatic congestion due to cardiac failure also causes abnormal liver function tests.
- Plasma albumin concentration – hypoalbuminaemia predisposes to both peripheral and pulmonary oedema.
- Thyroid function tests – hyperthyroidism and hypothyroidism may precipitate cardiac failure. Hypothyroidism can cause non-pitting oedema: myxoedema.
- Arterial blood gases (Table 7.4).
- D-dimer – a fibrin degradation product (elevated in pulmonary embolus). High sensitivity but low specificity, generating a lot of false positive results. Sometimes useful as a 'rule-out' test.
- C-reactive protein – elevated in inflammatory processes, such as pneumonia.

Table 7.4 Examples of arterial blood gas results in dyspnoeic patients*

	Examples	PO$_2$ (kPa)	PCO$_2$ (kPa)	pH
Normal ranges		10.5–13.5	4.5–6.0	7.35–7.45
Type 1 respiratory failure (hypoxaemia without hypercapnoea)	Left ventricular failure, pulmonary embolus	↓ (<8.0)	↓	– / ↑
Type 2 respiratory failure (hypoxaemia with hypercapnoea)	Chronic obstructive pulmonary disease, severe asthma with exhaustion	↓ (<8.0)	↑ (>6.0)	↓
Acute hyperventilation	Anxiety states	–	↓	↑

* The low pH in type 2 respiratory failure is secondary to acute retention of carbon dioxide. The high pH in acute hyperventilation results from a loss of carbon dioxide (respiratory alkalosis). The pH in type 1 respiratory failure may be increased (due to loss of carbon dioxide) or may be normal due to raised lactic acid levels/metabolic compensation.

Arterial blood gases

Arterial blood gases must be performed for all dyspnoeic patients at presentation. See Table 7.4 for examples of common findings.

Points to note:

- In acute conditions, such as acute LVF, pulmonary embolus, pneumothorax and early asthma – a respiratory alkalosis occurs (i.e., a low PCO$_2$ and a high pH). The kidneys have not yet compensated by excreting bicarbonate.
- Hypoxia – oxygen therapy causes the blood PO$_2$ to rise and the respiratory drive to fall, so ventilation is reduced and the blood PCO$_2$ rises. In asthma, exhaustion causes the ventilatory drive to fall off and the PCO$_2$ to rise; this precedes respiratory arrest and is an indication for artificial ventilation of the patient.
- COPD with chronic CO$_2$ retention – the pH is normal because metabolic compensation has occurred and bicarbonate levels rise as a result of renal retention of bicarbonate (this takes a few days to occur).
- Severe asthma with acute CO$_2$ retention – the pH falls as the PCO$_2$ rises as there has been insufficient time for metabolic compensation to occur.
- Metabolic acidosis can occur in liver and renal failure (with normal oxygen and normal or low carbon dioxide if compensating).

Electrocardiography

This might show:

- Ischaemic changes may be seen in patients with coronary artery disease.
- Sinus tachycardia with right axis deviation/anterior T wave inversion/right bundle branch block/S1Q3T3 pattern in patients who have a PE.
- Atrial fibrillation – may be seen secondary to any lung pathology or ischaemia.

COMMON PITFALLS

Despite the S1Q3T3 pattern (deep S wave in lead I, Q wave and inverted T wave in lead III) being seen as a classic finding in pulmonary embolism, it is not a particularly sensitive or specific test for PE by itself. The commonest ECG changes in pulmonary embolism are sinus tachycardia and anterior T wave inversion.

Chest radiography

Note the following:

- Cardiomegaly in cardiac failure – increased cardiothoracic ratio.
- Signs of pulmonary oedema – bat's wing shadowing, upper lobe blood diversion, Kerley B lines (Fig. 7.2).
- Focal lung consolidation in pneumonia (shadowing of a lung segment with an air bronchogram).
- Pleural effusion – suggests infection, malignancy or cardiac failure.
- Hyperexpanded lung fields in emphysema (ability to count more than six rib spaces over the lung fields); bullae may be seen in emphysema.

Upper lobe blood diversion

Peri-hilar shadowing

Diffuse interstitial shadowing

Enlarged heart

Fig. 7.2 Chest X-ray with features of pulmonary oedema.

- Presence of a pneumothorax – ask for a film in full expiration if this is suspected.
- Occasionally oligaemic lung fields in PE (but often appears normal).

Echocardiography

This may reveal:

- Left ventricular (LV) systolic dysfunction.
- Valve lesions.
- Ventricular hypertrophy and pulmonary hypertension.

Computed tomography

This is used to obtain detailed visualization of pulmonary fibrosis or small peripheral tumours that cannot be reached with a bronchoscope. CT pulmonary angiography (CTPA) is used to analyse blood flow in the pulmonary system and is the gold standard for identifying pulmonary emboli. It will also detect pulmonary oedema, consolidation or evidence of malignancy.

Urine tests

If there is no evidence of cardiac disease and the plasma albumin is low, consider urine testing. Nephrotic syndrome causes loss of at least 3 g protein in 24 hours. The albumin:creatinine ratio may be used to estimate proteinuria, avoiding the need for 24-hour collections.

Pulmonary function tests

These tests are used to investigate:

- Lung volumes – increased in COPD, reduced in restrictive lung disease.
- Flow-volume loop – scalloped in COPD.
- Carbon monoxide transfer – reduced in the presence of normal airway function in restrictive lung diseases.

Ultrasound

Consider ultrasound of the pelvis in patients with no evidence of cardiac, renal or liver disease and bilateral ankle oedema to investigate for venous thrombosis or a mass lesion causing external compression.

RECENT ONSET DYSPNOEA AT REST IN AN ILL PATIENT

If a patient is unwell with dyspnoea, this is a cardiopulmonary emergency requiring rapid diagnosis and treatment. It is necessary to distinguish between the following life-threatening causes:

- Acute LVF.
- PE.
- Tension pneumothorax.
- Life-threatening asthma.
- Pneumonia.

Acute left ventricular failure

The detailed management of acute LVF is discussed in more detail in Chapter 24. Classic signs of LVF can be seen and include:

- Severe dyspnoea.
- Central cyanosis.
- Patient sits upright.
- Bilateral basal fine end-inspiratory crepitations (in severe LVF the crepitations extend upwards to fill both lung fields).
- Hypotension secondary to poor LV output (common).
- Blood gases show hypoxia and often hypocapnoea due to hyperventilation. There is usually a metabolic acidosis as a result of poor tissue perfusion.

Treatment includes high-concentration inhaled oxygen via a mask and intravenous diuretic (furosemide). Current National Institute for Health and Care Excellence (NICE) guidance no longer advises routine use of opiates and nitrates in this situation.

Pulmonary embolus

This can present in a number of ways, for example:

- Severe dyspnoea.
- Collapse and syncope.
- Hypotension.
- Cardiorespiratory arrest (often with pulseless electrical activity or ventricular fibrillation).

If PE is suspected, anticoagulation should be commenced immediately with subcutaneous low-molecular-weight heparin (LMWH), novel oral anticoagulant or an intravenous heparin infusion.

Haemodynamic instability may suggest massive PE – thrombolysis may be administered or emergency pulmonary angiography carried out in an attempt to disrupt the embolus.

Other respiratory causes of breathlessness

Refer to Crash Course: Respiratory Medicine 5th Edition for more detail.

Pneumothorax

Pneumothorax may be an acute or chronic cause of dyspnoea. In pneumothorax, there is a connection between the pleural space and the atmosphere (via either the chest wall or the airways). This may be the result of trauma or rupture of bullae on the surface of the lung (may occur in emphysema, but also sometimes in young healthy patients).

Tension pneumothorax can occur if the air continues to accumulate in the pleural cavity, resulting in a progressive increase in pressure and displacement of the mediastinum away from the side of the lesion. This is characterized by the following clinical signs:

- Severe and worsening dyspnoea.
- Displaced trachea and apex beat. Hyperresonance on the affected side with reduced breath sounds.

- Progressive hypotension due to reduced venous return and therefore reduced filling of the right ventricle.
- Eventual collapse and cardiac arrest.

Treatment should be immediate, with insertion of a large-bore needle into the second intercostal space in the midclavicular line on the affected side to allow gas to escape spontaneously from the pleural cavity. A chest drain should then be inserted.

Acute asthma

Signs suggestive of a severe asthma attack include:

- The patient being unable to talk in full sentences due to dyspnoea.
- The patient sitting forwards and using accessory muscles of respiration.
- Tachycardia.
- Peak flow less than 50% of normal.
- Pulsus paradoxus – drop in systolic blood pressure of >10 mmHg on inspiration.

Hypercapnoea on blood gas analysis suggests exhaustion and respiratory arrest could be imminent – this may occur before severe hypoxia. The patient should be considered for intubation and artificial ventilation.

This is a medical emergency and appropriate treatment with oxygen therapy, nebulized bronchodilators, and intravenous hydrocortisone should be commenced immediately.

Pneumonia

There may be pyrexia or even signs of septic shock (e.g., hypotension, renal failure). Blood gases may reveal hypoxia. The chest radiograph might show consolidation. Radiographic changes can be deceptively mild in certain atypical infections.

Blood and sputum cultures should be taken (if possible) and antibiotic therapy according to local guidelines should be started as soon as possible.

● Chapter Summary

- There is a wide differential diagnosis in patients presenting with dyspnoea, including cardiac (e.g., LVF, ischaemic heart disease), respiratory (e.g., asthma exacerbation pneumothorax) and other pathologies (e.g., anxiety, anaemia).
- There is also a wide differential in patients presenting with ankle/leg oedema, including cardiac failure, hypoalbuminaemia, renal failure, hepatic failure and medication-related, as well as a number of other causes.
- Cardiac failure is the main diagnosis of concern in the patient who presents with dyspnoea and peripheral oedema. Detailed history-taking and examination is vital to establishing an accurate diagnosis.
- There are a number of life-threatening causes of dyspnoea and it is important to know how each of these should be investigated for (and subsequently managed).

Palpitation is the abnormal awareness of the heartbeat. Palpitations (multiple episodes of palpitation) may be rapid, slow or just particularly forceful beats occurring at a normal rate.

DIFFERENTIAL DIAGNOSIS

Palpitations may occur in a number of different disorders (Table 8.1). Any condition producing a change in cardiac rhythm, rate or stroke volume may result in palpitations.

Table 8.1 Differential diagnosis of palpitations

	Diagnosis
Arrhythmia	Bradycardia
	Sinus arrhythmia
	Sinus tachycardia
	Atrial fibrillation/flutter
	Atrial tachycardia
	Atrial/ventricular ectopic beats
	Supraventricular tachycardia
	Ventricular tachycardia
Non-arrhythmic cardiac causes	Septal defects
	Congestive heart failure
	Congenital heart disease
	Cardiomyopathy
	Valvular disease
Extra-cardiac causes	Anaemia
	Electrolyte abnormality
	Hypoglycaemia
	Fever
	Hyperthyroidism
	Hypovolaemia
	Pregnancy
	Phaeochromocytoma
Drugs and medications	Alcohol
	Caffeine and other stimulant drugs
	Sympathomimetic drugs (e.g., β-agonists, antimuscarinics, etc.)
	Nicotine
Psychiatric	Anxiety or depression
	Panic attacks

Some arrhythmias are of more concern than others and these are highlighted in red above. Adverse features to watch out for are shock, syncope, myocardial ischaemia or heart failure. Many of the other above causes of palpitations can also be severe or life-threatening, however, for instance profound anaemia or fever secondary to severe sepsis.

Rapid palpitations

Rapid palpitations may be either regular or irregular in rhythm. Regular palpitations may be a sign of:

- Sinus tachycardia.
- Atrial flutter.
- Atrial tachycardia.
- Supraventricular tachycardia (SVT).
- Ventricular tachycardia.

Irregular palpitations may indicate:

- Atrial fibrillation (i.e., with a fast ventricular response rate).
- Multiple atrial or ventricular ectopic beats.

CLINICAL NOTE

Remember, many patients presenting with palpitations do not have evidence of arrhythmia and many patients presenting with arrhythmia do not have palpitations!

Slow palpitations

Patients may describe these as missed beats or particularly forceful beats. After a brief pause in the heart rhythm the following beat is often more forceful due to longer ventricular filling time and therefore higher end-diastolic volume and higher stroke volume. Causes of slow palpitation may indicate:

- Ectopic beats with compensatory pauses.
- Atrioventricular (AV) block.
- Sick sinus syndrome.

Disorders causing increased stroke volume

An increase in stroke volume may be the result of:

- High-output states (e.g., anaemia, pregnancy, fever, thyrotoxicosis, etc.).
- Valvular lesions (e.g., mitral or aortic regurgitation).

HISTORY

When taking a history from a patient presenting with palpitations, aim primarily to answer the following questions:

1. What is the nature of the palpitations?

2. What is the likely underlying cause?
3. Do they represent a severe or life-threatening process?

This will help to structure your approach and present your findings in a logical manner.

Nature of the palpitations

Often it is helpful to ask patients to describe the palpitation by tapping it out themselves. This gives an idea of rate and rhythm (i.e., fast or slow, regular or irregular). Do the episodes involve single particularly forceful beats or longer runs of palpitations? Are the episodes paroxysmal (i.e., intermittent) or continuous in nature? Is the onset sudden or gradual?

Likely underlying causes of palpitation

Certain features of the history may be suggestive of the recognized causes of arrhythmia shown in Table 8.2.

CLINICAL NOTE

Hyperthyroidism is well recognized to predispose to palpitations, tachycardia and sometimes atrial fibrillation. It is somewhat less well recognized that *hypo*thyroidism can predispose to ventricular dysrhythmias.

Table 8.2 Features in the history that might suggest the cause of an arrhythmia

Cause of arrhythmia	Features in the history
Ischaemic heart disease	Exertional chest pain or breathlessness, history of myocardial infarction/coronary intervention or bypass grafting, Risk factors for coronary disease (see Chapter 12)
Thyroid disease	Tremor, excessive sweating, unexplained weight loss, lethargy, obesity
Valvular heart disease	History of rheumatic fever, previous valve surgery, previous intravenous drug use
Anaemia	Peptic ulcer disease, menorrhagia, recent operations
Proarrhythmic agents	Alcohol, caffeine, stimulant drugs, antiarrhythmic agents
Anxiety	Anxiety, paraesthesia in fingertips

Are the palpitations severe or life-threatening?

It is important to clarify whether palpitations are innocent or whether severe pathology is underlying (i.e., is the palpitation occurring in the context of heart failure, ischaemia or thromboembolic events?).

Is the palpitation associated with:

- Breathlessness, dizziness or syncope? This suggests cardiac output is compromised.
- Angina? This suggests the palpitations are causing (or perhaps being caused by) myocardial ischaemia.
- History of transient ischaemic attack, stroke or limb ischaemia? Certain arrhythmias (atrial fibrillation in particular) are associated with thromboembolic complications.

EXAMINATION

Examination is aimed towards identifying both signs of the underlying cause and any complications of palpitations. This is summarized in Fig. 8.1.

General observation

Look for:

- Cyanosis – suggestive of cardiac failure or lung disease (remember pulmonary embolus is a well-recognized cause of tachyarrhythmia).
- Dyspnoea – suggestive of cardiac failure or lung disease.
- Pallor – suggestive of anaemia.
- Fever – pyrexia, sweating, etc. may be suggestive of underlying infection (may precipitate arrhythmias, such as atrial fibrillation).
- Thyrotoxic or myxoedematous facies.

COMMON PITFALLS

Cardiac disease can both cause and be caused by disease in other systems, so do not get caught out and remember to thoroughly examine all systems.

Cardiovascular system

Pulse

Palpate the pulses to assess for rate, rhythm, volume and character for at least 15 s.

- Rate. Bradycardia can be associated with higher stroke volume due to a longer period for ventricular filling between beats. This may result in forceful beats. Tachycardia (of any cause) can predispose to awareness of palpitations.

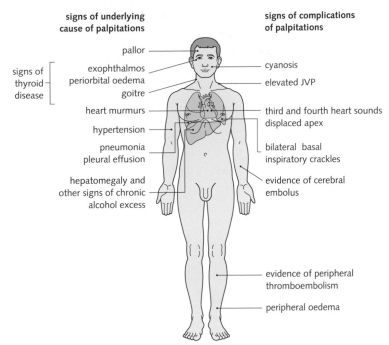

signs of underlying
cause of palpitations

signs of complications
of palpitations

pallor

cyanosis

signs of
thyroid
disease

exophthalmos
periorbital oedema
goitre

elevated JVP

heart murmurs

third and fourth heart sounds
displaced apex

hypertension

pneumonia
pleural effusion

bilateral basal
inspiratory crackles

hepatomegaly and
other signs of chronic
alcohol excess

evidence of cerebral
embolus

evidence of peripheral
thromboembolism

peripheral oedema

Fig. 8.1 Important points to note when examining a patient who has *palpitations*. *JVP*, Jugular venous pressure.

- Rhythm. Is the rhythm regular? If not, is it regularly irregular (as in some bigeminal rhythms or heart blocks) or irregularly irregular (as in atrial fibrillation)?
- Volume. A high-volume pulse (due to high-output states and aortic or mitral regurgitation) is most easily felt at the radial pulse. Volume may vary from beat to beat in certain rhythms, such as atrial fibrillation, due to variation in ventricular filling time and therefore stroke volume. In these cases, low-volume ventricular contractions may not conduct a palpable pulse to peripheral arteries. This is called a 'pulse deficit'. Radial pulse assessment may give an inaccurate reflection of the true heart rate, particularly in tachycardia. Assessment of rate at the cardiac apex is more accurate.
- Character. Abnormal character may suggest underlying valvular heart disease (see Chapter 10).

CLINICAL NOTE

Sinus arrhythmia is a term for sinus rhythm with a beat to beat variation in the P–P interval (interval between subsequent P waves). This usually occurs due to changes in vagal tone due to different stages of the respiratory cycle and is a normal physiological phenomenon most commonly seen in the young.

Blood pressure

Hypertension is a well-recognized cause of atrial fibrillation (and ischaemic heart disease). Pulse pressure may give information as to valvular causes of palpitation with a narrow pulse pressure suggesting aortic stenosis and a wide pulse pressure suggesting aortic regurgitation.

Jugular venous pressure

Jugular venous pressure may be elevated if the patient has congestive cardiac failure as a consequence of an uncontrolled tachycardia or has atrial flutter or fibrillation secondary to pulmonary embolism.

Apex beat

This may be displaced in the patient with left ventricular failure. The apex beat in hypertrophic cardiomyopathy is classically forceful in nature, with a double impulse if the left ventricular outflow tract is obstructed. Individuals with hypertrophic cardiomyopathy are more at risk of arrhythmia.

Heart sounds

A third or fourth heart sound may be heard. Mitral or aortic regurgitation are possible causes of high output state and may cause murmurs. A murmur of mitral stenosis may be heard as this condition leads to atrial dilatation and therefore increasing risk of atrial fibrillation.

Respiratory system

Bilateral basal inspiratory crepitations may be heard in patients with left ventricular failure. There may be signs of underlying chest infection, a common cause of palpitations.

Gastrointestinal system

Hepatomegaly and ascites may be signs of congestive cardiac failure or alcoholic liver disease. Alcohol is one of the commonest causes of tachyarrhythmias. Look for other signs of liver disease if this is suspected.

Limbs

Examine for:

- Peripheral oedema – may be a sign of congestive cardiac failure.
- Tremor – may be a sign of thyrotoxicosis or alcohol withdrawal.
- Brisk reflexes – seen in thyrotoxicosis.
- Abnormal neurology – may be a sign of previous cerebral embolus.

INVESTIGATIONS

Biochemical tests

The following tests may aid diagnosis:

- Serum electrolytes – deranged levels of potassium and calcium in particular can predispose to arrhythmia.
- Full blood count – look for anaemia or raised white cell count.
- Inflammatory markers – may be relevant if palpitations arise in context of sepsis.
- Thyroid function tests – palpitations may result from both hyperthyroid and hypothyroid states.
- Liver function tests – deranged in congestive cardiac failure or alcoholic liver disease.
- 24-hour urinary catecholamines – not routinely done but may be useful to exclude phaeochromocytoma in some cases.

Electrocardiography

12-lead electrocardiography

This may enable instant diagnosis if the palpitations are present at time of testing. However, if the palpitation is intermittent or paroxysmal, the ECG may be normal.

There may be signs of the cause of the palpitation on the ECG, for example ischaemia, or presence of a delta wave or short PR interval (as seen in some congenital causes of paroxysmal tachyarrhythmias, such as Wolff-Parkinson-White syndrome).

Ambulatory electrocardiography

Monitoring of the ECG for a longer period (e.g., 24 hours) may reveal paroxysmal arrhythmias. Patients press an alert button when they have symptoms, marking that period of the recording for review.

Longer-term monitors may be necessary to document infrequent episodes. This may involve external monitoring for a longer period or in some cases use of an implantable loop recorder. A loop recorder is a small subcutaneous ECG monitoring device that may be left in for 2 to 3 years.

COMMUNICATION

Ask about frequency of episodes; remember, a normal 24-hour recording does not exclude arrhythmia if the arrhythmia is paroxysmal and the patient has not had any symptoms when monitored.

Exercise electrocardiography

This test can be used to reveal exercise-induced arrhythmias. Examples of ECGs illustrating atrial fibrillation, atrial flutter and SVT are shown in Fig. 8.2.

Vagotonic manoeuvres

Such manoeuvres include:

- Valsalva manoeuvres – (e.g., blowing into a large syringe).
- Carotid sinus massage – there is a risk of stroke in patients with carotid artery disease (due to embolization of plaque) so avoid in the elderly and those with history of myocardial infarction, transient ischaemic attack or stroke.
- Diving reflex – this involves submerging the face in water (or applying a cold wet towel to the face). This is particularly effective in infants in whom the diving reflex is better preserved.

HINTS AND TIPS

A modified Valsalva manoeuvre has been shown to be much more effective for reverting supraventricular tachycardia to sinus rhythm. Position the patient semi-recumbent in the bed. Have him or her perform a Valsalva manoeuvre as normal, but immediately following the manoeuvre, the patient should be repositioned supine and legs passively raised. Recent evidence suggests this may be much more effective than standard Valsalva manoeuvres.

These manoeuvres act to increase vagal tone, which in turn increases the refractory period of the AV node. This enables differentiation between three common tachyarrhythmias that are sometimes indistinguishable on ECG recording:

- Atrial flutter.
- Atrial fibrillation.
- SVT.

Characteristic features of these tachyarrhythmias are listed in Table 8.3.

Adenosine administration

Adenosine is a purine nucleoside that acts to block the AV node. When administered intravenously, it will achieve complete AV block. Its half-life is very short (only a few seconds), so this effect is very short lived. Adenosine can be useful in both the diagnosis of arrhythmia (differentiation of tachyarrhythmias) and in terminating reentrant tachyarrhythmias involving the AV node (see Table 8.3).

Side effects of adenosine include bronchospasm, so avoid in asthmatics. In individuals with asthma, verapamil might be used as an alternative. Adenosine has a higher rate of minor adverse effects but verapamil is associated with higher risk of significant hypotension.

Fig. 8.2 Electrocardiograms illustrating atrial fibrillation, atrial flutter and supraventricular reentry tachycardia. A) Note the irregularly irregular rhythm (variable R-R), underlying 'fibrillation' (F) and absence of P waves preceding QRS complexes. B) Note a regular rhythm at a rate divisible into 300 (150 beats/min in this case). Sometimes underlying flutter (F) waves can be seen at a rate of 300 per min.

(Continued)

C Supraventricular reentry tachycardia

lead V1

lead V2

lead V3

X

Fig. 8.2, cont'd C) Note the fast, regular rhythm (usually 140–240 beats/min). P waves are present but not always easy to see, they may occur before or after the QRS (and are sometimes hidden by the QRS complex). Point X shows reversion to sinus rhythm, note the normal P wave preceding it.

Table 8.3 Characteristic features of atrial fibrillation, atrial flutter and supraventricular reentry tachycardia

	Atrial fibrillation	**Atrial flutter**	**Supraventricular tachycardia**
Rate	Any rate, pulse deficit may be present if fast	Atrial flutter rate is 300/min; the ventricular rate is usually divisible into this (e.g., 150 or 100 beats per minute) (due to 2:1 or 3:1 conduction)	140–260/min
Rhythm	Irregularly irregular	Regular	Regular
Response to adenosine/ Valsalva manoeuvre	Unnecessary – irregurlarly irregular rhythm should be recognisable. Adenosine can be dangerous if accessory pathway present	Slowing of ventricular rate reveals 'saw-tooth' flutter waves	Blocking the atrioventricular node may 'break' the reentry circuit, terminating the tachycardia

Chest X-ray

Chest X-ray may reveal evidence of heart failure, either as a direct cause of palpitations or as a result of cardiac decompensation secondary to arrhythmia.

Echocardiography

This may reveal valvular pathology, evidence of congenital heart disease or cardiomyopathy. Echocardiography enables evaluation of chamber size and of ventricular function, which may both be deranged due to arrhythmia.

Electrophysiological study

This is useful in investigating patients suspected of having tachyarrhythmias due to abnormal reentry pathways. The technique enables localization of the reentry circuit, which may then be ablated using a radiofrequency thermal electrode placed inside the heart.

Other investigations

Various other investigations may be required to identify a suspected cause of the palpitation, for example:

- Computed tomography pulmonary angiography – if a pulmonary embolus is likely.
- Coronary angiogram – if coronary artery disease is suspected.

PALPITATIONS IN THE UNWELL PATIENT

Many causes of palpitations can be severe or life threatening. In the patient presenting acutely unwell and complaining of palpitations, investigation and treatment is comprised of supportive treatments and treatment of the underlying cause of the palpitations. This may involve for instance:

- Blood transfusion in severe anaemia.
- Antibiotic treatment in sepsis.
- Fluid resuscitation in hypovolaemia.
- Glucose replacement in hypoglycaemia.
- Direct treatment of a primary arrhythmia.

Adverse features in patients with arrhythmia

The first thing to do when you see a fast heart rhythm is to establish the patient's clinical status. In the patient presenting with palpitations and an arrhythmic cause of their symptoms, there are a number of adverse features that, if identified, should be of particular concern:

- Shock – in this context shock is often used to indicate hypotension with a systolic blood pressure of <90 mmHg. The patient may also present with pallor, sweatiness, be peripherally shut down, confused or demonstrate altered consciousness. Remember that cardiogenic shock and arrhythmia may also occur together as the result of other cardiac problems, such as myocardial infarction.
- Syncope – transient loss of consciousness due to a global reduction in cerebral blood flow. Palpitations in the context of syncope suggest an 'unstable' arrhythmia that has resulted in impairment of cardiac output.
- Myocardial ischaemia – either as the patient reporting chest pain and/or electrocardiographic evidence of ischaemia.
- Heart failure – arrhythmias may cause pulmonary oedema, either with or without evidence of peripheral oedema.

These adverse features in conjunction with either a bradyarrhythmia or tachyarrhythmia represent a peri-arrest situation requiring rapid diagnosis and treatment to avoid deterioration.

CLINICAL NOTE

Many causes of shock are treated with fluid resuscitation. Fluid resuscitation in *cardiogenic* shock may, however, be detrimental as the heart is already struggling to pump the existing intravascular volume round the body. Additional fluid may predispose to pulmonary oedema.

Management of arrhythmia

If adverse features are occurring in the context of arrhythmia and palpitations, management is focused on treating the underlying arrhythmia.

For tachyarrhythmias in the unstable patient with a pulse, treatment usually involves synchronized direct current (DC) cardioversion. For bradyarrhythmias, the primary treatment is generally with chronotropes or pacing. Supportive treatments, such as oxygen, should always be given if indicated.

For more information about the treatment of arrhythmia (including in arrest and peri-arrest situations) see Chapter 15.

Chapter Summary

- History taking should be tailored to establish the nature of palpitations, the likely underlying cause and whether palpitations are serious or life threatening.
- There are a number of different causes of palpitations, most are benign but some are life threatening.
- It can often be difficult to document episodes of arrhythmia if they are happening very infrequently.
- Sometimes simple vagal manoeuvres can revert patients with tachyarrhythmias back to sinus rhythm and avoid the use of medical interventions.
- Patients presenting with palpitations and evidence of myocardial ischaemia, heart failure, shock or syncope are potentially peri-arrest and warrant urgent treatment.

Syncope | 9

Syncope is a loss of consciousness, usually due to a reduction in perfusion of the brain.

DIFFERENTIAL DIAGNOSIS OF SYNCOPE

Many conditions can give rise to syncope – this can occur due to numerous different pathologies (Table 9.1).

There are also a number of other conditions that may cause reduced (or loss of) consciousness, but are not true syncope as they are not due to a reduction in cerebral perfusion. These conditions include:

- Hypoglycaemia.
- Hypoxia.
- Epilepsy.
- Intoxication.

Certain other conditions may also resemble syncope, but there is no loss of consciousness, including psychogenic 'syncope', drop attacks, cataplexy, etc.

It is worth remembering these mimics of syncope in the patient who presents complaining of a faint or collapse.

CLINICAL NOTE

The term 'Stokes-Adams attack' is sometimes used to refer to a reduction in (or loss of) cardiac output and loss of consciousness due to transient arrhythmia (e.g., asystole, ventricular fibrillation, atrioventricular block).

HISTORY

The first differentiation to be made is between cardiac and non-cardiac (usually neurological) syncope (and to decide whether the event is syncope at all)!

COMMUNICATION

Patients may describe syncopal episodes in a number of different ways. Syncopal episodes may be referred to as fits, faints, funny turns, collapses, blackouts – it is important to pin down exactly what they mean!

It is often difficult to definitively diagnose the cause of collapse, but differentiation depends upon a detailed history of the episode of collapse with particular emphasis on the features outlined here.

The events preceding the collapse should be elucidated:

- Exertion – can precipitate syncope in hypertrophic cardiomyopathy (HCM) or aortic stenosis.
- Pain or anxiety or prolonged standing – in vasovagal syncope.
- Soon after standing – postural hypotension.
- Neck movements – aggravate vertebrobasilar attacks or carotid sinus hypersensitivity.

Speed of onset of collapse might be:

- Immediate with no warning – classic presentation of syncope due to arrhythmia.
- Rapid with warning – preceded either by lightheadedness (vasovagal) or by an aura (epilepsy).
- Gradual with warning – hypoglycaemia preceded by lightheadedness, nausea and sweating.

A collateral history (a witness account) of the syncope itself. This is vital; no history is complete without one:

- Patient lies still, breathing regularly – classic of arrhythmia (a prolonged episode can cause epileptiform movements secondary to cerebral hypoxia).
- Patient shakes limbs or has facial twitching, possibly associated with urinary incontinence and tongue biting – suggestive of epilepsy, but myoclonus can occur with vasovagal syncope.
- Patient becomes very pale and grey immediately before collapsing – vasovagal syncope.
- Patient becomes very pale and white following collapse and flushes red when regains consciousness – suggests a cardiac cause such as arrhythmia.

Table 9.1 Differential diagnosis of syncope (the more acutely life-threatening conditions are highlighted in red)

Classification	Examples	Notes
Cardiac arrhythmias	• Paroxysmal supraventricular or ventricular tachycardia (either idiopathic or secondary to long QT syndrome, Wolff-Parkinson-White syndrome, etc.) • Bradyarrhythmia – sinus bradycardia, complete or second-degree heart block, sinus arrest • Pacemaker/implantable cardioverter defibrillator dysfunction	Usually sudden onset and unprovoked, sometimes preceded by palpitations There may be a personal or family history of cardiac disease There may be abnormalities seen on a resting electrocardiogram
Structural cardiac disease	• Valve disease causing obstruction (e.g., aortic stenosis or pulmonary stenosis [rare]) • Hypertrophic cardiomyopathy (HCM) causing obstruction	May have associated murmur. Symptoms generally dependent on severity of underlying condition. May be associated with exertion. May have co-existing signs of heart failure
	• Acute coronary syndrome	Chest pain, nausea, sweating, breathlessness may be present ECG may show ST segment or T wave changes
	• Atrial myxoma	Most often due to mitral valve obstruction. May have an audible tumour 'plop'
Cardiopulmonary disease	• Pulmonary embolus	Acute breathlessness, chest pain, hypoxia ECG may show sinus tachycardia +/− evidence of right heart strain
	• Acute aortic dissection	Severe tearing chest pain, may radiate to the back, may be hypotensive/shocked
	• Pulmonary hypertension	Often asymptomatic, may cause breathlessness/lethargy
Neurally mediated (reflex)	• Vasovagal (e.g., due to stress, noxious stimuli, heat, etc.) • Situational (e.g., micturition, defaecation, post-exercise, needle phobia, sight of blood, etc.)	Very common, there may be preceding symptoms (dizziness, nausea, flushing, etc.) or obvious precipitant Often history of previous similar episodes
	• Carotid sinus hypersensitivity	May occur when rotating head, shaving, etc. May be precipitated by carotid sinus massage
Orthostatic (postural) hypotension	• Volume depletion (e.g., vomiting, diarrhoea, poor intake, blood loss) • Autonomic failure (e.g., due to drugs, alcohol, multisystem atrophy, diabetic neuropathy, etc.)	Syncope occurs shortly after standing up History may reveal underlying predisposing factors
Cerebrovascular/ miscellaneous	• Vascular steal syndromes	Precipitated by arm exercises
	• Neurogenic (transient ischaemic attack (TIA)/cerebrovascular accident (CVA)/subarachnoid haemorrhage/ vertebrobasilar disease)	Patient neurological examination may be abnormal May be severe headache in subarachnoid haemorrhage It is rare for TIA to cause syncope

The recovery of consciousness can also be characteristic. In general, if the patient:

• Feels normal soon after episode – a cardiac cause is more likely.

• Feels washed out and nauseated and takes a few minutes to return to normal – the cause is probably vasovagal.

• Feels very drowsy/confused and falls asleep soon after regaining consciousness – epilepsy (postictal state) is probable.

Past medical history

As always, a thorough history is needed:

- Any cardiac history is important – ischaemia may precipitate arrhythmias.
- A history of stroke or transient ischaemic attack (TIA) may suggest a cerebrovascular cause – this is rare.
- Diabetes mellitus may cause autonomic neuropathy and postural hypotension, whereas overly tight control of diabetes mellitus puts the patient at risk of hypoglycaemia.
- A history of head injury may suggest secondary epilepsy secondary to cortical scarring.

Drug history

Important points include the following:

- Antihypertensives and diuretic agents predispose to postural hypotension.
- Class I and class III antiarrhythmics may cause long QT syndrome and predispose to torsades de pointes. All antiarrhythmic agents may cause bradycardia leading to syncope.
- Some other drugs may also predispose to long QT syndrome (e.g., antiemetics, antipsychotics and antidepressants).
- Vasodilators precipitate syncope in pulmonary hypertension.

Family history

A family history of sudden death or recurrent syncope may occur in patients who have HCM or Brugada syndrome and also in those rare cases of familial long QT syndrome (Romano-Ward and Jervell Lange-Nielson syndromes).

Social history

Note that:

- Alcohol/benzodiazepine withdrawal (on a background of previous excess) is a risk factor for withdrawal fits.
- Smoking is a risk factor for ischaemic heart disease.
- Occupation is important in terms of the implications that diagnosis may have – for instance, certain diagnoses may bar from driving (discussed later).

EXAMINATION

The points to note on examination of the patient who has syncope are summarized in Fig. 9.1 and discussed in turn below. On inspection, look for any:

- Signs of shock – such as pallor or sweating.
- Neurological deficit suggestive of a cerebrovascular cause.

Cardiovascular system

On examination note the following:

- Pulse – any irregularity in rhythm and character of pulse (slow rising in aortic stenosis, jerky in HCM).
- Erect and supine blood pressures to detect postural hypotension (>20 mmHg drop in systolic blood pressure from lying to standing is diagnostic).

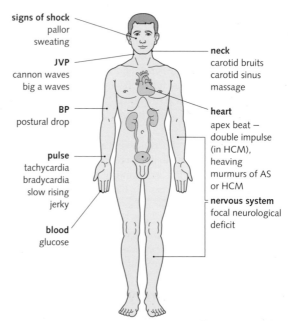

Fig. 9.1 Points to note on examination of a patient presenting with syncope. *AS*, Aortic stenosis; *BP*, blood pressure; *HCM*, hypertrophic cardiomyopathy; *JVP*, jugular venous pressure.

- Jugular venous pulse – cannon waves in complete heart block (due to the atrium contracting against a closed tricuspid valve); prominent 'a' wave in pulmonary hypertension.
- Apex beat – double impulse (HCM), heaving (aortic stenosis).
- Any murmurs.
- Carotid bruits – indicating carotid artery stenosis and possible cerebrovascular disease.
- Response to carotid sinus massage (may be indicated in some patients) – apply unilateral firm pressure over the carotid sinus with the patient in bed and attached to a cardiac monitor. Full resuscitative equipment should be easily accessible. Patients who have carotid sinus hypersensitivity will become very bradycardic or asystolic (sinus arrest). Do not test for this if patient has a carotid bruit, known carotid arterial disease or previous stroke.

Neurological system

This system should be fully examined to detect any residual deficit.

INVESTIGATIONS

First-line tests to exclude emergencies are shown in Table 9.2.

Blood tests

The following tests should be performed:

- Full blood count – anaemia may be secondary to haemorrhage, which will cause postural hypotension; leucocytosis is seen in sepsis and following seizure.
- Electrolytes and renal function – hypokalaemia predisposes towards arrhythmias.
- Calcium – hypocalcaemia is a cause of long QT syndrome.
- Cardiac biomarkers if suspicion of acute coronary syndrome – a myocardial infarction may cause sudden arrhythmia. Note that arrhythmia itself may cause moderate elevation in cardiac biomarkers.
- Blood glucose – both formal laboratory measurement and finger prick testing are of use. Finger prick testing is quick to perform and is particularly useful if done at the time of the syncopal episode.
- Lactate – raised in seizure and ischaemia.

Electrocardiography

This may show:

- Evidence of bradyarrhythmia or tachyarrhythmia – may be either overt ongoing arrhythmia or evidence that supports presence of paroxysmal rhythm

Table 9.2 First-line tests to exclude an emergency cause of syncope

Test	Diagnosis/ Notes
Electrocardiogram (ECG)	12-lead ECG provides rapid information – may provide evidence of arrhythmia, myocardial infarction, pulmonary embolus.
Blood testing	Including full blood count, urea and electrolytes, glucose – these investigations cover sepsis, haemorrhage, electrolyte abnormalities and hypoglycaemia as cause of syncope. Certain other tests may be indicated depending on clinical picture.
Continuous cardiac monitoring (e.g., on coronary care unit)	If paroxysmal arrhythmia is suspected.
Chest X-ray	May show oligaemia (pulmonary embolus), widened mediastinum (aortic dissection) or cardiomegaly (heart failure/cardiomyopathy).
CT scan	CT pulmonary angiography if pulmonary embolus is suspected. CT head if possible cerebral infarct/subarachnoid haemorrhage or other intracranial bleed.

disturbance (e.g., short PR interval and delta waves in Wolff-Parkinson-White syndrome).
- Heart block.
- A long QT interval.
- Evidence of ischaemia.
- Evidence of pulmonary embolus – sinus tachycardia is common. Other potential findings include ST depression/T wave inversion in V1–V4, II, III and aVF, right bundle branch block, right axis deviation or an 'S1Q3T3' pattern.

Ambulatory ECG monitoring

Ambulatory ECG monitoring (often referred to as Holter monitoring) is used to provide a continuous ECG trace (usually for 24 or 48 hours) to detect paroxysmal episodes of arrhythmia. Longer cardiac monitoring can be performed using implantable event recorders.

Chest radiography

On the chest radiograph there may be:

- Cardiomegaly – may suggest HCM or heart failure (potentially secondary to valvular abnormality).
- Oligaemic lung fields – suggestive of pulmonary embolus.
- Widened mediastinum – may indicate aortic dissection.

Echocardiography

This may reveal:

- Aortic stenosis or other valvular abnormalities.
- HCM.
- Atrial dilatation in supraventricular tachycardia.
- Ventricular abnormalities in ventricular arrhythmias or as the result of valvular abnormalities. Right ventricular abnormalities may be seen in pulmonary hypertension.

Other investigations

Other investigations that may be considered include:

- Tilt table testing – a non-invasive test where the patient is strapped to a table lying flat and then tilted to an angle of almost upright. Symptoms, blood pressure, heart rate are measured throughout this process. Simple tilt produces hypotension and possibly syncope in autonomic denervation. Prolonged tilt may provoke vasovagal syncope with bradycardia and hypotension.
- Electrophysiological (EP) study of the heart – consider if arrhythmia is strongly suspected, but not revealed by Holter monitoring.
- Electroencephalography (EEG) – this will assist in the diagnosis of epilepsy in selected patients.

SYNCOPE OF RECENT ONSET IN AN ILL PATIENT

This situation represents a medical emergency requiring rapid diagnosis and treatment. It is necessary in this situation to distinguish between life-threatening and more benign causes.

- Potentially life-threatening or more concerning causes of syncope are described in more detail later.

Cardiac causes

Aortic stenosis

Syncope is effort-induced as the left ventricular output is restricted by the outflow obstruction. The murmur is ejection systolic ('tight' or high frequency when critically stenosed) and the diagnosis of severe aortic stenosis is supported by the finding of a slow-rising carotid pulse and a heaving apex beat.

Electrocardiography may show left ventricular hypertrophy. Echocardiography reveals the stenotic valve, and assessment by Doppler velocity change through the valve may give an indication of the severity.

Tachyarrhythmias

Syncope due to supraventricular tachyarrhythmia (SVT) tends to occur only if the heart rate is extremely fast. Ventricular tachycardia is more likely than SVT to cause

syncope because it is accompanied by asynchronous ventricular contraction. If these arrhythmias are not prominent on ambulatory monitoring, they may be induced during electrophysiological testing.

Bradyarrhythmias

Syncope may occur secondary to a bradyarrhythmia if the cardiac output falls markedly as a consequence of the drop in rate. An ongoing bradyarrhythmia is easily detected on ECG (e.g., sinus bradycardia and second-degree or complete heart block). Some conditions, however, occur intermittently and the ECG may be normal after the syncopal episode; for example, heart block may occur intermittently with normal sinus rhythm between episodes.

Ambulatory ECG monitoring is, therefore, needed to capture these episodes. This may be difficult, if they are separated by long periods of time.

Acute coronary syndromes

Acute coronary syndromes may lead to syncopal episodes due to reduced cardiac output and hypotension as a result of myocardial function being impaired or arrhythmia. Patients may also complain of chest pain, sweating, breathlessness and nausea. ECG may show evidence of ischaemia/infarction.

Cardiomyopathies

Hypertrophic obstructive cardiomyopathy can give rise to syncope by obstructing left ventricular outflow on exercise or as a result of ventricular tachycardia or fibrillation. This arrhythmic 'sudden death syndrome' can also commonly occur in patients who have cardiomyopathy of other aetiologies (including arrhythmogenic right ventricular dysplasia and dilated cardiomyopathy).

Prolonged QT interval

This may be congenital or drug-induced, usually by psychiatric or class III antiarrhythmic drugs (e.g., amiodarone, sotalol). The syncope is caused by a self-limiting ventricular tachycardia characterized by a systematically rotating QRS vector (torsades de pointes). Tachycardia and syncope may be relieved by rapid ('overdrive') pacing or pharmacological sinus tachycardia (e.g., using isoprenaline). The resting non-arrhythmic ECG shows QT prolongation.

Brugada syndrome

Brugada syndrome is caused by a mutation in the gene coding for cardiac sodium channels. It is generally inherited in an autosomal dominant fashion so there may be a family history of syncope or sudden death. The typical finding is ST elevation followed by T wave inversion in leads V1–V3 of the resting ECG (Brugada sign). The patient presents with episodes of syncope caused by polymorphic VT, which may progress to VF and death if not terminated.

Circulatory causes

Hypovolaemia

This can present as postural hypotension (i.e., loss of consciousness on standing, relieved by lying flat). This occurs because the blood volume is inadequate, even with an intact baroreflex, to maintain arterial blood pressure in the face of gravity-dependent blood pooling. If this is due to acute haemorrhage, there are usually other obvious manifestations, such as trauma or haematemesis and melaena. However, large volume internal bleeding can sometimes be difficult to detect. With acute blood loss, the haemoglobin may be normal because there may not have been time for haemodilution to occur.

Septic shock

This causes similar effects by excessive vasodilatation, which prevents baroreflex compensation for postural-dependent blood pooling. However, the patient is usually obviously septic and febrile.

Aortic dissection

Injury to the innermost layer of the aorta (the intima) allows blood to enter and flow between the layers of the vessel wall, creating a false lumen. Patients may experience a severe, sudden onset, stabbing or tearing pain that sometimes radiates to the back. A widened mediastinum on chest X-ray in context of this type of pain should raise suspicion of aortic dissection; computed tomography (CT) scan can confirm the diagnosis. There are a number of complications that may co-exist with aortic dissection, including myocardial infarction (involvement of coronary arteries), aortic regurgitation, heart failure, ischaemia or infarction of other organs (e.g., stroke, mesenteric ischaemia, renal ischaemia). This is an emergency and, in some cases, warrants urgent surgical intervention.

Pulmonary embolism

Obstruction of pulmonary arteries by embolus enters into the differential diagnosis of all cardiovascular emergencies in which syncope is a feature. Chronic thromboembolism or primary pulmonary hypertension can also lead to postural hypotension because the resistance to right ventricular ejection is too high to allow adequate cardiac output when the filling pressure drops on standing. This results in reduced blood flow reaching the left side of the heart from the pulmonary artery and reduced left ventricular output as a result. CT pulmonary angiography (CTPA) may demonstrate pulmonary embolus if suspected.

Cerebrovascular causes

For full explanation of these syndromes, consult **Crash Course: Neurology**.

Stroke and transient cerebral ischaemia

TIA very rarely causes loss of consciousness, whereas the patient is unlikely to regain consciousness quickly after a sufficiently large major territory infarct or haemorrhage. You should be cautious about offering TIA as part of your differential diagnosis for syncope. Severe headache and/or neurological deficit in association with syncope may be indicative of subarachnoid haemorrhage.

Vertebrobasilar syndrome

This is caused by obstruction of the arteries to the posterior part of the brain (brain stem and cerebellum). The syncope may be preceded by vertigo or dizziness. This syndrome is often associated with cervical spondylosis. The vertebral artery becomes kinked on head movement as it travels through the distorted cervical vertebra, causing interruption to circulation.

Other neurological causes

For neurological causes without any cardiovascular aetiology, see **Crash Course: Neurology**. Remember epilepsy should always be kept in mind as a cause of collapse during history taking.

Metabolic causes

In the common situation of insulin-dependent diabetes mellitus, most patients are inadequately controlled, which leads to more rapid development of heart disease and autonomic neuropathy. Some patients will have overly tight control; these patients tend to experience episodes of loss of consciousness due to hypoglycaemia. However, hypoglycaemia can occur in any treated diabetic patient and may be precipitated by exercise or a reduction in food intake.

For more on metabolic causes of syncope see **Crash Course: Metabolism and Nutrition.**

HINTS AND TIPS

Cardiovascular syncope is always accompanied by hypotension. Syncope with normal blood pressure is likely to have a neurological, cerebrovascular or metabolic cause.

DRIVING REGULATIONS IN SYNCOPAL PATIENTS

Various diagnoses may disqualify the patient from driving for a period of time (see Table 9.3 for examples of exclusions). This may have serious implications for a patient's livelihood.

Table 9.3 Overview of current DVLA guidelines on driving after syncope/collapse/seizure

	Group 1 (cars, motorcycles)	Group 2 (HGVs, buses)
Arrhythmia (either atrial or ventricular), sinoatrial node disease, atrioventricular conduction defect	Must not drive if arrhythmia has caused or is likely to cause incapacity. May drive after condition is diagnosed and has been adequately treated for 4 weeks.	Must not drive if arrhythmia has caused or is likely to cause incapacity. May drive after condition is diagnosed, adequately treated for 3 months and left ventricular ejection fraction is >40%.
Congenital complete heart block	No restriction if asymptomatic. Must not drive if symptomatic until pacemaker implanted.	Must not drive until pacemaker implanted.
Pacemaker implantation (including box change)	Must not drive for 1 week.	Must not drive for 6 weeks.
Implantable defibrillator for arrhythmia associated with incapacity	Must not drive for 6 months post implantation and after any shock (or 2 years if shock or arrhythmia causes incapacity).	Permanently bars from driving group 2 vehicles.
First seizure	Must not drive for 6 months (longer if further seizure is deemed medically likely).	Must not drive for 5 years (longer if further seizure is deemed medically likely).
Epilepsy	May qualify for re-licensing if remains seizure-free for 1 year.	Must not drive until seizure-free for 10 years (without anti-epileptics) before re-licensing considered.

DVLA guidelines on fitness to drive are extensive and regularly updated. To fully describe current guidelines is outside of the scope of this book – for full guidelines visit: https://www.gov.uk/guidance/assessing-fitness-to-drive-a-guide-for-medical-professionals. Accurate as of July 2018.

● Chapter Summary

- Syncope is a transient loss of consciousness that is the result of reduced perfusion to the brain.
- The differential diagnosis of syncope is extensive and a detailed history (including a collateral history) is vital for diagnosis.
- There are a number of conditions that may mimic syncope (with or without loss of consciousness), including hypoglycaemia, epilepsy, hypoxia, etc.
- Syncope may be the presenting complaint for a number of different life-threatening pathologies, including episodes of arrhythmia (e.g., ventricular tachycardia/fibrillation/asystole), pulmonary embolism, myocardial infarction, stroke, etc.
- Episodes of syncope may have severe implications for an individual's eligibility to drive (and therefore also their occupation).

A heart murmur is a sound caused by turbulent blood flow, when the velocity of blood is disproportionate to the size of the orifice it is moving through. The presence of a murmur does not always indicate disease.

DIFFERENTIAL DIAGNOSIS OF A HEART MURMUR

Murmurs can arise at a valve or narrowing, across an abnormal communication within the heart or due to increased blood flow across normal structures:

- Left ventricular outflow obstruction – an example is hypertrophic cardiomyopathy (HCM).
- Septal defects – ventricular or atrial septal defects.
- Vascular disorders – coarctation of the aorta, patent ductus arteriosus, arteriovenous malformations (pulmonary or intercostal) and venous hum (cervical or hepatic).
- Increased cardiac output with normal anatomy (benign or innocent 'flow' murmur) – high-output states (e.g., anaemia, pregnancy, thyrotoxicosis).
- Increased flow across a normal pulmonary valve in atrial and ventricular septal defect.

HINTS AND TIPS

Cardiac sounds can be mistaken for murmurs. These include third and fourth heart sounds, midsystolic clicks (heard in mitral valve prolapse), metallic heart sounds and pericardial friction rubs. Other sounds not related to the heart (e.g., pleural rubs, venous hums) may be similarly confused.

Differential diagnoses of heart murmurs are shown in Table 10.1.

HISTORY

When taking a history from a patient who has a heart murmur, aim to answer the following questions:

- What is the possible aetiology of the murmur (e.g., infective endocarditis, valve lesion secondary to rheumatic heart disease, high-output state, etc.)?
- Are there any complications of valve disease (e.g., cardiac failure, exacerbation of ischaemic heart disease, arrhythmias, syncope, etc.)?

Presenting complaint

Many patients with murmurs may be asymptomatic. However, patients may present with a variety of symptoms, including:

- Shortness of breath – suggestive of cardiac failure; other features include orthopnoea, paroxysmal nocturnal dyspnoea, peripheral oedema, liver congestion and fatigue.
- Chest pain – may be due to left ventricular outflow obstruction in aortic stenosis or hypertrophic obstructive cardiomyopathy (HOCM), atypical chest pain (a feature of mitral valve prolapse) or coexistent ischaemic heart disease.
- Syncope – especially seen in patients who have left ventricular outflow obstruction (e.g., aortic stenosis or HOCM).
- Fever, rigors and malaise – common presenting complaints in patients who have infective endocarditis.
- Palpitations – for example, mitral valve disease is associated with atrial fibrillation.

Past medical history

Focus on possible causes of a murmur:

- Rheumatic fever in childhood.
- Previous cardiac surgery – mechanical prosthetic valves cause a metallic first or second heart sound. Both metal and tissue prosthetic valves frequently cause flow murmurs; however, they can also be complicated by regurgitation, thrombosis/stenosis or infective endocarditis.
- Previous myocardial infarction – may cause ventricular dilatation and consequent functional valve regurgitation, dysfunction of papillary muscle leading to valve regurgitation or a ventricular septal defect.
- Recent dental procedures or operations – may be a cause of infective endocarditis.
- Other medical conditions associated with valvular heart disease (see Table 10.1).

HINTS AND TIPS

The age of the patient is often helpful (e.g., aortic stenosis in an older patient is most likely degenerative, murmurs in young children are often congenital).

Table 10.1 Differential diagnoses of heart murmurs

Phase of cardiac cycle	Nature of murmur	Lesion	Causes
Systolic	Ejection systolic	Aortic stenosis (AS)	Senile degenerative calcification, calcification of congenital bicuspid valve, rheumatic fever, congenital valvular abnormality, congenital subvalvular stenosis, congenital supravalvular stenosis.
		Aortic sclerosis	Hardening of the valve without causing obstruction to flow. A precursor of aortic stenosis.
		Hypertrophic obstructive cardiomyopathy (HOCM)	Genetic mutations causing hypertrophy of cardiac muscle, which can, in the minority of cases, lead to left ventricular outflow tract (subvalvular) stenosis. If there is no murmur or obstruction, it is known as HCM.
		Increased flow across normal valve	Increased cardiac output (e.g., anaemia, pregnancy, thyrotoxicosis, sepsis, athletes, hypertension, large AV fistula, Paget disease, beriberi).
		Pulmonary stenosis (PS)	Congenital malformations (e.g., tetralogy of Fallot, Noonan syndrome, congenital rubella syndrome. Carcinoid syndrome).
		ASD	Congenital.
	Pansystolic	Mitral regurgitation (MR)	Functional MR due to dilatation of the MV annulus: LV aneurysm, dilated cardiomyopathy. Valvular: rheumatic fever, infective endocarditis, MV prolapse, chordal rupture (e.g., connective tissue disorder, such as Marfan syndrome), papillary muscle infarction, SLE (Libman-Sacks lesion).
		Tricuspid regurgitation (TR)	Functional due to RV dilatation (most common): chronic LV failure, RV infarction, pulmonary hypertension (e.g., cor pulmonale), Marfan syndrome. Valvular: rheumatic fever, infective endocarditis, congenital malformations (e.g., Ebstein's anomaly), carcinoid syndrome).
		VSD with left-to-right shunt	Congenital, acquired (e.g., septal infarct).
Diastolic	Early diastolic	Aortic regurgitation (AR)	Functional due to dilatation of valve ring or aortic root: cystic medial necrosis (Marfan syndrome), aneurysm, aortic dissection, syphilitic aortitis, hypertension, ankylosing spondylitis. Valvular: rheumatic fever, infective endocarditis, bicuspid aortic valve, degenerative, RA, SLE.
		Pulmonary regurgitation (PR)	Functional due to dilatation of valve ring: pulmonary hypertension, complication of MS (Graham Steell murmur), Marfan syndrome. Valvular: infective endocarditis, rheumatic fever, carcinoid, tetralogy of Fallot.
	Mid-diastolic	Mitral stenosis (MS)	Rheumatic fever (almost always), calcification, congenital.
		Tricuspid stenosis (TS)	Rheumatic fever (almost always), carcinoid syndrome, congenital.
		Austin Flint murmur	Regurgitant jet from AR impinges opening of mitral valve anterior leaflet.
		Left and right atrial myxomas	Tumour obstruction of valve orifice in diastole.
Continuous		PDA	Congenital (physiological in newborns, otherwise pathological).
		AV fistula	
		Cervical venous hum	
		Mixed AS and AR	As above.

ASD, atrial septal defect; *AV*, Arteriovenous; *LV*, left ventricular; *MV*, mitral valve; *PDA*, patent ductus arteriosus; *RA*, rheumatoid arthritis; *RV*, right ventricular; *SLE*, systemic lupus erythematosus; *VSD*, ventricular septal defect.

Medication history

Patients may be on anticoagulation for:

- Atrial fibrillation – this can cause decompensation from stable valvular disease or may be a consequence of valvular disease.
- Mechanical valve replacement – anticoagulation is mandatory due to increased risk of mechanical valve thrombosis or thromboembolism.
- Recent surgery – especially joint replacement.

Very rarely, valve fibrosis can be drug-induced (e.g., cabergoline, pergolide).

Family history

Ask about family history of cardiac problems or sudden death – as may occur for patients who have HCM.

Social history

Ask in particular about:

- Smoking – an important risk factor for atherosclerosis.
- Alcohol intake – if excessive, may result in dilated cardiomyopathy.
- History of drug abuse – intravenous uses increases infective endocarditis risk (especially right heart involvement), and prolonged MDMA use can induce valve fibrosis.

EXAMINATION

Figure 10.1 gives a summary of potential findings on examination of a patient who has a heart murmur.

General observation

Look for signs of cardiac failure (i.e., dyspnoea, cyanosis or oedema).

Look also for clues indicating the cause of the murmur:

- Anaemia – may cause a high-output state or be caused by infective endocarditis.
- Scars of previous cardiac surgery – median sternotomy, valvulotomy or other thoracotomy scars.

HINTS AND TIPS

Remember that the click of a mechanical prosthetic valve can often be picked up from the end of the bed! This can be a valuable clue and direct the rest of your examination in OSCEs. Prosthetic aortic valves are normally associated with a flow murmur. It is also interesting to note that if the valve is obstructed by clot or vegetation, the click may disappear.

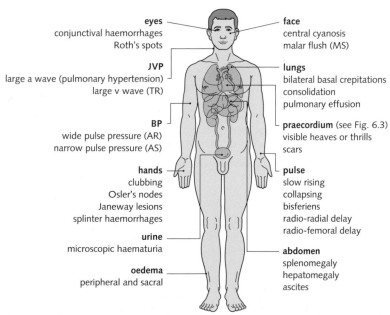

Fig. 10.1 Possible findings in a patient who has a heart murmur. *AS,* Aortic stenosis; *AR,* aortic regurgitation; *MS,* mitral stenosis; *TR,* tricuspid regurgitation.

Cardiovascular system

Hands

Look for peripheral stigmata of infective endocarditis:

- Splinter haemorrhages (small linear longitudinal haemorrhages under the nail or in the nailbed). More than five is considered pathological.
- Osler nodes (painful red-purple raised papules on pulps of fingers/toes, classically at the tips).
- Janeway lesions (non-tender erythematous or haemorrhagic flat lesions on the palms and soles, classically on the thenar eminence).
- Finger clubbing – develops late.

Pulse

Examine the pulse at both the radial site and the carotid artery. Abnormal pulses due to valvular disease include:

- Slow rising or plateau pulse in aortic stenosis.
- Collapsing or waterhammer pulse in aortic regurgitation or patent ductus arteriosus.
- Bisferiens pulse in severe mixed aortic valve disease.
- A jerky pulse in HOCM.

Radio-radial and radio-femoral delay can be found in aortic coarctation. This may be associated with a bruit heard over the back, which can be confused for a murmur.

Blood pressure

This may also give important clues:

- A narrow pulse pressure is a sign of severe aortic stenosis.
- A wide pulse pressure may be seen in aortic regurgitation, patent ductus arteriosus or high-output states.

Jugular venous pressure

Possible findings include:

- An elevated jugular venous pressure in congestive cardiac failure.
- Large 'a' waves (see Chapter 2) in pulmonary stenosis and pulmonary hypertension.
- Absent 'a' wave in atrial fibrillation.
- Cannon 'a' waves in complete heart block.
- Large 'v' waves – a sign of tricuspid regurgitation.

Precordium

Remember to look for surgical scars.
On palpation, possible abnormalities of apex beat include:

- Double apical impulse – due to HOCM or left ventricular aneurysm.
- Tapping apex beat – due to mitral stenosis.

- Heaving apex beat – due to aortic stenosis, HOCM or left ventricular hypertrophy.
- Displaced thrusting apex beat – due to aortic or mitral regurgitation or any sustained high-output state.

CLINICAL NOTE

It is easier to remember the correct association between murmurs and apex beat character if you bear in mind a heave is due to pressure overload, and a thrust is due to volume overload.

A parasternal heave can be felt with the hand along the left sternal edge and is a sign of right ventricular hypertrophy or strain. It may be felt in patients with mitral valve disease, pulmonary hypertension or lung disease (cor pulmonale).

If flow is very turbulent, a thrill (loud palpable murmur) may be felt with the fingertips on the chest wall in any of the areas where the corresponding murmurs are best heard. For locations of valve areas see Fig. 5.5.

When describing murmurs, consider:

1. Where in the cardiac cycle does it occur (systolic, diastolic or continuous)?
2. How loud is the murmur?
3. What quality does it have?
4. In which location is it best heard?
5. Does it radiate?
6. In which respiration phase is the murmur loudest?
7. Accentuation manoeuvres?
8. Are there any associated features?

COMMON PITFALLS

The volume of a murmur does not correlate with the severity of the lesion. For example, if left ventricular failure results from severe aortic stenosis, the ejection systolic murmur can become much quieter due to reduced cardiac output. However, the pitch of a murmur correlates with pressure gradient across the orifice – the higher the pressure, the higher the pitch.

After auscultating at the four main valve areas, if a systolic murmur is heard, the axilla and the carotid arteries should be auscultated with the diaphragm of the stethoscope for radiation. The murmur of mitral regurgitation often radiates to the axilla and the murmur of aortic stenosis classically radiates to the carotid arteries, although loud murmurs can sometimes be heard all over the precordium and in the axilla.

Diastolic murmurs (never innocent) can be quiet and difficult to hear and so may be augmented with certain manoeuvres:

- Rolling the patient onto his or her left-hand side brings the apex of the heart into contact with the chest wall and may make the murmur of mitral stenosis audible. Brief exercise by the patient can also make a mitral stenotic murmur louder.
- By asking the patient to sit forward and hold his or her breath in expiration, a murmur of aortic regurgitation can be heard better at the left sternal edge.

HINTS AND TIPS

Murmurs from valves on the left side of the heart (mitral and aortic) are louder on expiration. Those from the right side of the heart (tricuspid and pulmonary) are accentuated by inspiration.

A summary of murmur characteristics is shown in Table 10.2. The most commonly heard murmurs are aortic stenosis and mitral regurgitation.

CLINICAL NOTE

There are a number of eponymous signs that may be seen in the patient with aortic regurgitation:

- Quincke's sign – visible nailbed pulsation of blood. Sometimes called the 'lighthouse' sign because it almost flashes.
- Corrigan's sign – exaggerated carotid pulsation.
- De Musset's sign – head nodding.
- Duroziez's sign – diastolic femoral murmur.
- Traube's sign – 'pistol shot' femorals.
- Müller's sign – uvula pulsations.

The intensity of murmurs is graded from 1 to 6, from very quiet to very loud. It may not be wise to describe yourself as an expert in finals by describing a murmur as grade 1!

- Grade 1 – only audible in ideal conditions by an expert.
- Grade 2 – only audible in ideal conditions by a non-expert.
- Grade 3 – easily audible, no palpable thrill.
- Grade 4 – loud, associated with a thrill.
- Grade 5 – very loud with a thrill, audible with edge of the stethoscope partly off the chest.
- Grade 6 – audible without a stethoscope.

HINTS AND TIPS

Many students (and doctors!) find auscultation and interpretation of murmurs difficult. Don't worry – if you listen carefully to the cardiac cycle of every patient that you examine, you will get a feel for the range of normal sounds, and you will start to pick up abnormal sounds more easily.

Peripheral pulses

All peripheral pulses should be palpated. Radio-femoral (and occasionally radio-radial) delay may be found with coarctation of the aorta, and lower limb pulses may be reduced. There may be discrepancy in the blood pressure taken in each arm or between right arm and either leg.

Peripheral oedema

Pitting oedema may be elicited by applying firm pressure (for at least 10 seconds) with a finger. Be careful, this can be painful for the patient. Observe the patient's face as you press.

Respiratory system

Examine the chest carefully. Possible findings include:

- Bilateral basal fine end-inspiratory crepitations – suggests left ventricular failure and pulmonary oedema.
- Evidence of respiratory tract infection – sepsis may cause a high-output state, septic emboli from right-sided infective endocarditis can cause pneumonia.

Gastrointestinal system

Important findings include:

- Hepatomegaly or ascites, seen in right ventricular failure or biventricular failure.
- Splenomegaly, a feature of infective endocarditis.

INVESTIGATIONS

Blood tests

These include:

1. Full blood count – anaemia may be seen as a sign of chronic disease in a patient who has infective endocarditis and is also a cause of hyperdynamic state; a leucocytosis is also a feature of infective endocarditis.
2. Urea, creatinine and electrolytes – may be deranged in patients who have cardiac failure as a result of poor renal perfusion or diuretic therapy.

Table 10.2 Characteristics of murmurs

Timing	Lesion	**Best heard (valve area)** **Radiates to** **Accentuate with** **Quality**	Possible systemic features
Ejection systolic (crescendo–decrescendo)	Aortic stenosis	**B** Aortic **R** Carotids (often all over precordium including axilla) **Q** Harsh, high-pitch	Slow rising pulse Narrow pulse pressure Heaving non-displaced apex beat Ejection click Quiet or absent S2 (if severe) Reversed splitting of S2 (prolonged LV emptying) S4 May have LVF (S3, pulmonary oedema)
	Aortic sclerosis (*Asymptomatic*)	**B** Aortic **R** Classically does not radiate	No slow rising pulse Normal pulse pressure S2 normal or loud
	Hypertrophic obstructive cardiomyopathy	**B** Aortic and tricuspid for ESM Apex and tricuspid for PSM **A** Standing from squatting or Valsalva (↑gradient by emptying LV) **Q** High-pitch	Pulse jerky or normal upstroke Double apical impulse
	↑flow across normal valve	**B** Aortic **R** No radiation **Q** Soft	No other cardiovascular abnormalities
	Pulmonary stenosis (PS)	**B** Pulmonary and tricuspid **Q** High-pitch	Ejection click Wide splitting of or quiet S2 RV heave
	Atrial septal defect	**B** Pulmonary **Q** Very similar to PS	Fixed splitting of S2
Pansystolic	Mitral regurgitation	**B** Apex **R** Left axilla **A** Exercise **Q** Blowing	Quiet S1 Obliterated S2 S3 Thrusting, displaced apex beat Often AF Midsystolic 'click' and late systolic murmur in mitral valve prolapse
	Tricuspid regurgitation	**B** Tricuspid	Giant 'v' waves in jugular venous pressure (JVP) Pulsatile hepatomegaly May have thrusting RV impulse May have signs of RVF
	Ventricular septal defect	**B** Tricuspid **R** Right lower sternal border **Q** Loud and rough	Wide splitting of S2 Prominent RV impulse May have signs of cardiac failure or Eisenmenger syndrome

Early diastolic S_1 S_2 S_1	Aortic regurgitation	**B** Tricuspid **A** Leaning forward, breath held in expiration **Q** High-pitch	Bounding and collapsing pulse Wide pulse pressure S3 Thrusting, displaced apex Eponymous signs (see clinical note box) Systolic flow murmur (high flow) Austin Flint (mid-diastolic) murmur Bisferiens pulse (if severe)
	Pulmonary regurgitation	**B** Tricuspid and pulmonary	Wide splitting of S2 Hyperdynamic thrusting RV impulse
Mid-diastolic S_1 S_2 S_1	Mitral stenosis	**B** Apex (bell) **A** Roll onto left side, breath held in expiration Exercise **Q** Rumbling, low-pitch, presystolic accentuation if in sinus rhythm	Tapping non-displaced apex (palpable S1) Loud S1 Opening snap Often AF Pulmonary oedema If associated pulmonary hypertension, mitral facies/parasternal heave/loud P2/Graham Steell murmur (PR due to MS) May develop signs of RVF
	Tricuspid stenosis	**B** Tricuspid	Elevated JVP, with giant 'a' waves and slow 'y' descent May develop signs of RVF and pulsatile liver Often associated with other valvular lesions
Continuous S_1 S_2 S_1	Patent ductus arteriosus	**B** Second intercostal space below left clavicle; pulmonary and tricuspid **R** Left scapula **Q** Machinery-like, with late systolic accentuation	Large volume peripheral pulses Prominent apex beat May develop signs of cardiac failure or Eisenmenger syndrome

AF, Atrial fibrillation; JVP, jugular venous pressure; LV, left ventricle; LVF, left ventricular failure; MS, mitral stenosis; P2, pulmonary valve closure; PR, pulmonary regurgitation; RV, right ventricular; RVF, right ventricular failure; S1, first heart sound; S2, second heart sound; S3, third heart sound; S4, fourth heart sound.

3. Liver function tests – these may be abnormal in patients who have hepatic congestion secondary to cardiac failure.
4. Erythrocyte sedimentation rate (ESR) and C-reactive protein (CRP) – these are markers of inflammation or infection and are useful in monitoring treatment of infective endocarditis.
5. Blood cultures – this is crucial if infective endocarditis is suspected, in which case at least three sets should be taken before commencement of antibiotic therapy.

Urinalysis

Dipstick test of the urine should always be performed with new murmurs. Microscopic haematuria is a common finding in patients who have infective endocarditis.

Chest radiography

This may reveal an abnormal cardiac shadow (e.g., large left atrium and prominent pulmonary vessels in mitral stenosis, enlarged left ventricle in mitral or aortic regurgitation or the abnormal aortic shadow in coarctation).

Abnormality in the lung fields (e.g., pulmonary oedema, pulmonary effusion) may also be seen as a complication of left-sided valvular disease.

Electrocardiography

The 12-lead ECG may give useful information:

1. Atrial fibrillation may be a sign of mitral valve disease.
2. P mitrale (broad bifid P waves) may be seen if there is left atrial enlargement as a result of mitral stenosis, and if this is severe, it may also result in pulmonary hypertension and P pulmonale (peaked P waves) due to right atrial enlargement.
3. Left ventricular hypertrophy and strain pattern may be seen in aortic stenosis, HCM aortic regurgitation or mitral regurgitation.
4. Right ventricular hypertrophy may be a sign of mitral or pulmonary stenosis.
5. AV block may be seen in infective endocarditis due to aortic root abscess formation.

Echocardiography

Transthoracic echocardiography

Transthoracic echocardiography is the most widely used imaging technique for murmurs and is frequently the key investigation for valvular disease. It enables the valves to be visualized, and Doppler echocardiography assesses the direction of flow and velocity of flow (used to derive pressures) across valves. Vegetations may be seen, although infective endocarditis cannot be ruled out without transoesophageal echocardiography as it is more sensitive. Left ventricular function and pulmonary artery pressure can be estimated. The presence of a ventricular septal defect or patent ductus arteriosus may be visualized using echocardiography but may rarely require cardiac catheterization to more accurately assess the abnormality and shunt volume.

Transoesophageal echocardiography

Transoesophageal echocardiography is very useful because it gives detailed information on structures that are difficult to see using transthoracic echocardiography. Examples of its uses include:

1. Detection of vegetations.
2. Assessment of prosthetic valves.
3. Detailed evaluation of the mitral valve before mitral valve repair.

Cardiac magnetic resonance imaging

This can be useful to more accurately delineate anatomy. It can outline the size of aortic root in aortic regurgitation, to demonstrate congenital malformations (e.g., aortic coarctation) and occasionally is helpful to assess the degree of valve stenosis.

Cardiac catheterization

Before valve replacement this is performed to obtain information about the:

1. Presence of coexisting coronary artery disease.
2. Direct measurement of the degree of pulmonary hypertension in patients who have mitral valve disease.

Catherization can directly measure the severity of the left-to-right shunt in patients who have ventricular or atrial septal defects.

PRESENTING YOUR FINDINGS

Murmurs crop up regularly in exams. The most frequently tested in OSCEs are aortic stenosis, mitral regurgitation, infective endocarditis, prosthetic valves, aortic regurgitation and adult congenital heart diseases; however, other murmurs may be examined.

When presenting a murmur, describe it using a system such as below.

- Timing.
- Intensity.
- Position (of stethoscope AND patient) where heard loudest.

- Radiation.
- Quality.
- Systemic features – include complications, such as heart failure, infective endocarditis or prosthetic valve failure.

For example, you might say: The most obvious abnormality is an early diastolic murmur of grade 2 intensity. It is heard loudest in the tricuspid area with the patient sitting forward and does not radiate. The murmur is accentuated by the patient holding his breath in expiration. It is a decrescendo high-pitched murmur and is associated with a collapsing pulse, a displaced thrusting apex beat, a third heart sound and bibasal crepitations. There are no stigmata of infective endocarditis, and he is a tall thin gentleman with a high-arched palate. These features are consistent with aortic regurgitation potentially due to Marfan syndrome and complicated by a degree of left ventricular failure. However, the patient does not look distressed or unwell.

● Chapter Summary

- When taking a history with murmurs in mind, remember to look for potential causes.
- Examination of murmurs includes the entire cardiovascular system and other systems that may explain non-cardiac causes of murmurs.
- Remember to take three to six sets of blood cultures before administering antibiotics if infective endocarditis is suspected.
- If a cardiac cause of murmur is suspected, echocardiography is the first imaging investigation of choice and frequently the only imaging that is required.
- Using a systematic approach will assist in diagnosing the most likely causes of a murmur and help you with a polished presentation.

Atherosclerosis 11

Atherosclerosis is a progressive, inflammatory disease of large- and medium-sized arteries. It is characterized by focal accumulation of lipid in the vessel intima with an associated inflammatory and smooth muscle infiltrate. It is thought that atherosclerosis is present to some degree in all adults. The consequences of atherosclerosis, which include ischaemic heart disease, peripheral vascular disease and cerebrovascular disease, are estimated to account for 45% of deaths in Europe and 31% of global deaths in 2015.

PATHOGENESIS

The pathogenesis of atherosclerosis is often described by the response to injury hypothesis. This states that chronic damage to the vascular endothelium and the associated endothelial dysfunction are the key events in initiating the process. The steps involved in development of atherosclerosis are shown in Fig. 11.1 and include:

1. Endothelial dysfunction: chronic endothelial cell injury can occur as a result of cigarette smoking and high levels of cholesterol (particularly LDL), leading to metabolic dysfunction and structural changes. Damage activates endothelial cells, upregulating inflammatory adhesion molecules (e.g., ICAM-1), promoting monocyte and platelet adhesion. This upregulation is also caused by altered gene expression at sites where the pattern of blood flow is altered, such as bends and bifurcation in vessels. Injury increases permeability to lipids and LDL, allowing their accumulation in the intima.

2. Formation of a fatty streak: monocytes adhere to the endothelium, migrate into the intima and differentiate into macrophages. Local oxidation of LDL attracts macrophages and once in the intima, macrophages take up the oxidized LDL and become foam cells. Platelets adhere to activated endothelial cells or areas of denuded matrix and become activated. Activated platelets, activated endothelial cells and macrophages release platelet-derived growth factor stimulating smooth muscle cell migration from the media to the intima.

3. Development of lipid plaque: smooth muscle proliferation and an increase in extracellular matrix occur in the intima. Additional cytokines and growth factors produced by activated macrophages and platelets promote additional monocyte and smooth muscle infiltration. Lipid may also be released from dying foam cells, contributing to extracellular free lipid pools.

4. Advanced plaques: an advanced atherosclerotic plaque consists of a lipid-rich 'core' and a fibrous 'cap'.

Fig. 11.1 The stages in the development of an atherosclerotic plaque, from the initial endothelial damage through to an advanced plaque. (A) Endothelial dysfunction. (B) Formation of the fatty streak. (C) Development of a lipid plaque. (D) Advanced atherosclerotic plaque (*LDL*, low-density lipoprotein).

The core of the lesion (which can become necrotic) consists of free lipid, macrophages, smooth muscle cells and cellular debris. The fibrous cap is composed primarily of collagen and lies over the core, beneath the endothelium.

A stable advanced atherosclerotic plaque, such as that depicted here, is likely to remain asymptomatic for years. Initially, as the plaque expands it causes remodelling of the media allowing the vessel to increase its diameter, accommodating the plaque without compromising the vessel lumen. The degree to which this occurs varies greatly. In the absence of this remodelling, the plaque will grow, protrude into the lumen and progressively decrease lumen size. It will only become apparent when the luminal diameter is not sufficient to allow adequate organ perfusion.

> **CLINICAL NOTE**
>
> Clinically significant atherosclerosis may remain silent for years, and the first manifestation is often myocardial infarction.

The stability of the plaque is dependent on the strength and thickness of the fibrous cap, which relies on the balance between inflammation and repair. If this balance is disturbed and inflammation predominates, the cap may become thinner and less stable, and one of the following may occur (Fig. 11.2):

1. Plaque erosion: this occurs when there is damage to the endothelium overlying the plaque. This exposes the prothrombotic subendothelial connective tissue, causing platelet adhesion and formation of a thrombus on the surface of the plaque, which can occlude the lumen. The sequence of events in thrombus formation is shown in Fig. 11.3.
2. Plaque rupture/fissure: this occurs in advanced plaque when deep fissures form in the plaque allowing blood to flow into the plaque. A thrombus then forms within the plaque causing it to expand and occlude the vessel lumen.

Atherosclerotic plaques create areas of weakness in vessel walls, which also predisposes to aneurysm formation.

CLASSIFICATION OF ISCHAEMIC HEART DISEASE

Ischaemic heart disease (IHD) is the manifestation of atheromatous disease affecting one or more of the epicardial coronary arteries. Classification is shown in Table 11.1.

If an atherosclerotic plaque grows slowly, over months, collateral vessels may develop and protect the myocardium from acute insult in the original vessel. A faster rate of vessel occlusion and a greater degree of vessel occlusion by thrombus will increase the severity of clinical presentation.

Stable angina is the chronic manifestation of coronary artery disease and results from coronary artery stenosis due to stable atherosclerotic plaques.

Unstable angina (UA) occurs if occlusion is incomplete or very short-lived. Myocardial infarction occurs when myocytes die (necrosis) due to myocardial ischaemia. Irreversible damage occurs from between 20–40 minutes after vessel occlusion. The evolution of infarcted myocardium is depicted in Fig. 11.4. The area of myocardium affected depends on the vessel involved. ECG changes allow assessment of the area involved (see Fig. 13.5). The area of

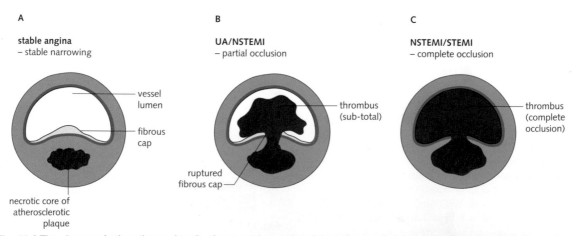

Fig. 11.2 The changes in the atherosclerotic plaque and associated thrombus underlying each of the manifestations of coronary artery disease. (A) Stable angina: atherosclerotic plaque with solid fibrous cap reducing the vessel lumen size. (B) UA/NSTEMI: erosion or rupture of fibrous cap with partially occlusive thrombus formation. (C) NSTEMI/STEMI: erosion or rupture of fibrous cap with complete vessel occlusion by thrombus (*NSTEMI*, non-ST elevation myocardial infarction; *STEMI*, ST elevation myocardial infarction; *UA*, unstable angina).

A

The continuous endothelial layer prevents circulating platelets from coming into contact with the prothrombotic subendothelial components
- von-Willebrand factor (VWF)
- Collagen

The intact endothelium prevents activation of platelets by secretion of nitric oxide and prostacyclin.

B

Subendothelial VWF tether platelets on platelet surface receptor GPIb – IX – V. Firm adhesion to subendothelial collagen via GPVI activates the platelet and stimulates release of ADP and synthesis of thromboxane A_2 (TXA_2).

C

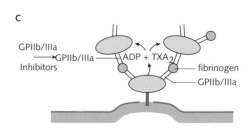

Binding of GPVI also induces expression and activation of platelet integrin GPIIb/IIIa, which binds to fibrinogen. The ADP and TXA_2 released activate other platelets, inducing expression of GPIIb/IIIa and allowing platelet cross linking via fibrinogen. Activation of platelets causes further release of ADP and TXA_2 causing a positive feedback effect.

D

The aggregation of platelets provides a prothrombotic surface for the clotting/coagulation cascade. The coagulation cascade (**D**) results in formation of fibrin which forms a mesh around and between the aggregated platelets. This end result is a clot.

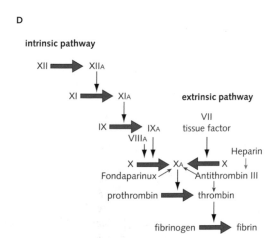

Fig. 11.3 Platelet activation, thrombosis and the coagulation cascade (*ADP*, adenosine diphosphate; *GP*, glycoprotein; *NO*, nitric oxide; *PGI*, prostacyclin; *TXA₂*, thromboxane A₂; *VWF*, von-Willebrand factor;). *Red arrows* – inhibitory action. *Green arrows* – enhancing action.

Table 11.1 Classification of ischaemic heart disease in order of increasing severity. This outlines the pathological intracoronary finding, resulting damage, presentation and initial investigation findings

Coronary artery disease			
		Acute coronary syndromes	
		Myocardial infarction	
Stable angina	**Unstable angina**	**NSTEMI**	**STEMI**
Constant stenosis Ischaemia without necrosis	Dynamic stenosis Ischaemia without necrosis	Obstruction to flow Cardiomyocyte necrosis	Obstruction to flow Cardiomyocyte necrosis
Predictable effort-dependent symptoms	Unpredictable/worsening symptoms	Prolonged symptoms, can occur at any time	Prolonged symptoms, can occur at any time
May have reversible ECG changes No biomarker rise	May have reversible ECG changes No biomarker rise	May have irreversible ECG changes Biomarker rise	ST elevation in the distribution of the coronary artery affected Biomarker rise

ECG, Electrocardiogram; NSTEMI, non-ST elevation myocardial infarction; STEMI, ST elevation myocardial infarction.

time	macroscopic appearance	microscopic appearance
0–12 hours	not visible	infarcted muscle appears uncoloured on staining with nitroblue tetrazolium due to loss of oxidative enzymes; non-infarcted muscle stains blue
12-24 hours	pale with blotchy discolouration	infarcted muscle is brightly eosinophilic with intercellular oedema
24–72 hours	dead area appears soft and pale with a slight yellow colour	infarcted area excites an acute inflammatory response neutrophils infiltrate between dead cardiac muscle fibres
3–10 days	hyperaemic border develops around the yellow dead muscle	organization of infarcted area replacement with vascular granulation tissue
weeks to months	white scar	progressive collagen deposition infarct is replaced by a collagenous scar

Fig. 11.4 Morphological changes occurring following myocardial infarction

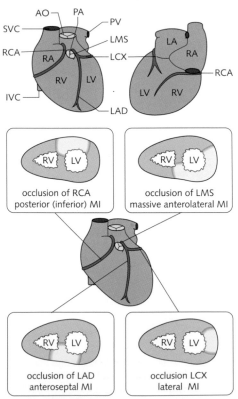

Fig. 11.5 Site of myocardial infarction and associated vessel involvement (*Ao*, aorta; *IVC*, inferior vena cava; *LA*, left atrium; *LAD*, left anterior descending; *LCX*, circumflex coronary artery; *LMS*, left main stem; *LV*, left ventricle; *MI*, myocardial infarction; *PA*, pulmonary artery; *PV*, pulmonary vein; *RA*, right atrium; *RCA*, right coronary artery; *RV*, right ventricle; *SVC*, superior vena cava).

infarction following occlusion of each of the major vessels is shown in Fig. 11.5.

Clinically, acute plaque changes can manifest as one of three acute coronary syndromes, in order of increasing severity:

1. UA: angina of increasing severity or at rest without evidence of myocardial necrosis.
2. Non-ST elevation myocardial infarction (NSTEMI): new onset chest pain with biochemical evidence of myocardial necrosis but no ST segment elevation on ECG.
3. ST elevation myocardial infarction (STEMI): acute chest pain, often associated with autonomic symptoms, such as sweating or vomiting, with biochemical evidence of myocardial necrosis and ST segment elevation or new left bundle branch block on ECG. This is usually associated with complete occlusion of the coronary artery and significant myocardial necrosis.

● Chapter Summary

- Atherosclerosis is a progressive inflammatory disease; early evidence of it can be found even in our twenties.
- It is the pathological basis of ischaemic heart disease, cerebrovascular disease and peripheral arterial disease, which are major causes of mortality.
- Slow stable progression may lead to collateral vessel formation and a degree of compensation.
- Acute plaque events may lead to acute coronary syndrome, ischaemic stroke, acute limb ischaemia or acute mesenteric ischaemia.
- Early ECG and biomarker measurement will identify and differentiate the acute coronary syndromes.

Risk factors for atherosclerosis and its associated conditions can be broken down into 'modifiable' and 'non-modifiable' as follows:

Non-modifiable

1. Age: increased age increases the number and severity of atherosclerotic lesions.
2. Sex: men are affected to a much greater extent than women, until the menopause when the incidence in women increases.
3. Genetic predisposition: a family history of atherosclerotic disease is a strong risk factor even when known genetic diseases such as familial hypercholesterolaemia are excluded.
4. Existing coronary artery disease.

Modifiable

1. Smoking.
2. Hypertension.
3. Diabetes mellitus.
4. Dyslipidaemia.

Other, less important factors involved in the development of atherosclerosis include a sedentary lifestyle, a diet high in saturated fat and obesity. Rare contributing factors include thrombophilias (e.g., antiphospholipid syndrome) or other hypercoagulable states (e.g., essential thrombocythaemia), atrial fibrillation and drugs promoting a prothrombotic state.

RISK PREDICTION AND PRIMARY PREVENTION OF ISCHAEMIC HEART DISEASE

1. Primary prevention aims to reduce a person's risk of developing ischaemic heart disease. It involves treating seemingly healthy individuals, many of whom may never go on to develop the disease.
2. Secondary prevention targets risk factors in a person with known coronary disease, who clearly has a higher risk and will likely receive greater benefit from treatments to prevent progression and future events.

Clinically significant coronary disease may be asymptomatic for many years, but may present unexpectedly with myocardial infarction or sudden death. Diminishing this risk is the aim of population-wide and individual-based primary prevention.

Those with higher risk have potentially more to gain from risk reduction, as the same intervention with fixed relative risk reduction will result in a greater absolute risk reduction. For those who are at high risk, lifestyle interventions and pharmacological measures are directed at controlling risk factors such as hypertension, hypercholesterolaemia, poor glycaemic control and obesity.

Although specific approaches to smoking cessation are beyond the remit of this book, it is important to encourage cessation at every encounter, in primary prevention as well as at every stage of coronary artery disease. Opportunistic brief interventions to give advice are shown to be effective, although the most successful may be unfortunately after disease has manifested. All health professionals should be involved. Positive encouragement, advice on the complications of smoking and information about self-help groups should all be made available to smokers. Smoking-cessation clinics (which often work on a self-referral basis) are now commonplace.

In-depth information regarding diabetes and its management can be found in Crash course general medicine.

The following sections will concentrate on dyslipidaemias and hypertension.

Risk calculation

To guide doctors as to who will benefit most from primary prevention measures and pharmacological treatment, various risk stratification models have been developed to estimate an individual's risk of developing cardiovascular disease. This is most pertinently applied to treatment decisions in dyslipidaemia. The first of these was the Framingham risk prediction chart (Fig. 12.1).

The Framingham model was developed in the USA and is less applicable to the UK population. Simple-to-use online risk prediction calculators have been developed and validated in the UK to guide decisions surrounding primary prevention. These take into account many of the major risk factors such as age, sex, smoking, lipid levels and blood pressure (BP), even incorporating postcodes to take into account the index of multiple deprivation score. In England and Wales, the QRISK score (now updated to QRISK3) stratifies risk using a broadened range of factors. In Scotland, the ASSIGN score is used.

Calculators should not be applied if the patient already has other conditions that place them at high risk and would qualify for treatment of these factors in their own right. These include type 1 diabetes, hypertension with target organ damage, chronic kidney disease (CKD) and familial hypercholesterolaemia. Some calculators may also underestimate risk if there are additional risk factors which cannot be inputted (e.g., HIV treatment, serious mental health problems, medications that cause dyslipidaemia, autoimmune and systemic inflammatory disorders).

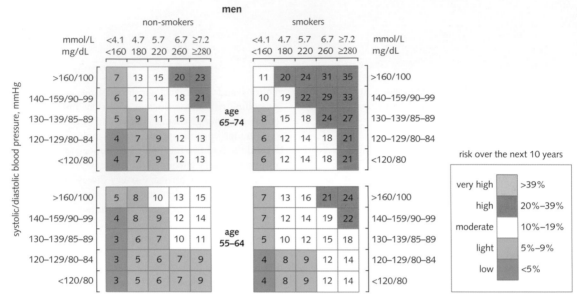

Fig. 12.1 A sample of the Framingham charts for estimating a patient's risk of developing cardiovascular disease.

LIPIDS AND THE CARDIOVASCULAR SYSTEM

Lipid transport and metabolism and targets of lipid modifying drugs

The insolubility of lipids in plasma means a special transport mechanism is required. This is provided by lipid–protein complexes known as lipoproteins. The apolipoproteins (protein component of lipoproteins) also act as receptors for cell surface proteins, which determine the destination of different lipoproteins. Low-density lipoprotein (LDL) is the main lipoprotein involved in the transport of cholesterol. Fig. 12.2 shows the main transport pathways for dietary lipids (exogenous) and for lipids from the body's stores (endogenous).

It is thought that apolipoprotein A is a prothrombotic lipoprotein that is particularly involved in coronary artery disease, while high levels of high-density lipoprotein (HDL) are protective. The classification of lipoproteins is outlined in Table 12.1.

Hyperlipidaemia

Hyperlipidaemia can be classified as hypertriglyceridaemia (raised triglycerides), hypercholesterolaemia (raised cholesterol) or hyperlipoproteinaemia (raised lipoproteins). In reality there may be combinations of each. Although these classifications are useful, they must be used with care because, although hypercholesterolaemia is a risk factor for development of atherosclerosis, it is increasingly apparent that the balance between LDL (damaging) and HDL (pro-

tective) may be more important than the absolute levels. As a result, some people prefer the term 'dyslipidaemia', as it refers to derangement of lipids rather than simply an increase. LDL cholesterol is the most helpful primary treatment target.

> **HINTS AND TIPS**
>
> In patients with high cholesterol, lipids can be deposited in the subcutaneous tissues. Common sites include the skin around the eyes (xanthelasma) and in tendons (tendon xanthomata), and premature (<45 year) corneal arcus (around the corneal margin) may be seen.

Management of hyperlipidaemia

Hyperlipidaemia can be treated with lifestyle interventions or pharmacologically. Lifestyle interventions should include reduction of calorific intake, saturated fats and dietary cholesterol. Reduction of alcohol consumption and regular exercise are also beneficial. The clinical efficacy of supplements of omega-3 fats (present in fish oils) is currently unproven.

The National Institute for Health and Care Excellence (NICE) recommends that patients who have coronary artery disease should have total cholesterol maintained under 4 mmol/L with low-density lipoprotein (LDL) maintained below 2 mmol/L. Lipid-lowering therapy should be offered to all patients irrespective of their cholesterol as part of a secondary prevention strategy.

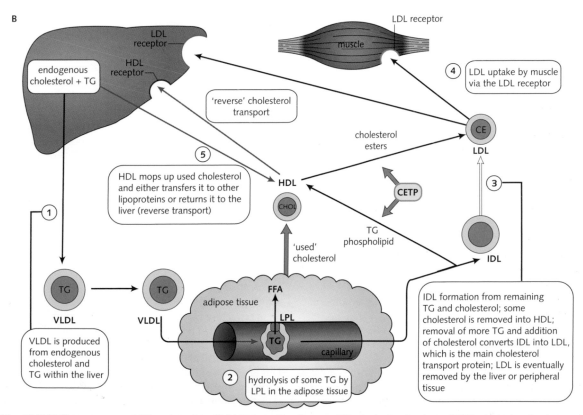

Fig. 12.2 (A) Exogenous and (B) endogenous lipid transport pathways, *CE,* cholesterol esters; *CETP,* cholesterol ester transfer protein; *CM,* chylomicron; *FFA,* free fatty acid; *HDL,* high-density lipoprotein; *IDL,* intermediate-density lipoprotein; *LDL,* low-density lipoprotein; *LPL,* lipoprotein lipase; *TG,* triacylglycerol; *VLDL,* very low-density lipoprotein.

Table 12.1 Classification of lipoproteins

Particle	Source	Predominantly transports
Chylomicron (CM)	Gut	Triacylglycerol
Very low-density lipoprotein (VLDL)	Liver	Triacylglycerol
Intermediate-density lipoprotein (IDL)	Catabolism	Cholesterol
Low-density lipoprotein (LDL)	Catabolism	Cholesterol
High-density lipoprotein (HDL)	Catabolism	Cholesterol
Lipoprotein A	Liver, gut	—

In primary prevention, there is no universally accepted level at which drug therapy should be started and the decision is usually based on assessment of overall risk of cardiovascular disease. NICE guidelines for lipid-lowering therapy in primary prevention have recently changed. They now recommend starting treatment in patients with a 10-year cardiovascular risk of >10% (previously >20%) using validated risk calculators.

If cholesterol levels are very high, this should prompt taking a family history and consideration of familial hypercholesterolaemia. This not only confers increased risk to the individual but also young family members and should prompt genetic counselling and consideration of treatment.

CLINICAL NOTES

FAMILIAL HYPERCHOLESTEROLAEMIA
Lipid levels are mostly determined in a polygenic pattern, although a number of monogenic lipid disorders exist. Familial hypercholesterolaemia is the most common and strongly correlated to coronary artery disease. Estimated frequency is >1/500 in the population; it confers an increased risk of coronary artery disease of at least 10-fold, and this can be dramatically reduced by treatment.

Simon Broome diagnostic criteria in adults:

(a) Total cholesterol >7.5 mmol/L or LDL cholesterol >4.9 mmol/L

(b) Tendon xanthomatas in patient or first- or second-degree relative

(c) DNA-based evidence of a mutation in LDL receptor, apo B-100 or PCSK9

(d) Family history of myocardial infarction <50 years in second-degree relative or <60 years in first-degree relative

(e) Family history of raised cholesterol >7.5 mmol/L in first- or second-degree relative.

Definite familial hypercholesterolaemia is defined as (a) plus one of (b) or (c), and possible familial hypercholesterolaemia is defined as (a) plus one of (d) or (e).

Secondary causes of dyslipidaemia are less well known than secondary causes of hypertension but make a contribution in a significant proportion of the population. Common causes include excess alcohol, uncontrolled diabetes, hypothyroidism, cholestatic liver disease and nephrotic syndrome. Medication causes include antipsychotic medication, corticosteroids and some immunosuppressant drugs. If treatment of these causes if possible, antihypertensives may not be required.

Drugs used to lower cholesterol

Statins (e.g., simvastatin, atorvastatin)
Statins are β-hydroxy-β-methylglutaryl coenzyme A (HMG-CoA) reductase inhibitors. HMG-CoA reductase is the rate-limiting step in cholesterol synthesis. When inhibited, the liver compensates for the decreased cholesterol synthesis by increasing LDL receptor expression, which decreases plasma levels of LDL. Statins are the first-line drug for high cholesterol, can reduce cholesterol by more than 50% and have been repeatedly demonstrated, to reduce mortality in both primary and secondary prevention of cardiovascular disease. In addition to their cholesterol lowering effects, statins have an anti-atherosclerotic effect, reducing the inflammatory activity within atherosclerotic plaques (and thus strengthening the fibrous cap) and reducing the size of plaques. The main side-effects include reversible myositis and disturbed liver function tests.

Ezetimibe
This is an orally acting selective inhibitor of cholesterol absorption. It may be used alone or in combination with a statin in refractory cases. It can lower cholesterol by a further 15% to 20% when taken in addition to a statin.

PCSK9 inhibitors
This new class of drugs targets the PCSK9 protein involved in the control of the LDL receptor. The two monoclonal antibodies available, alirocumab and evolocumab, are subcutaneous injections, administered usually every 2 weeks. They can lower LDL cholesterol levels by over 50%; however, currently they are only available for use in certain high-risk cases of familial hypercholesterolaemia or mixed dyslipidaemia where maximal tolerated doses of statins have not achieved sufficient cholesterol reduction.

Bile acid binding resins (e.g., colestipol and colestyramine)

Cholesterol is the initial substrate for synthesis of bile acids. These drugs bind bile acids in the intestine, forming insoluble complexes, increasing excretion of bile acids. To replenish bile acid levels, cholesterol is utilized for bile acid synthesis, thus reducing plasma cholesterol levels. This removes LDL cholesterol from circulation; however, these drugs can aggravate hypertriglyceridaemia.

Drugs used to lower triglyceride levels

Fibrates

Gemfibrozil reduces lipolysis of triglycerides in adipose tissue, leading to decreased hepatic production of very low-density lipoprotein (VLDL). Bezafibrate causes decreased VLDL and decreased triglycerides, but it may increase LDL. Fibrates are used mainly in familial hyperlipidaemia. Gemfibrozil does not increase LDL but increases the risk of myopathy from statins; therefore it should not be co-prescribed.

HYPERTENSION

Hypertension is not only a major risk factor for myocardial infarction and heart failure, but also cerebrovascular disease, peripheral vascular disease, renal failure, cognitive decline and premature death. To reduce the risk of these, it is important to diagnose and adequately treat hypertensive patients.

Definition of Hypertension

Normal BP increases with age and varies throughout the day according to factors such as stress and exertion. There is also an underlying diurnal variation, with the lowest blood pressure occurring at around 4 AM. In the population, there is a skewed normal distribution.

The definition of hypertension is therefore somewhat arbitrary, and cardiovascular disease risk increases with increasing BP even within the normal range. Current British Hypertension Society guidelines define hypertension as above 140/90 mmHg in adults. In some patients, diastolic BP may be normal whilst systolic BP is raised. This is known as isolated systolic hypertension.

In some people BP can be consistently higher when measured at their GP or clinic, otherwise known as 'white coat hypertension'. Diagnosis is now recommended with multiple BP readings away from the clinical environment, e.g., ambulatory BP measurement or home BP measurement, as this is shown to correlate better with BP-related clinical outcomes.

Classification and causes

Hypertension is classified according to severity and its underlying cause.

Severity of hypertension

Optimal BP is thought to be less than 120/80 mmHg. The normal range includes up to 130/85 mmHg, and levels up to 140/90 mmHg in the clinical environment are considered high normal. If either systolic or diastolic levels are consistently higher, the patient is hypertensive (Table 12.2).

Causes of hypertension

Primary (essential) hypertension accounts for around 95% of hypertensive patients; the precise aetiology is unknown, but it is probably multifactorial. Either increased cardiac output or total peripheral resistance will increase blood pressure.

Predisposing factors include:

1. Age (blood pressure rises with age).
2. Genetic susceptibility.
3. High salt intake.
4. Obesity.
5. Physical inactivity.
6. Excessive alcohol intake.

Secondary hypertension accounts for the remaining 5% of cases (Table 12.3). Here, hypertension arises as a result of another disease process, such as:

1. Renal: parenchymal damage (e.g., acute glomerulonephritis, renal vasculitis) can cause an increase in BP. Atherosclerosis in the renal arteries causing renal artery stenosis also causes hypertension by decreasing renal perfusion, stimulating the renin–angiotensin system. Renal damage is both a cause and consequence of hypertension.

Table 12.2 Severity of hypertension

Hypertension	Clinic readings		ABPM/HBPM	
	Systolic	Diastolic	Systolic	Diastolic
Grade 1 (Mild)	≥140	≥90	≥135	≥85
Grade 2 (Moderate)	≥160	≥100	≥150	≥95
Grade 3 (Severe)	≥180	≥110	No need to verify with ABPM	

ABPM, Ambulatory blood pressure monitoring; *HBPM*, home blood pressure monitoring

Table 12.3 Causes of secondary hypertension

Mechanism	Pathology
Renal	Renal parenchymal disease (e.g., chronic atrophic pyelonephritis, chronic glomerulonephritis), renal artery stenosis, renin-producing tumours
Endocrine	Acromegaly, hypo- and hyperthyroidism, hypercalcaemia, adrenal cortex disorders (e.g., Cushing disease, Conn syndrome, congenital adrenal hyperplasia), adrenal medulla disorders (e.g., phaeochromocytoma)
Vascular disease	Coarctation of the aorta
Other	Hypertension of pregnancy, carcinoid syndrome
Increased intravascular volume	Polycythaemia (primary or secondary)
Drugs	Alcohol, oral contraceptives, monoamine oxidase inhibitors, glucocorticoids
Psychogenic	Stress

2. Endocrine.
   (a) Primary hyperaldosteronism (e.g., Conn syndrome): causes salt and water retention, increasing blood volume, preload and thereby cardiac output.
   (b) Phaeochromocytoma: catecholamine–releasing tumour of the adrenal medulla.
3. Coarctation of the aorta: a narrowing of the aorta, usually just distal to the left subclavian vein, increases resistance to flow through the aorta and can result in upper limb hypertension and lower limb normo- or hypotension.
4. Pregnancy: hypertension occurs during 10% of first pregnancies.
5. Drugs: the oral contraceptive pill causes hypertension in approximately 5% of women. Other drugs such as stimulants, nonsteroidal antiinflammatory drugs (NSAIDs) and interestingly liquorice, can play a role.

HINTS AND TIPS

Identifying secondary hypertension is of great clinical significance because treatment of the underlying cause may be possible. In younger patients with less risk factors present, more effort should be made to find an underlying cause. Secondary causes are also more likely to cause hypertension refractory to antihypertensives or hypertensive emergencies. However, a wide range of possible causes exist, so it is essential to look carefully and keep an open mind.

Effects of hypertension of the vessels

Hypertension not only accelerates atherosclerosis, but it also results in characteristic changes to arterioles and small arteries – known as arteriolosclerosis. All these changes are associated with narrowing of the vessel lumen. Changes in hypertension include:

1. In arteries: muscular hypertrophy of the media, reduplication of the external lamina and intimal thickening.
2. In arterioles: hyaline arteriosclerosis (protein deposits in wall) – this can lead to hypertensive kidney disease.
3. In vessels of the brain: microaneurysms (Charcot–Bouchard aneurysms) can occur, thought to increase the risk of haemorrhagic stroke.

Complications of hypertension

1. Atherosclerosis: hypertension increases the risk of developing clinically significant atherosclerotic plaques. This increases the risk of stroke, peripheral vascular disease and myocardial infarction.
2. Renal damage: gradual development of renal dysfunction occurs in hypertension, especially if it is poorly controlled. The pattern of renal disease caused by hypertension is often referred to as hypertensive nephrosclerosis.
3. Cardiac: the increased afterload caused by the raised blood pressure increases left ventricular work and causes left ventricular hypertrophy (LVH). This can lead to heart failure.
4. Arrhythmia: the risk of atrial fibrillation is increased in hypertensive individuals.
5. Retinal damage: retinal haemorrhages and papilloedema (in advanced stages) cause visual disturbances.

Clinical features

History

Most hypertensive patients are entirely asymptomatic, and in essential hypertension, no obvious cause can be found; therefore this can affect compliance with therapy, which may have unwanted side-effects. Occasionally in hypertension, patients may complain of headaches, tinnitus, recurrent epistaxis, dizziness, fainting or visual disturbance. It is rare for these to be truly attributable to hypertension.

HINTS AND TIPS

There is no correlation between symptoms and severity of hypertension in the vast majority of patients. However, symptoms can be severe in accelerated hypertension.

The aim of history taking is to look for secondary causes, identify any complications of hypertension that have already developed and look for concomitant risk factors that increase future risk of complications.

Secondary causes (Table 12.4):

- Repetitive episodes of palpitations, sweating, headaches, anxiety or collapse may indicate the possibility of a phaeochromocytoma. Although symptoms are episodic, hypertension may be persistent.
- Paroxysmal muscle weakness and tetany may suggest hyperaldosteronism.
- Weight loss or gain, tremor, hair loss, heat intolerance or feeling cold may suggest the presence of thyroid disease.
- Weight gain, weakness, acne, hirsutism, headache, emotional lability, new development of diabetes and reproductive dysfunction may suggest Cushing syndrome.

Complications of hypertension:

- Heart failure: dyspnoea, orthopnoea or ankle oedema.
- Ischaemic heart disease: episodic ischaemic chest pain.
- Cerebrovascular disease: previous unilateral motor/sensory deficit, speech disturbance and/or visual disturbance.
- Peripheral vascular disease: intermittent claudication, rest pain and ulceration.

Past medical history

In a condition with many varied causes, it is helpful to find out about all previous illnesses and operations.

Secondary causes:

1. Any reason for chronic corticosteroids (such as asthma, chronic obstructive pulmonary disease (COPD) or autoimmune disease) may lead to Cushing syndrome.
2. Renal failure may be caused by recurrent urinary tract infections, especially in childhood, or previous urinary tract obstruction.
3. Previous thyroid surgery.

Risk factors:

1. Dyslipidaemia.
2. Diabetes is a concomitant risk factor for ischaemic heart disease. It can also lead to diabetic nephropathy, which may contribute to hypertension.
3. Renal parenchymal disease, diagnosed or otherwise, is important to identify, as it alone increases risk of cardiovascular conditions and is an indication for BP control without other risks.
4. Myocardial infarction (MI) or stroke in the past – any existing vascular disease will put the patient at much higher risk of future vascular complications.

Drug history

Take a careful history of all drugs being taken which may increase BP:

1. Prescribed drugs e.g., oral contraceptives and steroids.
2. Even nasal or eye drops containing vasoconstrictors can cause systemic effects.

3. Over-the-counter analgesics (e.g., NSAIDS).
4. Unexpected substances such as liquorice can cause apparent mineralocorticoid excess.

Ask about previous treatment for hypertension – a high BP reading may be after the patient has decided to stop taking antihypertensives or stopped treatment due to side effects (e.g., postural hypotension). If hypertension has been refractory to multiple treatments at good dose, there should be a search for secondary causes and the patient should be referred for specialist input.

Family history

Primary hypertension is a multifactorial disease with both genetic and environmental inputs. A family history of hypertension is therefore not an uncommon finding. Some secondary causes of hypertension have a genetic component:

1. Adult polycystic kidney disease is an autosomal dominant condition associated with hypertension, renal failure and cerebral artery aneurysms.
2. Phaeochromocytoma may occur as part of a multiple endocrine neoplasia syndrome (MEN 2, autosomal dominant) associated with medullary carcinoma of the thyroid and hyperparathyroidism.

A family history of ischaemic heart disease is another risk factor for ischaemic heart disease.

Social history

Social factors that may contribute to hypertension:

- Alcohol.
- Smoking.
- Diet: high salt intake.
- Lack of exercise.
- Stimulants e.g., cocaine and amphetamine.

Examination

Important points when taking the blood pressure manually:

1. The patient should be seated comfortably – preferably for 5 min before measurement in a quiet warm setting.
2. Use the correct cuff size – if too small, it will cause a spuriously high reading.
3. Whilst palpating the brachial artery, inflate the cuff. The point at which the pulse becomes impalpable is roughly equal to the systolic blood pressure.
4. Deflate the cuff and now place your stethoscope over the brachial artery. Inflate the cuff to 20 mmHg above the estimated systolic pressure.
5. Systolic blood pressure is recorded as the point during bladder deflation where regular sounds start to be heard (Korotkoff phase I).
6. Diastolic blood pressure is recorded as the point at which the sounds disappear (Korotkoff phase V). In children and pregnant women, muffling of the sounds is used as the diastolic blood pressure (Korotkoff phase IV).

Table 12.4 Summary of important causes of secondary hypertension

Causes	Renal parenchymal disease	Renal artery stenosis	Primary hyperaldosteronism	Phaeochromocytoma	Cushing syndrome
History	Obstruction or urinary tract infections, haematuria, family history of polycystic kidney disease	Fibromuscular dysplasia: early onset hypertension Atherosclerotic stenosis: hypertension of abrupt onset, resistant to treatment, flash pulmonary oedema	Episodes of muscle weakness, tetany, family history of early onset hypertension and cerebrovascular events	Paroxysmal hypertension, episodes of headache, sweating, palpitations, pallor, collapse, family history of phaeochromocytoma	Rapid weight gain, polyuria, polydipsia, psychological disturbance
Examination	Enlarged palpable kidneys in polycystic kidney disease	Abdominal bruit	Arrhythmias if severe hypokalaemia	Signs of neurofibromatosis (e.g., café-au-lait spots, neurofibromas)	Cushingoid features
Investigations	Decreased GFR, protein or blood or WCC in the urine, may have hyperkalaemia	Size discrepancy between kidneys on ultrasound, rapid renal function decline spontaneously or in response to ACEi	Hypokalaemia, metabolic alkalosis, incidental discovery of adrenal masses	Incidental discovery of adrenal (or extra-adrenal) masses	Hyperglycaemia
Diagnostic tests	Renal ultrasound, further renal investigations	Renal Duplex Doppler ultrasound, further detailed renal artery imaging	Aldosterone-renin ratio, adrenal CT/MRI, selective adrenal venous sampling	Urinary metanephrine collection, CT/MRI abdomen and pelvis	24-hour urinary cortisol, dexamethasone suppression test, adrenal/pituitary/chest imaging for source

ACEi, ACE inhibitor; *CT*, computed tomography; *GFR*, glomerular filtration rate; *MRI*, magnetic resonance imaging; *WCC*, white cell count.

As with the history, when performing the examination in hypertension (Fig. 12.3) look for signs of:

1. An underlying cause of hypertension.
2. Target-organ/end-organ damage (i.e., LVH, cardiac failure, ischaemic heart disease, peripheral artery disease, cerebrovascular disease, renal impairment and hypertensive retinopathy).
3. Co-existent risk factors for ischaemic heart disease.

Signs consistent with secondary hypertension:

- Features of Cushing syndrome: round face, interscapular and supraclavicular fat pads, abdominal obesity, proximal myopathy, easy bruising, striae, acne, hirsutism, acanthosis nigricans.
- Skin stigmata of neurofibromatosis (associated with phaeochromocytoma).
- Polycystic kidneys may be palpable.
- Renal artery bruits may be heard in renovascular hypertension.
- Auscultation of precordial or chest murmurs (aortic coarctation, aortic disease, upper limb arterial disease).
- Diminished and delayed femoral pulses (aortic coarctation, aortic disease, lower limb arterial disease).
- Left-right arm BP difference (subclavian artery stenosis, uncommonly aortic coarctation).

- As secondary hypertension has many possible causes, thoroughly examine all systems and remember to look out for signs of thyroid disease, acromegaly, etc.

Signs of end-organ damage:

- Retina: fundoscopic abnormalities as below.
- Brain: motor or sensory deficits, speech disturbance.
- Carotid arteries: disease may cause bruits and is a risk factor for stroke.
- Heart: heart rate, elevated JVP, third or fourth heart sound, heart murmurs, arrhythmias, heaving apical impulse, pulmonary crepitations, peripheral oedema.
- Peripheral arteries: absence, reduction or asymmetry of pulses, poor perfusion and cold extremities, atrophic changes, ischaemic skin lesions.
- Kidneys: peripheral oedema, signs of anaemia or uraemia, fistulae, transplanted kidneys.
- Abdominal aortic aneurysm can be a sign of generalized atherosclerosis, but this is rarely looked for in practice.

Signs of other risk factors for ischaemic heart disease:

- Diabetes: fingertip black lancet marks, lipohypertrophy at insulin injection sites, insulin pump.
- Tendon xanthomata, xanthelasma.
- Obesity.

Additional notes on cardiovascular examination

When examining the pulse, remember:

1. Rate – tachycardia or bradycardia may be found in underlying thyroid disease.

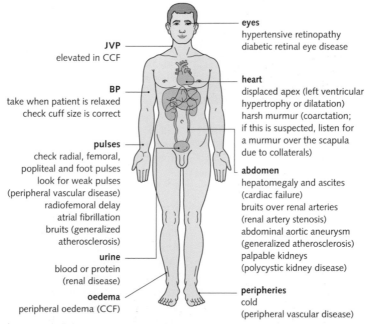

Fig. 12.3 Important clinical findings in hypertensive patients. This illustration is only a guide and there are many other possible findings. *BP*, Blood pressure; *CCF*, congestive cardiac failure; *JVP*, jugular venous pressure.

2. Rhythm – atrial fibrillation may occur as a result of hypertensive heart disease.
3. Symmetry – compare the pulses; radial-femoral delay with unequal blood pressures between the upper and lower limbs point towards coarctation.

Bear in mind:

1. In aortic coarctation, continuous or systolic murmurs may be heard in the left infraclavicular area or below the left scapula; however, there may be a continuous hum from collaterals in a range of areas. 85% of cases have an associated bicuspid valve and this may cause an ejection click. There may also be a fourth heart sound (S4) if the heart has become hypertrophied and non-compliant.
2. Hypertensive heart disease – look for LVH (e.g., heaving apex beat) leading onto heart failure, atrial fibrillation or ischaemic heart disease.

COMMON PITFALLS

Left ventricular hypertrophy is due to pressure overload and results in a non-displaced, heaving apex beat. This should not be confused with the displaced thrusting apex beat secondary to volume overload (e.g., mitral regurgitation) and dilatation of the left ventricle.

Eyes

RED FLAG

Patients exhibiting grade III or IV hypertensive retinopathy have a hypertensive emergency and need urgent treatment.

A detailed examination of the fundi looking for hypertensive retinopathy provides valuable information about the severity of the hypertension (Fig. 12.4). Table 12.5 highlights the features of the different grades of hypertensive retinopathy on ophthalmoscopy.

HINTS AND TIPS

Look for features of both hypertensive and diabetic retinopathy on examination as diabetes may be undiagnosed.

Fig. 12.4 Stages of hypertensive retinopathy. (A) Grade II, showing silver wiring *(SW)* and arteriovenous nipping *(AVN)* where an artery crossing above a vein causes apparent compression of the underlying vein. (B) Grade III, showing evidence of haemorrhages *(H)* and exudates *(E)*. (C) Papilloedema – the optic disc *(OD)* is swollen and oedematous – a sign of a hypertensive emergency.

Investigations

The investigations listed in Table 12.6, should be performed at presentation in all hypertensive patients to look for evidence of end-organ damage, identify possible secondary hypertension and as a measure of response to treatment. For example, LVH (Fig. 12.5) should gradually regress once hypertension has been successfully controlled.

Table 12.5 Grades of hypertensive retinopathy

Grade	Features
I	Narrowing of the arteriolar lumen occurs giving the classic 'silver wiring' effect
II	Sclerosis of the adventitia and thickening of the muscular wall of the arteries leads to compression of underlying veins and 'arteriovenous nipping'
III	Rupture of small vessels leading to haemorrhages and exudates
IV	Papilloedema (plus signs of grades I–III)

Table 12.6 Investigations for hypertension

Investigations	Notes
Blood tests	Renal function and electrolytes, blood lipid profile, blood glucose/HbA1c
Urine dipstick	Microscopic haematuria or proteinuria
ECG	Can provide evidence of LVH (i.e., R wave in V5 >25 mm, deep S wave in V1 >25 mm, tallest R wave in V5 or V6 added to S wave in V1 >35 mm, R wave in AVL >11 mm, lateral T wave inversion)
Consider echocardiogram	LVH, usually concentric in nature (i.e., left ventricular wall thickness >1.1 cm); performed routinely at some centres because LVH is thought to be a valuable indicator of prognosis

LVH, Left ventricular hypertrophy

Investigation of Secondary Hypertension

If the patient is at high risk of having secondary hypertension, then further investigations are indicated. Criteria may include:

1. Younger people (e.g., under 40 years).
2. Symptoms of an underlying cause (e.g., phaeochromocytoma – sweating, dizzy spells, tachycardia).
3. Signs of an underlying cause (e.g., differential blood pressure between arms, hypokalaemia or Cushingoid/acromegalic appearance).
4. Symptoms and signs of hypertensive emergency (i.e., blood pressure >180/110 mmHg, grade 3 or 4 hypertensive retinopathy or cardiac failure at a young age).
5. Hypertension refractory to 3 antihypertensives.
6. A sharp decline in renal function (reduction in estimated glomerular filtration rate of >25% or increase in creatinine of >30%) after initiation of angiotensin-converting enzyme (ACE) inhibitor or angiotensin II receptor antagonist. The kidney in renal artery stenosis is heavily dependent upon increased levels of angiotensin II to provide adequate blood pressure (and maintain renal perfusion); this is prevented by administration of ACE inhibitors/angiotensin II receptor antagonists.

The following screening tests will exclude most causative conditions:

1. Aldosterone:renin ratio to exclude primary hyperaldosteronism. This may be due to a single adenoma (Conn syndrome) or bilateral adrenal hyperplasia.

Fig. 12.5 Electrocardiographic features of left ventricular hypertrophy (LVH). Note the cardinal features indicating LVH: R wave in V5 or V6 plus S wave in V1 exceeds seven large squares; T wave inversion in lateral leads V4–V6.

2. 24-h urine protein and creatinine clearance to exclude marked renal pathology.

3. Plasma free metanephrines and 24-h urinary fractionated metanephrines to exclude phaeochromocytoma.

4. 24-h urine 5-hydroxy indole acetic acid (5HIAA) or plasma chromogranin A to exclude carcinoid syndrome.

5. 24-h urine cortisol excretion and dexamethasone suppression test to exclude Cushing disease.

6. Renal ultrasound may reveal overt structural abnormality (e.g., bilateral small kidneys in chronic renal parenchymal disease, enlarged polycystic kidneys, phaeochromocytoma, asymmetrical kidneys in renal artery stenosis).

7. If coarctation is suspected, a chest X-ray (CXR) may demonstrate rib notching (specific but often incidental finding) and cardiomegaly. Coarctation may be confirmed on echocardiography or contrast-enhanced computed tomography (CT)/magnetic resonance imaging (MRI).

8. CT or MR angiogram to exclude renal artery stenosis if there is a high index of suspicion.

See further condition specific investigations in Table 12.4.

Management

Hypertension is a common disorder. If left untreated, multiple organ systems can be damaged as outlined previously, which is reduced by adequate blood pressure control. As patients are often asymptomatic, they are less likely to comply with drug regimens or follow-up visits to their doctor.

COMMUNICATION

Explain to patients that hypertension can be well treated with medications, but, untreated, hypertension can have serious complications. They may not experience symptoms even if their blood pressure is elevated, so it is important to continue with their treatment even if they feel well. Discuss all treatment options, including lifestyle advice, and if using medicines, discuss their effects and common side effects.

Identifying and stopping contributors to hypertension are important, such as prescribed medicines (e.g., the contraceptive pill, NSAIDs), over the counter medicines and drugs of abuse.

All other risk factors for ischaemic heart disease should be sought and treated in these patients.

The 2011 NICE/British Hypertension Society guidelines (reviewed 2014) for hypertension suggest:

1. Use non-pharmacological measures in all hypertensive and borderline hypertensive people.

2. Initiate antihypertensive drug treatment in people with severe hypertension, stage 2 hypertension or stage 1 hypertension in patients less than 80 years old who have target organ damage, diabetes, cardiovascular disease, renal disease or a 10-year cardiovascular risk score of ≥20% (see later).

3. Optimal blood pressure treatment targets are <140/90 mmHg in patients <80 years, or <150/90 mmHg in patients ≥80 years.

Non-pharmacological management

Non-pharmacological management may decrease blood pressure sufficiently to prevent the need for drug therapy in patients with mild hypertension or may avoid multiple hypertensives.

The following lifestyle interventions are recognized:

1. Weight loss (losing 10 kg weight may reduce BP by 10 mmHg).

2. Reduction in alcohol consumption (currently, the maximum recommended weekly intake is 14 units for both men and women).

3. Reduction in salt intake.

4. Diet low in fat with five portions of fruit and vegetables a day.

5. Regular exercise.

Pharmacological management

The choice of antihypertensive agents in newly diagnosed patients should be guided by the British Hypertension Society algorithm, shown in Fig. 12.6.

Choice of therapy may also be influenced by co-existing disease. These agents may be used alone or in combination to achieve good blood-pressure control. Remember, compliance is likely to be better if once-daily preparations are used and polypharmacy is avoided (i.e., the drug regimen is kept as simple as possible by using a higher dose of a single agent before adding another drug).

Angiotensin-converting enzyme inhibitors

ACE inhibitors (e.g., ramipril) inhibit the conversion of angiotensin I to angiotensin II by ACE (Fig. 12.7). They also inhibit breakdown of bradykinin (a vasodilator) by ACE. When started, renal function and electrolytes should be monitored. They should not be used to treat patients with severe renal artery stenosis because inhibition of angiotensin II production will prevent the efferent arteriolar constriction that maintains glomerular filtration in the presence of renal artery stenosis.

Angiotensin II receptor antagonists

Angiotensin II receptor antagonists (e.g., losartan) inhibit angiotensin II from binding to its receptor. They are useful in patients treated with ACE inhibitors who develop a dry cough (due to elevated bradykinin).

Calcium channel blockers

Calcium channel antagonists block voltage-gated calcium channels in myocardium and vascular smooth muscle. This

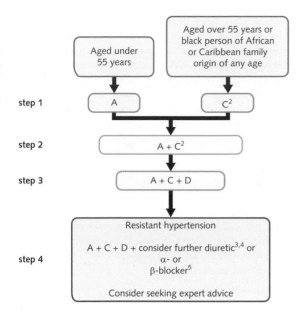

step 1

step 2   A + C²

step 3   A + C + D

step 4

Resistant hypertension

A + C + D + consider further diuretic³,⁴ or
α- or
β-blocker⁵

Consider seeking expert advice

A: ACE inhibitor or low-cost angiotensin II receptor blocker (ARB)¹

C: Calcium channel blocker (CCB)

D: Thiazide-like diuretic

Fig. 12.6 British Hypertension Society guidelines for management of hypertension.
¹ Choose a low-cost ARB.
² A CCB is preferred but consider a thiazide-like diuretic if a CCB is not tolerated or the person has oedema, evidence of heart failure or a high risk of heart failure.
³ Consider a low dose of spironolactone⁴ or higher doses of a thiazide-like diuretic.
⁴ At the time of publication (September 2017), spironolactone did not have a UK marketing authorization for this indication. Informed consent should be obtained and documented.
⁵ Consider an alpha- or beta-blocker if further diuretic therapy is not tolerated or is contraindicated or ineffective.

Fig. 12.7 Action of angiotensin-converting enzyme (ACE) inhibitors and angiotensin II (A_{II}) receptor antagonists. A_I, Angiotensin I; A_{II}, angiotensin II; AT_1, angiotensin II receptor type 1; B_2, activated bradykinin-activated by endothelial cell; *BK*, bradykinin; *NO*, nitric oxide; PGI_2, prostacyclin.

causes a decrease in myocardial contractility, electrical conductance and vascular tone. Calcium antagonists interfere with the action of various vasoconstrictor agonists (e.g., noradrenaline/norepinephrine, angiotensin II, thrombin). Due to their negative inotropic effect, they are contraindicated in systolic dysfunction.

The dihydropyridine calcium antagonists, amlodipine and nifedipine, act peripherally on arterioles, relaxing arteriolar vascular smooth muscle and causing vasodilatation. The dihydropyridine calcium channel blockers do not slow the heart rate.

The non-dihydropyridine calcium channel blockers, verapamil and diltiazem, decrease heart rate and therefore are rarely used for hypertension alone.

Diuretics

Usually a thiazide-type diuretic (e.g., bendroflumethiazide) is used. These inhibit sodium reabsorption in the distal renal tubule, which causes increased salt and water excretion, decreasing blood volume and thus decreasing blood pressure. Thiazide diuretics also have a direct vasodilator effect, further reducing blood pressure. Although loop diuretics (e.g., furosemide) produce a more marked diuresis, they are not used in hypertension. The important side-effect to be aware of is hypokalaemia (which increases the risk of arrhythmia); if serum potassium is disproportionately low with low drug doses and sodium is high-normal, this should raise suspicion of primary hyperaldosteronism. Other side effects include hypercalcaemia, hyperglycaemia and hyperuricaemia. Thiazide-like diuretics (e.g., indapamide, chlorthalidone), which have similar mechanisms of action and side effects to thiazides, are preferred to conventional thiazides by NICE guidelines since 2011.

α-Blockers

α-Blockers (e.g., doxazosin) are antagonists of α-adrenoceptors. There is postsynaptic blockade of $α_1$-adrenoceptors, which prevents sympathetically mediated vascular smooth muscle contraction and leads to vasodilatation. They cause a decrease in total peripheral resistance and thus a decrease in blood pressure. Doxazosin is often used for labile (catecholamine-mediated) hypertension. Blockade of α-receptors also prevents sympathetically mediated release of renin in the kidneys.

Side-effects of α-blockers include postural hypotension caused by loss of sympathetic vasoconstriction, particularly marked following the first dose.

β-Blockers

β-Blockers were previously first-line but are used rarely for hypertension alone now, as they are less effective and often less well tolerated. If other agents are contraindicated, they may be considered in younger people. β-Blockers are antagonists of β-adrenoceptors. They block sympathetic activity in the heart ($β_1$), peripheral vasculature ($β_2$) and other tissues, including the bronchi ($β_2$). In the heart, this results in a decrease in heart rate and myocardial contractility, which reduces cardiac output and blood pressure.

The effect of β-blockers on the peripheral vasculature leads to a loss of β-mediated vasodilatation, causing an unopposed α-vasoconstriction. This may initially cause an increase in vascular resistance, elevating blood pressure, but, in long-term use, the vascular resistance returns to pre-treatment levels. Some β-blockers can preferentially act on β_1-adrenoceptors, being more cardioselective; however, even these drugs have some blocking effect on the β_2-adrenoceptor. Types of β-blockers include:

1. Propranolol, atenolol (act on β_1, β_2).
2. Metoprolol, bisoprolol (selective β_1-blockers).

The main side-effects of β-blockers are bronchoconstriction and bradycardia. Be cautious in people with asthma or COPD as they may exacerbate symptoms.

HINTS AND TIPS

The use of β-blockers alone for phaeochromocytoma can result in severe hypertension due to the unopposed action of noradrenaline on the α-receptors.

A summary of these and other agents is given below (Table 12.7).

Follow-up

Follow-up is as important as the initial treatment. Patients should be seen on a yearly basis, involving:

1. Examination to look for evidence of end-organ damage – especially cardiovascular system and retinas.
2. Urinalysis.
3. Blood tests for urea, creatinine and electrolytes – these may be deranged due to renal damage secondary to hypertension or to drug therapy or both.
4. ECG and/or echocardiography if there are concerns.
5. Screen for risk factors for ischaemic heart disease (i.e., blood lipid profile and blood glucose) and lifestyle advice if necessary.

Hypertensive emergencies and urgencies

If blood pressure is very quickly raised to extremely high levels, this may result in rapid organ damage over hours to weeks. This is a hypertensive emergency, a rare event that requires same-day hospital assessment and immediate monitored treatment. Hypertensive emergencies are also known as accelerated or malignant hypertension, although these are older and less specific terms. If there is not yet organ damage, this is referred to as hypertensive urgency and should be treated promptly with oral agents.

Any cause of hypertension can cause a hypertensive emergency; however, it is more common with secondary hypertension, especially phaeochromocytoma and renal causes. There are no absolute levels of hypertension associated with symptoms or organ damage; however, levels required are usually beyond the grade 3 hypertension cut-off.

End-organ damage may include hypertensive encephalopathy, cerebrovascular infarct or haemorrhage, acute left ventricular failure, hypertensive retinopathy, aortic dissection, renal failure, microangiopathic haemolytic anaemia and eclampsia.

Symptoms tend to be non-specific and vary by organ affected and include headache, nausea and vomiting, visual disturbance, altered level of consciousness, seizures, neurological deficit, chest pain and oliguria.

Examination should seek:

- Secondary causes.
- End-organ damage:
  - Cardiovascular.
  - Neurological.
  - Retinopathy.

Investigations include:

- Blood tests: full blood count (FBC), clotting screen, urea and electrolytes (U&Es), liver function tests (LFTs), thyroid function tests (TFTs).
- Urinalysis: protein, blood.
- ECG: LVH, left atrial (LA) enlargement.
- CXR: LVH, cardiac failure.
- Other tests for organ damage if suspected.
- Tests for secondary causes.

Urgent admission to a high-dependency unit (HDU)/ICU is required for hypertensive emergencies, for continuous monitoring of BP and controlled gradual BP reduction. Rare cases may require additional procedures (e.g., intracranial pressure monitoring if intracranial pressure is increased or dialysis in renal failure). The rate of BP reduction and agents used depends on the specific organ damaged. Generally, the goal is to lower BP slowly to prevent sudden drops that may prompt ischaemia. There are two main exceptions: in aortic dissection, if tolerated, rapid BP lowering is preferred to minimize the tendency for dissection to extend; and in acute ischaemic stroke when there should generally be no intervention to BP unless there is a strong indication, in case reduction worsens cerebral perfusion and brain injury.

Malignant hypertension is an old term which reflects the historic prognosis, where mortality was 80% in the first year and 5-year survival was close to zero. Now, prognosis is markedly improved, with better blood pressure control and survival is approximately 80% at 5 years.

Table 12.7 Overview of drugs used to treat hypertension

Class of drug	Examples	Indications	Precautions/ contraindications	Adverse effects
Diuretics	Thiazides (e.g., bendroflumethiazide), thiazide-like diuretics (e.g., indapamide, chlorthalidone)	Mild hypertension or in conjunction with other agents for more severe hypertension	Thiazides exacerbate diabetes mellitus; all diuretics should be avoided in patients who have gout if possible	Hypokalaemia, dehydration, exacerbation of renal impairment, gout
Antiadrenergic agents	β-Blockers (e.g., atenolol, propranolol, bisoprolol, metoprolol)	Moderate to severe hypertension (note that they are antianginal)	Asthma, cardiac failure, severe peripheral vascular disease	Postural hypotension, bradycardia, bronchospasm, fatigue, impotence, cold extremities, nightmares
	α-Blockers (e.g., prazosin, doxazosin)	Moderate to severe hypertension	Postural hypotension	Postural hypotension, headache
	Centrally acting agents (e.g., methyldopa)	Moderate hypertension (safe during pregnancy)	Depression, phaeochromocytoma, acute porphyria	Postural hypotension, allergic reactions, drowsiness, galactorrhoea, gynaecomastia, haemolytic anaemia
Calcium channel blockers	Nifedipine, amlodipine	Moderate hypertension* (note that they are antianginal)	Cardiac failure, heart block (second- or third-degree) – these are contraindications mainly for verapamil and diltiazem	Postural hypotension, headache, flushing, ankle oedema
Angiotensin-converting enzyme inhibitors	Ramipril, captopril, enalapril, lisinopril, perindopril	Moderate to severe hypertension, especially with cardiac failure	Renal artery stenosis, pregnancy	Postural hypotension, dry cough (in approx. 10%), rash, angioedema, renal failure, hyperkalaemia, loss of taste
Angiotensin-II receptor blockers	Candesartan, losartan, valsartan	Moderate to severe hypertension, especially with cardiac failure	Renal artery stenosis, pregnancy	Postural hypotension, renal failure, hyperkalaemia
Vasodilators	Hydralazine	Moderate to severe hypertension	Severe tachycardia, systemic lupus erythematosus	Postural hypotension, headache, lupus-like syndrome
	Sodium nitroprusside (as an intravenous infusion)	Hypertensive emergency	Compensatory hypertension, severe vitamin B12 deficiency	Weakness, cyanide toxicity if drug not protected from light

*Diltiazem and verapamil are less commonly used for hypertension because they have a more pronounced action on heart muscle and conductive tissues, respectively. Diltiazem is used predominantly for angina; verapamil for its antiarrhythmic effects.

Chapter Summary

- Optimal control of the risk factors for ischaemic heart disease is clearly required after ischaemic events (secondary prevention). In primary prevention, the threshold of pharmacological management is best determined by validated online risk calculators in most cases, but these calculators are not used in target organ damage, type 1 diabetes, CKD and familial hyperlipidaemia, as these are indications for treatment in their own right.
- Effective risk factor management is reliant upon patient education and participation.
- Dyslipidaemia can usually be well-controlled with statins or additional agents, and the mainstay of treatment is statins.
- Hypertension is common and often asymptomatic.
- Ambulatory or home BP monitoring is often important to accurately diagnose hypertension to prevent unnecessary long-term treatment and more frequent primary care follow-up.
- History, examination and investigation aims to identify secondary causes, existing complications of hypertension and coexistent cardiovascular risk factors.
- Pharmacological choices depend on age, ethnicity, co-morbidity and tolerance.
- Hypertensive urgencies require urgent assessment and oral treatment, but hypertensive emergencies require ICU or HDU management.

Ischaemic heart disease, also known as coronary artery disease (CAD), is the leading cause of death in the Western world and contributes to significant morbidity. The pathogenesis and clinical classification is described in Chapter 11 and includes stable angina and the acute coronary syndromes (ACS).

Causes of angina and ACS can be split into causes of reduced perfusion and increased demand. Exacerbating factors include the reduced oxygen content of blood reaching the myocardium.

Reduced perfusion:

1. Intra - coronary:
   - Atheromatous stenosis of coronary arteries (most common).
   - Thrombosis within coronary arteries.
   - Dissection of coronary arteries (may occur with aortic dissection or during angiography).
   - Spasm of normal coronary arteries (Prinzmetal angina).
   - Coronary arteritis in vasculitis (e.g., polyarteritis nodosa, Kawasaki syndrome).
   - Emboli as a result of atrial fibrillation (AF)/ mechanical valves/infective endocarditis etc., (rare).
2. Extra - coronary:
   - Severe aortic valve disease. (Remember angina is the first of the classic triad of symptoms to present.)
   - Hypertrophic cardiomyopathy.
   - Hypertension.
   - Microvascular angina (angina and evidence of exercise-induced ischaemia without obstructive atherosclerotic CAD).

Increased demand:

1. Increased cardiac output – exercise, stress, thyrotoxicosis, tachyarrhythmia etc.
2. Increased cardiac work required to maintain an adequate output (severe aortic stenosis).
3. Increased peripheral vascular resistance (hypertension).
4. Hypertrophy, either secondary to aortic stenosis or hypertension or as a primary defect as in hypertrophic cardiomyopathy.

Decreased blood oxygen content:

1. Severe anaemia.
2. Decreased oxygen saturations.

STABLE ANGINA

Angina pectoris is a symptom complex, primarily of central chest discomfort on exertion, relieved by rest. This is caused by coronary arterial insufficiency leading to intermittent myocardial ischaemia. Ischaemia occurs when the oxygen and nutrient demand is greater than its supply.

CLINICAL NOTE

Myocardial oxygen demand is very high, being about 8 mL O_2/min per 100 g and can increase up to fivefold during exercise. Even at rest, the coronary circulation receives 3%–5% of the total cardiac output, 10 times the average blood flow per gram of tissue. In angina, the stenosed vessel is unable to accommodate the necessary increase in blood flow during exertion, causing ischaemia and chest pain which subsides at rest when demand reduces. As a rule of thumb, it is said that the stenosis will need to reduce cross-sectional area of the vessel lumen by 70% before it produces symptoms.

The most common cause by far is atherosclerosis in one or more of the coronary arteries, producing predictable reversible ischaemic symptoms, and the rest of this chapter will focus on this.

Clinical Features of Angina

Angina means 'choking' and pectoris means 'of the chest'. Angina is largely a clinical diagnosis, based on the history.

Angina is classically a 'heavy', 'crushing', 'aching' or 'band-like' pain across the centre of the chest. The pain may radiate to the arm, neck or jaw. Patients may deny pain but describe a 'tightness' or 'discomfort'. Other precipitating factors include cold air and after a meal. Dyspnoea is often associated with chest pain. Angina equivalent, described as exertional dyspnoea without pain and relieved rapidly at rest or with nitrates, is rare but can occur in those at risk of neuropathy (e.g., elderly, diabetics).

Typical angina fulfils all of the following criteria (Diamond classification):

1. Substernal chest discomfort of characteristic quality and duration.
2. Provoked by exertion or emotional stress.
3. Relieved by rest and/or nitrates within minutes.

If only two of these criteria are fulfilled, it is termed *atypical angina*, and if one or none of the criteria are fulfilled, it is classified as non-cardiac chest pain.

Important points to note when diagnosing angina:

1. Oesophageal pain can also be relieved by nitrates.
2. Atypical chest discomfort, especially if it is related to effort, could still be angina.
3. Silent ischaemia is more common in patients with diabetes or the elderly who have autonomic neuropathy.

Typically, stable angina equates to predictable brief symptoms on exertion. However, as the coronary artery narrowing worsens, the amount of exertion required to produce angina reduces and the pain may occur even at rest or on minimal exertion. If this occurs over a short period of time, it may be termed *crescendo* or *unstable angina* (see Acute Coronary Syndromes, later). If pain continues even beyond rest, consider myocardial infarction (MI).

RED FLAG

A sudden worsening of exertional angina may be due to rupture of an atheromatous plaque in the coronary artery, which causes a steep decrease in its luminal diameter, and may even cause intermittent occlusion of the vessel. This condition may progress to myocardial infarction.

Obvious clinical signs are frequently absent in patients with angina alone. Signs to help diagnosis may relate to:

- Risk factors:
  - Hypertension.
  - Hypercholesterolaemia: premature corneal arcus (age <45), xanthelasma, xanthomata. If these are found, consider familial hypercholesterolaemia (see Chapter 12).
  - Diabetes mellitus: fingertip blood glucose measurement marks, lipodystrophy, insulin pump.
  - Smoking: odour, nicotine staining.
- Co-existent arterial disease (increases the likelihood of CAD):
  - Carotid bruits.
  - Peripheral arterial disease.
  - Cerebral vascular disease.
- Conditions which cause decompensation of angina:
  - Anaemia: pallor, including conjunctival.
  - Thyrotoxicosis: fine tremor, eye signs, goitre, AF.
- Heart failure as a result of ischaemic heart disease:
  - Raised jugular venous pressure (JVP) or peripheral oedema.
  - Cardiomegaly or third heart sound.
  - Bibasal crepitations.
- Other causes of angina:
  - Arrhythmia.
  - Aortic valve disease.
  - Hypertrophic cardiomyopathy.

Investigation of Angina

The investigation of patients presenting with chest pain is explained in detail in Chapter 6. The following investigations may be considered in a patient with angina:

1. Resting electrocardiogram (ECG): usually normal between episodes. During an attack, there may be ST segment depression and inverted T waves. Occasionally, evidence of previous infarction may be seen unexpectedly.
2. Exercise ECG: useful for confirming the diagnosis and risk stratification of CAD. Patients have a continuous ECG trace recorded while undergoing a standardized exercise protocol on a treadmill (the Bruce protocol) until myocardial ischaemia is provoked, determined by ST depression of more than 1 mm or chest pain. Horizontal or down-sloping ST depression greater than 1mm is a marker of disease severity, especially at low workload. However, if the symptoms only occur at high workload, exercise testing may not reveal any symptoms or ECG changes. Exercise ECG is not feasible in patients who cannot use the treadmill (e.g., due to severe arthritis).
3. Myocardial perfusion scanning: this relies on the principle that when the myocardium is stressed (either by exercise or pharmacologically with a positive inotrope, such as dobutamine), uptake of a radionucleotide tracer will be increased in line with the increase in perfusion. However, areas of myocardium which have impaired perfusion (due to stenosis in the arteries supplying them) will not exhibit increased uptake in response to stress.
4. Stress echocardiography (e.g., with dobutamine): reversible wall motion abnormalities may suggest an area of myocardium that is less well perfused when stressed. Decreased ejection fraction may be found as a complication.
5. Computed tomography (CT) coronary angiography: improvements in the spatial resolution of CT scanning have allowed it to be used in the assessment of CAD. It can detect stenosis in the coronary arteries and also the degree of calcification within the walls of the vessels, which has been shown to correlate with the degree of stenosis. Flow limitation may be calculated.
6. Coronary angiography (Figs 13.1 and 13.2): assesses the patency of the coronary vasculature by demonstrating the location and extent of coronary

Fig. 13.1 Coronary angiograms of normal (A) left and (B) right coronary arteries, each taken in two perpendicular views. (Courtesy Newby DE, Grubb NR. *Cardiology: an illustrated colour text.* Edinburgh: Elsevier, 2005.)

Fig. 13.2 Coronary angiogram of a patient with a severe coronary stenosis *(arrow)*. (Courtesy Newby D E, Grubb N R. *Cardiology: an illustrated colour text.* Edinburgh: Elsevier, 2005.)

artery stenosis. This is the most specific and sensitive test of coronary artery anatomical lesions and, as such, is the gold standard for diagnosis. It is important to remember that coronary angiography is invasive and there is a small risk of morbidity and mortality associated with the procedure. Coronary angiography is used first-line in patients who are clinically deemed to be high-risk, and in patients of lower risk following a positive non-invasive investigation result or a possible false negative and if symptoms are not controlled medically.

The choice between investigation modalities may depend on local availability and patient characteristics. Current National Institute for Health and Care Excellence (NICE) guidelines recommend CT coronary angiography in patients with possible angina. Patients with known CAD and possible angina should be assessed by stress imaging (stress echocardiogram, nuclear perfusion scan or magnetic resonance perfusion imaging).

Management of Angina Pectoris

As you can see, angina can be a result of other disease (e.g., severe aortic stenosis) and treatment should target any underlying cause. Treatment of exacerbating factors, such as severe anaemia, may resolve symptoms. However, management of standard stable angina involves addressing simultaneously:

1. Management of any modifiable risk factors.
2. Secondary prevention.
3. Management of the angina itself.

Management of risk factors

The main risk factors are described in Chapter 12. Any modifiable risk factors should be sought and treated to reduce the risk of disease progression, MI and death. This is also essential for risk stratification, and high-risk patients may benefit from more intensive preventative strategies.

1. Smoking: encourage cessation at every stage of management.
2. Hypertension: diagnose, encourage lifestyle modification, use medication if required, monitor if target achieved.
3. Diabetes: encourage good glycaemic control with dietary control and medication.
4. Hypercholesterolaemia: once angina secondary to CAD is diagnosed, medication is part of the secondary prevention strategy and should be offered to all, but lifestyle measures will still make a significant difference.

Secondary prevention

1. Aspirin: reduces platelet aggregation, to lower the risk of future MI and death, and should be offered to all as part of secondary prevention.
2. Statin: irrespective of cholesterol concentration, all patients should be maintained on a statin. The dose and intensity of the statin will depend on the baseline cholesterol concentration.
3. Angiotensin converting enzyme (ACE) inhibitors: this should be given to all patients and especially those with hypertension, left ventricular (LV) dysfunction, prior MI or diabetes mellitus.

Treatment of the angina

Treatment strategies for angina aim to restore the balance between myocardial supply and demand by increasing blood supply, and thereby oxygen supply, to the ischaemic myocardium and by decreasing the oxygen demand of the myocardium (Fig. 13.3).

Increasing blood supply can be achieved by:

1. Decreasing heart rate: coronary artery flow occurs primarily during diastole. Decreasing heart rate prolongs diastole, allowing more time for perfusion of the myocardium.
2. Dilating coronary arteries: this may be of more benefit in angina due to coronary artery spasm as stenosed coronary arteries are likely to be already maximally vasodilated by endogenous metabolic vasodilators (such as adenosine).

Decreasing the oxygen demand of the myocardium can be achieved by:

1. Decreasing heart rate.
2. Decreasing contractility.
3. Decreasing preload.
4. Decreasing afterload.

Antianginal drugs

Organic nitrates—Organic nitrates, such as glyceryl trinitrate (GTN), relax vascular smooth muscle cells by producing nitric oxide, which increases levels of cGMP and brings about potent dilatation. Nitrates mediate their effects by:

1. Dilatation of venous capacitance vessels (predominant effect). This causes pooling of blood in the venous system which:
   (a) Reduces the preload of the heart and, according to Starling's law, decreased preload leads to decreased cardiac output, thereby decreasing myocardial work.
   (b) Decreases arterial blood pressure, thus reducing the afterload.

Fig. 13.3 Balance of myocardial oxygen supply and demand in ischaemic heart disease, and the rationale for the use of antianginal therapies. (Courtesy Newby DE, Grubb NR. *Cardiology: an illustrated colour text.* Edinburgh: Elsevier, 2005.)

2. Dilatation of coronary arteries: nitrates have a direct vasodilatory effect on coronary arteries at high doses, increasing myocardial perfusion.

GTN is usually administered sublingually to avoid first-pass metabolism and its effects last around 30 minutes. These come as tablets (short shelf-life) or a spray (shelf-life 3 years). Tolerance develops to the effects of GTN if used regularly over 2 or 3 days and patients should be aware of this. It can be used to relieve an attack or can be taken pro-phylactically to prevent an attack.

Longer acting nitrates include isosorbide mononitrate and isosorbide dinitrate, and require a 'nitrate-free' interval overnight to prevent tolerance. These can come in oral tablet form, or transdermal patches or cream, where the location of application should be varied.

Nitrate side effects include postural hypotension and sometimes a reflex tachycardia as the body attempts to maintain blood pressure, and very occasionally syncope. More common side effects are headache and facial flushing.

β-Blockers (e.g., atenolol, metoprolol)—These drugs block sympathetic stimulation of the heart, leading to:

1. Decreased contractility (negative inotropic effect) and decreased oxygen demand.
2. Decreased heart rate (negative chronotropic effect), decreased oxygen demand and prolonged diastole, increasing duration of coronary blood flow.

They are also effective antihypertensive agents, and in some patients can perform a dual role, simplifying drug therapy.

Remember that β-blockers are contraindicated in:

1. Unstable cardiac failure.
2. Bradyarrhythmia.
3. Asthma (blockade of bronchial β_2-receptors causes bronchoconstriction, but chronic obstructive pulmonary disease without bronchospasm may not be a contraindication).

Side effects include:

1. Tiredness.
2. Postural hypotension – especially in elderly patients (who should start on a small dose initially).
3. Loss of sympathetic response to hypoglycaemia – use a more cardioselective agent.
4. Nightmares – use a non–fat-soluble agent (e.g., atenolol).
5. Male impotence.

HINTS AND TIPS

Many drugs of the same class have similar suffixes to their names. For example, most β-blockers end in '-olol' (e.g., propranolol, atenolol, metoprolol). This is useful when identifying the class of an unfamiliar drug.

Calcium channel blockers—These drugs block L-type Ca^{2+} channels in the heart and arteriolar smooth muscle:

1. Blockade of myocardial Ca^{2+} channels (greatest with non-dihydropyridine agents, verapamil and diltiazem) decreases heart rate and myocardial contractility, thereby decreasing myocardial oxygen demand. These medications also decrease electrical conductance and therefore are class IV antiarrhythmics.
2. Blockade of Ca^{2+} channels in vascular smooth muscle (greatest with dihydropyridine agents, such as nifedipine and amlodipine):
   (a) Peripheral vasodilatation decreases arterial blood pressure, decreasing afterload and myocardial work.
   (b) Direct dilatation of coronary arteries, increasing myocardial perfusion.

Nifedipine may be beneficially combined with β-blockers to minimize the side effect of reflex tachycardia. This occurs less with amlodipine and combination with β-blockers is safe. These both have additional antihypertensive effects. As amlodipine and nifedipine mainly affect peripheral vessels, side effects include flushing, headache and ankle oedema, but these are less of a problem with diltiazem and verapamil.

Verapamil predominantly inhibits conduction through the atrioventricular (AV) node, decreasing heart rate. It also exerts a negative inotropic effect, decreasing myocardial contractility. Diltiazem acts both on the heart and on the arterioles, decreasing heart rate and causing vasodilatation. Avoid verapamil or diltiazem in combination with β-blockers because of the risk of heart block and profound bradycardia. However, they may be useful single agents if β-blockers cannot be used due to excessive bronchoconstriction. Diltiazem can be a good antianginal agent, and verapamil can be useful in angina but is mainly used as an antiarrhythmic.

Nicorandil—Nicorandil is a potassium channel agonist that affects adenosine triphosphate (ATP)-dependent K^+ channels in vascular smooth muscle, causing hyperpolarization and vasodilatation. It affects both veins and arteries, thus reducing both preload and afterload. Nicorandil also has a nitrate component, in that it is a nitric oxide donor. Nicorandil is not used first-line but is an alternative to nitrates when tolerance occurs and if β-blockers and Ca^{2+} antagonists are contraindicated. Side effects are generally similar to nitrates, and include headache and flushing. Other side effects include gastrointestinal ulceration. Tolerance does not occur. They are contraindicated in hypotension or heart failure.

Ivabradine—This is a newer sinoatrial (SA) node modulator. It acts as an antagonist at the I_f ion channel, which inhibits the pacemaker potential in the SA node, slows the rate of depolarization and reduces heart rate (contraindicated in bradycardia). As it does not have the other effects of β-blockers and calcium channel blockers, it has additional benefits in heart failure. It is ineffective in patients with AF.

Ranolazine—This affects late sodium currents in myocardial cells, reducing intracellular calcium through the sodium-calcium exchanger, improving myocardial relaxation and coronary blood flow. This occurs independently of heart rate; therefore it can be used safely in combination with drugs that lower heart rate. It prolongs QT interval and is contraindicated in patients at risk of QT prolongation.

CLINICAL NOTE

ANTI-ANGINAL DRUGS

Drug choice depends on co-morbidities and contraindications, and the simplest combination sufficient to control symptoms should be used. A possible plan of action is:

1. Prescribe all patients aspirin 75mg daily and a statin if no contraindication.
2. Prescribe all patients a GTN spray and advise them to use it for the relief of angina or prior to any activity which is known to bring angina on.
3. Prescribe a β-blocker if not contraindicated.
4. Control hypertension and diabetes (may affect choice of other agents).
5. If β-blockade fails to control the symptoms or is contraindicated, there is a choice to start either a calcium antagonist (be prepared to add a long-acting nitrate if the effect is still insufficient) or to prescribe nicorandil, which has effects similar to those produced by a combination of calcium antagonist and nitrate. Avoid rate-limiting calcium antagonists in combination with β-blockers as there is a risk of precipitating heart block and bradycardia.
6. However, there is not much evidence that using multiple antianginal drugs is beneficial; therefore revascularisation is considered if a combination of two appropriate drugs have not controlled symptoms sufficiently.

Interventional treatments

There are two main ways of mechanically improving myocardial blood supply:

- Percutaneous coronary intervention (PCI).
- Coronary artery bypass graft (CABG).

Coronary angiography is used to help decide which revascularisation technique to use.

Percutaneous coronary intervention—PCI describes a number of procedures to relieve stenosis in the coronary arteries performed by insertion of a catheter, via the radial or femoral artery, under local anaesthetic and light sedation.

Percutaneous treatment options for CAD include:

1. Balloon angioplasty: an inflatable balloon is passed into the affected coronary artery and inflated within the stenosis, compressing it and expanding the lumen.
2. Metal stents: a balloon-mounted metallic stent is positioned within the stenosis, expanding the vessel walls and restoring vessel patency. Stents decrease the need for re-intervention when compared with balloon angioplasty but the stents can stimulate a proliferative response of the vascular smooth muscle. This proliferative response causes scar tissue deposition that can lead to narrowing of the expanded lumen (termed *restenosis*). This usually occurs within 3 to 6 months of implantation. Attempts to overcome this have led to the use of drug-eluting stents, which are coated with immunosuppressive agents.

Stents are highly thrombogenic and can cause blood clots to form, occluding the artery. This risk of thrombosis is ameliorated by the use of intravenous heparin at the time of PCI, and dual anti-platelet therapy, i.e., aspirin indefinitely and a $P2Y_{12}$ receptor (often 3-12 months, length dependent on thrombosis and bleeding risk). Glycoprotein IIb/IIIa receptor inhibitors may also be used in high-risk cases. See Table 13.1 and Chapter 11, **Fig. 11.3**.

Table 13.1 Antiplatelet agents used to prevent thrombosis following angioplasty ± stenting

Class of drug and examples	Action	Side effects
Aspirin	Irreversible inactivation of cyclooxygenase 1 within platelets – potent reduction of platelet aggregation.	Gastritis, including ulcer formation and bleeding, bronchospasm, renal impairment, rashes.
$P2Y_{12}$ antagonist (clopidogrel, ticagrelor, prasugrel)	Inhibits the platelet ADP receptor $P2Y_{12}$, preventing initiation of thrombus formation.	Haemorrhage, diarrhoea, nausea, neutropenia, hepatic dysfunction.
Glycoprotein IIb/IIIa receptor inhibitors (tirofiban, eptifbatide, abciximab)	Inhibits the binding of fibrinogen to GP IIb/IIIa receptors, thus inhibiting platelet aggregation. Given as an infusion at the time of the procedure, and only usually when thrombotic complications occur.	Thrombocytopenia, haemorrhage.

ADP, Adenosine diphosphate.

Complications of PCI:

These include major adverse effects such as:

1. MI – secondary to thrombosis, spasm of the coronary artery, or dissection of the coronary artery by the balloon.
2. Coronary artery perforation.
3. Stroke.
4. Rarely, death.

Less severe, but more common adverse effects such as:

1. Arrhythmias.
2. Contrast reactions (allergy and nephrotoxicity).
3. Haemorrhage or infection at the puncture site.

Coronary artery bypass graft—This is a major operation performed under general anaesthetic. Via median sternotomy to access the heart, the patient's own veins and/or arteries are reattached to bypass the stenosis in the coronary arteries. The vessels commonly used include the internal mammary artery, which is directly anastamosed distal to the stenosis, and the radial artery of the forearm and the long saphenous vein of the leg, which are anastamosed proximally to the aorta and distally beyond the stenosis. Arterial grafts have much better long-term patency than vein grafts.

The procedure is traditionally performed with the patients on a cardiopulmonary bypass machine that oxygenates the blood and the heart is stopped using cooling and cardioplegic solutions. In recent years, however, some surgeons have been performing this procedure on beating hearts using a specialized instrument to immobilize the area around the anastamosis (so-called 'off-pump' CABG).

CABG is usually indicated in patients with left main stem disease or triple-vessel disease, while patients with single- or double-vessel disease are usually treated with PCI. Generally, although CABG is associated with higher short-term mortality and morbidity, the need for subsequent re-intervention is less than with PCI, and overall long-term mortality is reduced.

Complications of coronary artery bypass grafting:

1. Death – mortality rates of approximately 1%.
2. Myocardial infarction, stroke and peripheral thromboembolism.
3. Wound infection.
4. Complications related to cardiopulmonary bypass – they include clotting and pulmonary abnormalities, and impaired cognitive function.

Minimally invasive CABG (MICABG) is a newer technique that involves a smaller incision, usually a left anterior minithoracotomy. The left or right internal mammary artery is used to graft the occluded vessel, which is generally the left anterior descending artery because this is within easy reach. Cardiopulmonary bypass is avoided; instead, the heart is slowed using β-blockers and a small immobilising instrument.

CLINICAL NOTE

PCI vs. CABG

Advantages of PCI over CABG:

1. Avoids major surgery, general anaesthesia and cardiopulmonary bypass, and the associated higher initial mortality.
2. Quicker healing and a shortened hospital stay.
3. Patients who have clotting disorders or who have recently had thrombolysis can be treated in an emergency.
4. If PCI is unsuccessful, CABG can still be performed (whereas a second CABG operation carries a much higher risk).

Disadvantages of PCI compared to CABG:

1. Not all patients will have CAD that is amenable to PCI. Patients with complex coronary disease, such as stenosis of the left main stem, multivessel disease and chronically occluded vessels, may be better served by CABG.
2. Thrombosis can occur at the site of stenting. Additionally, approximately 10% of patients who have had PCI will develop 'in-stent restenosis' (ISR). This rate is higher in diabetic patients, and those with smaller calibre or longer segments of stent. ISR can be treated by further PCI. The rate of early ISR has been reduced by the introduction of drug-eluting stents, but late ISR is increased and requires longer dual anti-platelet therapy, yet the need for revascularisation after PCI is still higher than after CABG. Long-term mortality is also lower with CABG.
3. Although it may provide symptomatic relief, there is no clear evidence that PCI confers any prognostic benefit over medical therapy in stable angina.

ACUTE CORONARY SYNDROMES

The pathophysiological basis and classification of ACS are described in full in Chapter 11.

In unstable angina, the patient typically presents with a sudden increase in exertional angina, with symptoms on minimal exertion or at rest; the pain usually subsides with rest and nitrates. In contrast to MI, there is no permanent change to the ECG or evidence of myocardial damage (elevation of the cardiac biomarker, high-sensitivity troponin).

Reminder:

1. Unstable angina due to coronary arterial thrombosis – there is rupture of an atheromatous plaque in the coronary artery, which causes a marked decrease in luminal diameter. The condition may progress to full infarction without urgent treatment. Patients should be treated as with NSTEMIs (risk assessed, started on NSTEMI treatment and admitted to hospital). This is an increasingly uncommon condition with the advent of high-sensitivity troponin assays.

2. Non-ST-elevation myocardial infarction (NSTEMI) – there is necrosis caused by thrombotic coronary artery occlusion in which the myocardial cell death is confined to the endocardial layers (not full thickness). Usually, this occurs because the occluded artery is relatively small, is a side branch or there is some collateral flow around the occluded vessel.

3. ST-elevation myocardial infarction (STEMI) – this represents a developing full-thickness MI, which can lead to arrhythmia, death or leave the patient with severe heart failure. This is a common ECG to see in Finals as making the diagnosis and rapidly instigating management is absolutely crucial. Delayed intervention leaves dead muscle, which shows as permanent Q waves on the ECG (see Fig. 13.4). Remember that new LBBB with prolonged cardiac chest pain should also be treated as acute STEMI with urgent primary PCI or thrombolysis.

Clinically, acute MI is defined by acute increase and/or fall of troponin, with at least one value raised above the 99th percentile of the upper reference limit, and at least one of the following:

- Symptoms consistent with ischaemia (lasting >20 mins).
- New, or presumed new, significant ST-T wave changes or left bundle branch block (LBBB) on 12-lead ECG (Fig. 13.4).
- New, or presumed new, pathological Q waves on ECG.
- New, or presumed new, loss of viable myocardium or regional wall motion abnormality on imaging.
- Intracoronary thrombus on angiography.

Criteria for established MI includes:

- New pathological Q waves in the absence of another cause.

- Imaging findings of regional wall motion abnormality in the absence of another cause.
- Pathological findings of healed or healing MI.

As raised troponin can be seen in other conditions, terminology for myocardial infarction has evolved over recent years. MI is now classified as below:

- Type 1: Injury related to primary myocardial ischaemia (spontaneous myocardial infarction, usually secondary to atheroma, STEMI and NSTEMI)
- Type 2: Injury related to supply/demand imbalance of myocardial ischaemia ('troponitis' – caused by myocardial stretch/damage: spasm, embolism, tachycardias, hyper/hypotension, anaemia, pulmonary oedema)
- Type 3: Myocardial infarction resulting in death when biomarker values are unavailable.
- Type 4: (a) Peri-angioplasty (>5× upper limit of normal); (b) secondary to stent thrombosis
- Type 5: related to CABG (>10× upper limit of normal).

Clinical Features of ACS

History

See Chapter 6 for more detail. In MI, the history provides clues about the likelihood and severity of the infarction. The time of onset is crucial to determine appropriate therapy. Ongoing chest pain suggests ongoing ischaemia and requires urgent treatment.

Classically, the main presenting complaint is of chest pain, usually:

1. Severe.
2. Lasts at least 20 mins.
3. Tight, crushing, heavy or band-like in nature.
4. Retrosternal in location.
5. May radiate to the left arm, throat or jaw.
6. Associated features include sweating, nausea and breathlessness.

Elderly and diabetic patients may have relatively little pain but may present with features of LV failure (profound breathlessness) or syncope.

Important features include a history of angina or intermittent chest pain, including increase in severity or frequency in the few weeks preceding this event. The patient may have a history of previous MI or of cardiac intervention, such as angiography, PCI or CABG. Find out if the patient is already on medications for CAD.

Fig. 13.4 (A) ECG showing acute anterior ST elevation myocardial infarction. (B) ECG 24 h after anterior STEMI, showing evolving ST changes and development of Q waves.

Ask about any bleeding risks because this will affect further management.

Determine how many of the risk factors for ischaemic heart disease are present: smoking, hypertension, diabetes mellitus, hypercholesterolaemia and positive family history.

Examination

The patient is often extremely anxious, distressed and restless; they may be in severe pain. Tachypnoea/increased work of breathing suggests pulmonary oedema, as does the presence of pink frothy sputum. The patient may be pale, clammy and sweaty with a reduced capillary refill time, or confused and oliguric, suggesting cardiogenic shock. Look for scars of previous surgery.

The pulse may be rapid secondary to anxiety or LV failure. In inferior MIs, there is often bradycardia and AV block, as a result of ischaemia of the AV node, or due to increased vagal tone secondary to ischaemia.

The blood pressure may be raised (pre-existing hypertension or raised due to anxiety). If there is cardiogenic shock, the blood pressure may be low.

The JVP may be elevated in cases of congestive cardiac failure or in pure right-ventricular infarction.

Examination of the precordium may reveal the following:

1. A displaced diffuse apex in cases of LV failure.
2. Rarely with anterior infarction, a paradoxical systolic outward movement of the ventricular wall may be felt parasternally.
3. The murmur of mitral regurgitation or ventricular septal defect – may occur as a new murmur due to rupture of the papillary muscle or ventricular septum, respectively.
4. A pericardial rub – if a delayed presentation, MI may be complicated by pericarditis, which is also a differential diagnosis.

5. Additional heart sounds – third or fourth heart sounds may be heard in MI and suggest LV failure.

Auscultate the lung bases; bilateral crepitations may suggest LV failure. Peripheral oedema may suggest right ventricular (or bi-ventricular) failure. It is most important to determine if there is any sign of LV impairment or cardiogenic shock, as these require urgent treatment.

Investigation of ACS

As you can see from the definitions, early ECG and measurement of cardiac biomarkers are the most urgent investigations to determine suitable treatment.

Electrocardiography

The ECG is a main diagnostic test in acute MI. It is important to have a thorough knowledge of the ECG appearances of different types of MI (see Chapter 3 and Figs 13.4–13.6). Delay in the diagnosis wastes precious time, as treatment should be given as soon as possible for maximum benefit – 'time is muscle'!

HINTS AND TIPS

Posterior MI can be missed, and can be seen as ST depression in the anterior leads with a dominant R wave and upright T waves. Flip the ECG upside down, looking through the back of the paper – the anterior ST depression of posterior MI looks like an anterior STEMI when looked at from behind.

A

Figure showing: aorta, pulmonary artery, circumflex coronary artery, LAD (runs down in line with the interventricular septum), 1st diagonal branch, left ventricle, right ventricle, superior vena cava, left main stem, right coronary artery

B

Location of MI	ECG changes
Anterior (LAD)	ST elevation in leads V1–4
Inferior (RCA or circumflex coronary artery)	ST elevation in leads II, III, aVF
Lateral (circumflex coronary artery)	ST elevation in leads V4–6
Posterior (RCA or circumflex coronary artery)	Prominent R wave in V1 and V2 with ST depression (mirror image of anterior MI)
Anterolateral (proximal LAD) above diagonal branch	ST elevation V1–6
Right ventricular infarction (suspect in inferior or posterior MI)	Consider right-sided ECG using lead V1 (as normal), leads V3–6 placed on the right side, limb leads as normal

Fig. 13.5 (A) Location of coronary arteries. Note the left anterior descending (LAD) coronary artery branch supplies the anterior aspect of the heart (the left ventricle and the septum), the right coronary artery (RCA) usually supplies the inferoposterior aspect and the circumflex supplies the lateral part of the left ventricle. **(B)** ST elevation in leads.

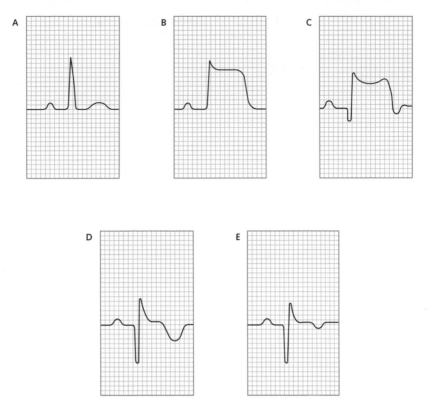

Fig. 13.6 Evolution of ECG changes following transmural myocardial infarction. (A) Normal ECG. (B) Acute ST elevation ('the current of injury'). (C) Progressive loss of R wave, developing Q wave, resolution of the ST elevation and terminal T-wave inversion. (D) Deep Q waves and T-wave inversion. (E) Old or established infarct pattern; the Q wave tends to persist but the T-wave changes become less marked. The rate of evolution is variable but, in general, stage B appears within minutes, stage C within hours, stage D within days and stage E after several weeks or months. (Courtesy Prof Newby, copied from Walker B, Colledge NR, Ralston S, Penman I (eds): *Davidson's Principles and Practice of Medicine.* 22nd ed. Elsevier; 2014, Fig. 18.71.)

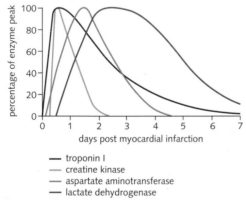

Fig. 13.7 Schematic profile of the release of cardiac enzymes and markers. (Courtesy Newby DE, Grubb NR. *Cardiology: an illustrated colour text.* Edinburgh: Elsevier, 2005, p.93.)

In ST elevation MI (STEMI), ST elevation or new LBBB must be present to make the diagnosis. Fig. 13.6 shows ST segment elevation and the subsequent changes seen on ECG in the days/weeks following a STEMI:

1. ST segment elevation – this is due to full-thickness myocardial injury and may appear within minutes of the onset of infarction; it is almost always present by 24 hours. The criteria for acute thrombolysis are a good history and ST segment elevation >1 mm in two or more consecutive limb leads, or >2 mm in two or more consecutive chest leads. Reciprocal ST segment depression may be present at the same time and represents the mirror image of the ST elevation as seen from the opposite side of the heart.
2. The ST elevation resolves and the T waves begin to invert.
3. Q waves develop within 24–72 h of MI.

HINTS AND TIPS

Persistent elevation of ST segments after 1 week is unusual, and usually indicates either re-infarction or a left ventricular aneurysm.

If there is LBBB, it is important to find an old ECG to compare – if it is new, this may represent an MI.

In unstable angina/non-STEMI (NSTEMI), ST segment depression and T wave inversion (similar to during an attack of angina) may be present. Be aware that in these cases, the ECG may also be completely normal.

Blood tests

Biochemical markers of myocyte necrosis

Myocyte necrosis can be detected biochemically by measuring levels of cardiac enzymes (creatine kinase-MB and lactate dehydrogenase) but these days, the diagnosis is nearly universally made by measuring cardiac troponin T or I. A rise in these markers suggests myocardial necrosis and therefore infarction (Fig. 13.7). NSTEMI may suggest a smaller area of infarction than STEMI; however, markers can be significantly elevated in NSTEMI. This is in contrast to unstable angina, where dynamic ischaemia does not result in cell loss.

Other causes of myocardial injury can cause a raised troponin level, such as:

1. Myocarditis.
2. Takotsubo cardiomyopathy.
3. Tachyarrhythmia.
4. Massive pulmonary embolism.
5. Critical illness (e.g., shock, sepsis).
6. Renal failure.

Renal function and electrolytes

These are important in all patients who have MI. Renal function may be deranged or may worsen due to poor renal perfusion in cardiogenic shock. Hypokalaemia may predispose to arrhythmias and may need to be corrected because acute MI is in itself a proarrhythmogenic condition.

Blood glucose

Diabetes mellitus should be controlled intensively after MI and all patients who have diabetes mellitus benefit from close blood glucose monitoring and management. However, hypoglycaemia should be avoided as this is associated with worse outcomes.

Full blood count

Anaemia may worsen angina. There is often a leucocytosis after acute MI.

Serum cholesterol

This should be measured within 24 hours of an MI; hypercholesterolaemia is a risk factor for MI and needs to be treated. Cholesterol level falls to an artificially low level 24 hours after MI, so after this time, a true reading can only be obtained 2 months after the MI.

Chest radiography

This should be performed on all patients who have acute MI. Points to note are:

1. Signs of pulmonary oedema – signify the need for heart failure treatment.
2. An enlarged heart – suggests chronic cardiac failure or tamponade.
3. Widening of the mediastinum – suggests possible aortic dissection, either as a differential diagnosis or in conjunction with MI, and an absolute contraindication for thrombolysis.

Echocardiography

Echocardiography is not an urgent investigation, but it is important to evaluate ventricular function following an acute MI. Complications of MI may be found which may alter management, such as mural thrombus, mitral regurgitation as a result of papillary muscle infarction, myocardial/septal rupture and pericardial effusion. It may occasionally demonstrate signs of right heart strain, which could alternatively suggest that a large volume pulmonary embolus is the cause of the chest pain and associated troponin rise.

Management of ACS

ACS is a medical emergency. You must know its acute management, and it is one of the few occasions in an exam when you will be expected to know the doses of drugs given.

Immediate management of all patients with ACS should be the administration of analgesia (usually morphine titrated to effect aspirin, a $P2Y_{12}$ antagonist (clopidogrel 300 mg or ticagrelor 180 mg) and a β-blocker (explained later). It is important to treat hypoxia with oxygen, but oxygen is not currently recommended for non-hypoxic patients routinely as there is evidence of possible harm. Morphine reduces pain and anxiety, which is not only important in making the patient more comfortable but may indirectly decrease O_2 demand by reducing heart rate and blood pressure. Remember to give an antiemetic together with morphine to prevent the common side effect of nausea/vomiting. The subsequent management is dependent on the presence of ST elevation and is shown in the algorithm in Fig. 13.8; however, remember to follow the guidelines in your local hospital.

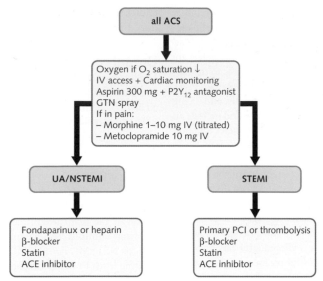

Fig. 13.8 Algorithm for the treatment of acute coronary syndromes. ACE, Angiotensin converting enzyme; ACS, acute coronary syndromes; GTN, glyceryl trinitrate; IV, intravenous; NSTEMI, non-ST elevation myocardial infarction; PCI, percutaneous coronary intervention; STEMI, ST elevation myocardial infarction; UA, unstable angina.

HINTS AND TIPS

The following are useful ways to remember immediate management of suspected ACS.

TIME is of the essence. Urgent investigations and actions:

T - troponin

I - IV access

M - monitor

E - ECG (urgently!)

The mnemonic 'MONA greets all patients' can be helpful to remember immediate management, although always use ABCDE first, at B check for hypoxia and administer O_2 if required, and for ACS give antiplatelets and nitrates urgently:

M - morphine and antiemetic

O- oxygen

N - nitrates

A - aspirin and $P2Y_{12}$ antagonist

In the context of cardiac chest pain, ST segment elevation on the 12-lead ECG usually signifies complete occlusion of a proximal coronary artery. If untreated, myocardial necrosis commences within 30 min, affecting full myocardial thickness within 6 hours. Forty percent of patients die before reaching hospital. Once ECG confirms STEMI, arrange urgent cardiology review for primary angioplasty where available; otherwise, consider thrombolysis if there are no

contraindications and admission to the coronary care unit. Treat new LBBB with cardiac chest pain as STEMI.

In NSTEMI or unstable angina, arrange a cardiology review and admit for ongoing specialist care and likely inpatient coronary angiography.

Drugs used in the immediate treatment of ACS

Preventing thrombus extension

Antiplatelet agents aim to prevent further activation and aggregation of platelets, reducing the likelihood of expansion of the thrombus occluding the affected coronary artery. A number of agents are available (see Table. 13.1).

HINTS AND TIPS

When thinking about antiplatelet agents, consider at which stage of the platelet thrombus formation they act. Both aspirin and $P2Y_{12}$ antagonists are given to patients with ACS because they inhibit the process of platelet aggregation at two points, and thus have a greater effect than one type of drug alone.

Aspirin—Aspirin is the most important antiplatelet drug in the treatment of CAD and reduces mortality in ACS. It irreversibly inhibits the enzyme cyclooxygenase (COX) which is involved in the synthesis of the potent platelet activator thromboxane A_2 from arachidonic acid. Inhibiting COX also blocks the synthesis of PGI_2, an inhibitor of platelet function. However, endothelial cells produce PGI_2, and are able to produce more COX enzyme (which platelets are unable to do as they have no nucleus). This leads to the balance shifting towards production of the anti-platelet PGI_2. In ACS, 300 mg aspirin should be given initially, and 75 mg daily thereafter. Side effects are relatively few and include an increased risk of bleeding due to inhibited platelet function and gastric irritation leading to stomach ulcers.

$P2Y_{12}$ antagonists—Clopidogrel is a thienopyridine derivative which blocks the $P2Y_{12}$ component of the adenosine diphosphate (ADP) receptor on platelet cell membranes. The blockade of this receptor prevents fibrinogen binding to the platelet and inhibits platelet aggregation. This is irreversibly modified by clopidogrel and prasugrel, and reversibly modified by ticagrelor. Clopidogrel has been the standard addition to aspirin for years for all ACS patients (300 mg loading dose, then 75 mg daily); however, newer agents have been developed. Ticagrelor (180 mg loading dose, then 90 mg twice daily) is now recommended as an initial treatment with aspirin in all guidelines (e.g., SIGN 2016), and prasugrel may be considered as an alternative in some high-risk groups.

GPIIb/IIIa inhibitors—The glycoprotein IIb/IIIa platelet receptor on activated platelet membranes binds fibrinogen, von Willebrand factor and other adhesive molecules. GPIIb/IIIa inhibitors inhibit this binding and thereby inhibit platelet aggregation and thrombus formation. Examples include tirofiban, abciximab and eptifibatide. These drugs are only used in ACS for high-risk patients and those undergoing urgent PCI.

Anticoagulant agents—All patients with unstable angina or NSTEMI should receive a pentasaccharide (fondaparinux), low molecular weight heparin, or, if renal function does not allow these, unfractionated heparin.

Immediate antianginal therapy

Nitrates—Nitrates are a useful early ACS treatment, they decrease cardiac workload (through venodilatation and peripheral artery vasodilatation) as well as directly causing coronary artery vasodilatation. In ongoing ischaemia, IV nitrate infusions can be a helpful bridge to coronary angiography. Remember that as they can reduce blood pressure, hypotension is a contraindication and close monitoring should be provided.

β-Blockers—Administration of β-blockers decreases heart rate and myocardial work. They have been demonstrated to be beneficial in patients following ACS and should be continued long term. Commencement is contraindicated if the patient has acute heart failure, bradycardia or hypotension. Avoid if the patient has asthma.

Calcium channel blockers—These decrease myocardial work and dihydropyridines can be added to a β-blocker if chest pain is ongoing. If β-blockers are not tolerated, verapamil or diltiazem would be a better choice as they do not cause rebound tachycardia and reduce the heart rate.

Urgent reperfusion therapies

Urgent restoration of coronary blood flow (reperfusion) prevents further LV damage and improves prognosis in STEMI. The amount of myocardium that can be salvaged falls exponentially with time, the greatest benefit being within 3 hours of symptom onset, and modest benefit beyond 12 hours.

Primary PCI

Primary PCI describes the situation when PCI is the initial definitive therapy to relieve the blockage and allow reperfusion of the myocardium, and thrombolytic agents have not been administered. There is no benefit from primary PCI for NSTEMI. For STEMI, immediate angioplasty with stenting leads to better outcomes than thrombolysis, and it should be considered if within 12 hours of chest pain onset and it can be delivered within 2 hours of possible thrombolytic therapy. When thrombolysis has been unsuccessful and PCI is performed, this is called rescue PCI.

Thrombolytic therapy

Thrombolytic (fibrinolytic) therapy is used to break down the thrombi that cause MI and allow reperfusion of the affected area. These agents achieve this by converting plasminogen to the fibrinolytic enzyme plasmin, which breaks down the fibrin mesh that binds a thrombus together (fibrinolysis). They are only used in STEMI within 12 hours of onset, when primary PCI is not available within 2 hours and must be administered by a senior doctor after careful assessment for the presence of contraindications. The administration of thrombolytic agents (except streptokinase) should be followed by an infusion of heparin for 48 hours to prevent recurrent thrombus formation and ischaemic events.

Thrombolytic agents include:

1. Tissue plasminogen activators (tPA), e.g., alteplase, tenecteplase, reteplase: these are the primary agents of choice for thrombolysis.
2. Streptokinase: rarely used in clinical practice now. Streptokinase cannot be used repeatedly as antibodies are generated which may induce anaphylaxis on subsequent exposure.

Important contraindications to thrombolysis (discuss each case with a senior clinician):

1. Previous intracranial haemorrhage or stroke of unknown origin at any time.
2. Recent ischaemic stroke (within 6 months).
3. Central nervous system damage/tumour/AV malformation.
4. Recent head injury/major trauma/surgery/bleeding.
5. Known bleeding disorder.
6. Suspected aortic dissection.

7. Non-compressible punctures in the last 24 hours.
8. Relative contraindications include prolonged or traumatic resuscitation, pregnancy and refractory hypertension.

Non-acute management

Complications after MI

After the patient is admitted, daily history, examination and observations aim to identify the development of complications. Cardiogenic shock would indicate a severe complication, such as myocardial rupture, unstable arrhythmia or significant heart failure. Patients with recurrent angina after ACS are high-risk, and timely angiography should be considered. Symptoms or signs of heart failure are treated, and any deterioration should prompt reconsideration of the cause and a search for new complications.

Sudden death (within 6 hours of symptom onset) occurs in 25% of patients following STEMI, usually as a result of arrhythmia. Therefore a cardiac monitor is applied to all patients initially, and continued until the patient is deemed stable. In those who survive this initial period, MI can lead to a number of acute and chronic complications, detailed in Table 13.2. The major ones include:

1. Heart failure: infarcted myocardium is unable to contract effectively.

Table 13.2 Complications of an acute myocardial infarction

Time frame	Complication
Early (0–48 hours)	Arrhythmias – VT, VF, SVT, heart block Cardiogenic shock due to left or right ventricular failure
Medium term (2–7 days)	Arrhythmias – VT, VF, SVT, heart block Pulmonary embolus (4–7 days) Rupture of papillary muscle (3–5 days) Rupture of interventricular septum (3–5 days) Free wall rupture (3–5 days) *Note:* Rupture of the above structures usually presents with acute cardiac failure and progresses rapidly to death; some patients may survive after surgery
Late (weeks to months)	Arrhythmias – VT, VF, SVT, heart block Cardiac failure Dressler syndrome (3–8 weeks) Left ventricular aneurysm (after several weeks to months) Mural thrombosis and systemic embolization

SVT, supraventricular tachycardia; VF, ventricular fibrillation; VT, ventricular tachycardia.

2. Arrhythmia: this can be any arrhythmia, although ventricular fibrillation (VF) is likely the cause in many patients who die suddenly following STEMI.
3. Myocardial rupture: this can be either the free wall of a ventricle or the interventricular septum and can be rapidly fatal without emergency surgical intervention.
4. Mitral regurgitation: owing to infarction and subsequent rupture of the papillary muscles.
5. Pericarditis: this can occur a few days after infarction (peri-infarction), and weeks to months later as an immunological phenomenon called Dressler syndrome.

Heart Block after MI—Ischaemic injury can occur at any point in the conducting system – the SA node, the AV node or anywhere from the bundle of His downwards.

AV block is commonly associated with inferior MI. This is due to ischaemia of the AV node, and usually recovers with reperfusion. However, if there is high degree AV block with clinical compromise, temporary pacing may be required.

Anterior MI may cause heart block if there is marked septal necrosis (indicating a large anterior MI), and will usually require a permanent pacemaker (see Chapter 15).

Cardiogenic Shock after Myocardial Infarction—Patients with cardiogenic shock due to a reversible cause such as MI may be treated with an intraaortic balloon pump. This is an infrequent bridging measure. The balloon sits in the descending aorta and, using the ECG for timing, inflates during diastole. This forces blood back to the coronary arteries and forward to the renal arteries, increasing perfusion of the heart and kidneys. The benefit of this treatment is unclear and the priority is usually to perform an angiogram and revascularize the patient as soon as possible.

Secondary prevention

- Antiplatelet therapies are continued. Usually this is lifelong aspirin, and in patients who have had a drug-eluting stent, generally a $P2Y_{12}$ antagonist for between 3 months and 1 year.
- High potency statin (regardless of measured cholesterol), as statins give benefit to MI regardless of cholesterol level.
- Long-term β-blockers potentially reduce recurrent infarction and may improve mortality, especially if there is significant LV dysfunction.
- ACE inhibitors confer greatest benefit in those with LV dysfunction, but can have an effect on ventricular remodelling, prevent heart failure and improve mortality. Additional benefit may be gained from aldosterone antagonists (e.g., spironolactone, eplerenone) if there is reduced ejection fraction after an MI.

Further management

Implantable cardioverter defibrillators are beneficial in patients with severely reduced ejection fraction after MI.

Early mobilization (after 48 h) is instituted to prevent venous stasis.

Follow-up care with a cardiologist is provided, and access to cardiac rehabilitation. This consists of:

1. Smoking cessation. This reduces the rate of recurrent MI by two-thirds to three-quarters. It is the single most important intervention (including medication) in reducing risk of recurrent MI. Where necessary, psychological and pharmaceutical support should be provided to improve rates of smoking cessation.
2. Dietary advice, particularly emphasizing the value of fish and olive oil, and fresh fruit and vegetables. Carbohydrate restriction for non–insulin-dependent diabetes mellitus and insulin resistance. Calorie restriction for patients who have diabetes mellitus or who are obese.
3. Advice on medications, their role in improving prognosis, and the importance of compliance.
4. Progressively increasing exercise level to incorporate rapid walking on a daily basis if possible. Group gym sessions may help some patients by encouraging exercise and giving psychological support to each other.
5. Advice from a clinical psychologist on how to cope with the illness.
6. A subsequent support group may be continued as long as each individual patient finds it helpful.

DVLA guidelines state that Group 1 drivers (most drivers) cannot drive for at least 1 week if they have been successfully treated with angioplasty, or 4 weeks if not (as long as ejection fraction is >40%). Group 2 drivers (large goods vehicles or passenger-carrying vehicles) cannot drive for 6 weeks and will require assessment before relicensing, and cannot renew a group 2 license if ejection fraction is <40%.

Chapter Summary

- Stable angina occurs due to myocardial demand exceeding supply as a result of a fixed stenosis. There are many possible exacerbating factors.
- If the diagnosis is in doubt, the choice of investigation depends on the likelihood of CAD and the patient's symptoms and co-morbidities.
- If two antianginal drugs have not sufficiently controlled symptoms of stable angina, consider revascularisation.
- Acute coronary syndrome is a medical emergency.
- Urgent ECG is essential to identify STEMI early, and troponin should be sent quickly as the result will take time to return.
- Manage ACS with an A–E approach and remember to apply the cardiac monitor early as many deaths occur due to early arrhythmia.
- STEMI is treated with emergency primary PCI if possible, or thrombolysis if the patient cannot be transferred to a PCI centre within 2 hours of the possibility of thrombolysis.
- In ACS, give antiplatelets as soon as possible to reduce mortality rates.

Heart failure (cardiac failure) is the clinical syndrome that arises when the heart is unable to maintain sufficient tissue perfusion to meet the metabolic demands of the body's tissues, despite normal filling pressures. Heart failure is a serious condition with a very poor prognosis: 20%–30% of patients will die within 1 year and 60% will be dead within 5 years. This is a worse prognosis than many cancers.

Heart failure can affect the left and right ventricles individually or both together. If left untreated, left-ventricular failure (LVF) will lead to right-ventricular failure (RVF) due to high right-ventricular pressure load.

PATHOPHYSIOLOGY OF HEART FAILURE

In the normal heart, during exercise and other stresses, there is an increased adrenergic stimulation of the myocardium and cardiac pacemaker tissue resulting in tachycardia and increased myocardial contractility.

Venoconstriction shifts blood to the central compartment resulting in an increased end-diastolic volume of the left ventricle, resulting in stretching of the myocytes. This stretch causes an increase in myocardial performance – as predicted by the Frank-Starling law (Fig. 14.1).

In most patients with heart failure, there is decreased stroke volume due to impairment of systolic function (contractility) of the left ventricle. The ejection fraction is usually reduced (<50%); this is sometimes called low-output heart failure or heart failure with reduced ejection fraction. In this situation, the reduction in myocardial contractility means the Starling curve is shifted downwards such that stroke volume is reduced for any given end-diastolic pressure (EDP).

Low output heart failure can also be caused by diastolic dysfunction in situations where ventricular filling is impaired. This limits the end-diastolic volume (EDV) and thus

Fig. 14.1 Relationship between end-diastolic volume and stroke volume in normal and failing myocardium (Frank-Starling relationship). In heart failure, reduced contractility reduces stroke volume for a given filling volume.

stroke volume and cardiac output. In diastolic dysfunction, ventricular compliance is usually decreased and the relationship between EDV and EDP becomes non-linear. As a result, the Starling curve is no longer valid. The relationship between EDV and stroke volume, however, is still valid. In this situation, EDV is reduced, restricting stroke volume, but the ejection fraction is preserved. This is sometimes referred to as heart failure with preserved ejection fraction. Simplistically, this is a situation where enough blood cannot get into the heart to be pumped around the body to maintain a satisfactory cardiac output.

Causes of heart failure

The most common cause of heart failure (in high-income countries) is systolic failure as the result of myocardial damage, due to:

- Ischaemic heart disease – an infarcted segment of ventricle is unable to contract effectively, decreasing systolic function; see Chapter 13.
- Myocarditis/cardiomyopathy – see Chapter 17.

Sometimes there is no initial abnormality of myocardial function, but cardiac failure occurs due to increased cardiac workload, as seen in:

- Hypertension – chronically increased afterload leads to compensatory left ventricular hypertrophy.

This increases myocardial oxygen demand and impairs diastolic filling due to decreased ventricular compliance.

- Valvular heart disease – can cause both pressure overload (aortic stenosis) and volume overload (aortic or mitral regurgitation) in the left ventricle, decreasing efficiency.
- 'High-output' cardiac failure – excessive demand on the heart; this may be either acute or chronic. Common causes include thyrotoxicosis, sepsis and chronic anaemia. Rarer causes include Paget disease of bone, arteriovenous malformations, high-flow arteriovenous dialysis fistulae, phaeochromocytoma and beriberi.

These processes most commonly affect the left ventricle (LV), but isolated failure of the right ventricle (RV) can occur in some circumstances. Remember that the most common cause of RVF is LVF. Causes of isolated RVF include:

- Right ventricular myocardial infarction (MI).
- Cor pulmonale: this is RVF due to disease of the pulmonary vasculature. It can be caused by recurrent pulmonary emboli, primary pulmonary hypertension or any respiratory disease in which there is persistent widespread hypoxic pulmonary vasoconstriction, such as chronic obstructive pulmonary disease (COPD). All of these conditions increase pulmonary vascular resistance causing pressure and volume overload of the right ventricle.

Decreased right ventricular output limits left ventricular preload and thus left ventricular stroke volume – this can bring about the same signs and symptoms as those that occur when the left ventricle is primarily affected.

HINTS AND TIPS

Remember, it is always necessary to identify the underlying pathology responsible for heart failure, so that a targeted treatment regimen can be employed.

Compensatory mechanisms

When stroke volume and cardiac output are reduced due to either systolic or diastolic dysfunction, there are a number of compensatory changes (Fig. 14.2) that occur to attempt to restore cardiac output and maintain tissue perfusion. These changes are successful initially. The decrease in stroke volume reduces arterial blood pressure, causing unloading of the arterial baroreceptors. This brings about a number of changes including:

- Increased sympathetic and decreased parasympathetic outflow to the heart, increasing heart rate and contractility (this process is limited in a diseased myocardium).
- Increased sympathetic outflow to peripheral vasculature causing vasoconstriction to increase total peripheral resistance (TPR), limiting venous pooling and increasing venous return.
- Decreased renal blood flow and increased sympathetic outflow to the kidneys increases release of renin. Renin-angiotensin-aldosterone system (RAAS) activation causes further peripheral vasoconstriction and promotes salt and water retention in the kidneys.
- Antidiuretic hormone (ADH) secretion is increased from the posterior pituitary, increasing renal water reabsorption.

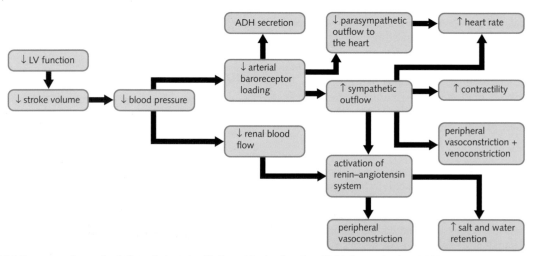

Fig. 14.2 Compensatory adaptations to impaired left ventricular function (*LV*, left ventricular; *ADH*, antidiuretic hormone).

These changes increase circulating volume and cardiac filling pressures, which increases stroke volume (by virtue of Starling's law), as well as increasing heart rate and TPR, which together maintain arterial blood pressure and tissue perfusion. In the early stages, these changes compensate for impaired cardiac function and the clinical features of heart failure may be minimal.

The vicious cycle of heart failure

As systolic dysfunction progresses and these compensatory mechanisms persist and intensify, they become maladaptive, accelerate disease progression and bring about the clinical syndrome of heart failure (Fig. 14.3):

- Persistent RAAS activation and ADH release causes further fluid retention. Initially in place to increase filling pressures to maximize stroke volume, filling pressures become excessive and stroke volume decreases due to excessive stretch of the myocytes. This moves the heart onto the downward part of the Starling curve.
- Increased filling pressures and ventricular pressures cause congestion in the pulmonary circulation and alveolar oedema (due to LV backpressure) and in the systemic veins causing peripheral oedema (due to RV backpressure).
- Excessive filling pressures cause dilatation of the ventricular walls. As the ventricles distend, the afterload increases. Dilatation can also cause disruption of the atrioventricular (mitral and tricuspid) valve annulus, leading to valvular regurgitation.
- The persistent tachycardia reduces the duration of diastole and thus the duration of coronary blood flow. With the increase in contractility, myocardial oxygen demand is increased while oxygen delivery is reduced. These two factors combined may cause myocardial ischaemia, further impairing function.

- Persistently high levels of angiotensin II, aldosterone and catecholamines leads to left ventricular remodelling, with changes in cardiac metabolism, myocardial thinning and fibrosis.

HINTS AND TIPS

A dilated heart is generally indicative of chronic rather than acute heart failure. The dilation does not have time to occur if failure is a purely acute process.

CLINICAL FEATURES

The symptoms and signs of cardiac failure vary depending upon a number of factors:

- Severity of heart failure.
- Which ventricle is involved (isolated right heart failure is less common and a pulmonary cause should be excluded).
- Age of the patient.

Regardless of the cause of heart failure, it is possible to predict the effects if the mechanics of pump failure are considered. The effects can be divided into forward and backward effects.

Forward effects

Forward effects refer to the failure of the pump to provide an adequate output. This applies to the left ventricle resulting in:

- Poor renal perfusion predisposing to prerenal failure.
- Poor perfusion of extremities resulting in cold extremities.

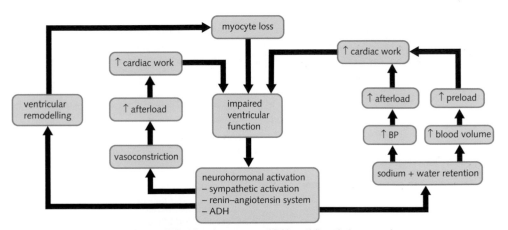

Fig. 14.3 The vicious cycle of heart failure (*BP*, blood pressure; *ADH*, antidiuretic hormone).

Table 14.1 Signs and symptoms of left and right ventricular failure and general signs and symptoms that might be seen in either. Often patients have a combination of left AND right ventricular impairment.

	Left ventricular (LV) failure	Right ventricular (RV) failure	General
Symptoms	• Dyspnoea due to pulmonary oedema. • Orthopnoea. • Paroxysmal nocturnal dyspnoea. • Wheeze (due to pulmonary oedema).	• Dyspnoea due to poor pulmonary perfusion. • Ankle swelling. • Anorexia, nausea, abdominal discomfort (due to hepatic congestion). • Nocturia.	• Fatigue. • Palpitations. • Exercise intolerance. • Dizziness.
Signs	• Bibasal pulmonary crackles. • Pleural effusions (usually bilateral but if unilateral, tend to be right sided). • Murmur of mitral regurgitation.	• Elevated jugular venous pressure. • Pitting bilateral peripheral oedema (ankle +/− sacral). • Hepatic enlargement and ascites. • Murmur of tricuspid regurgitation.	• Pale peripheries. • Tachycardia (either sinus tachycardia or arrhythmia). • Low-volume pulse. • Hypotension. • Additional heart sounds (S3 +/− S4). • Cachexia.

• Secondary changes in skeletal muscle structure leading to weakness and fatigue.

• Hypotension.

Forward failure of the right ventricle results in reduced pulmonary flow leading to dyspnoea and underfilling of the left ventricle resulting in hypotension and so on (as above).

Backward effects

Failure of the right and left ventricles results in congestion of the systemic and pulmonary venous systems, respectively, leading to systemic and pulmonary oedema. In the case of systemic oedema, this tends to be dependent (legs if walking, sacrum if bed-bound) but liver congestion and ascites may also occur.

HINTS AND TIPS

Although dividing heart failure into left ventricular failure and right ventricular failure seems complicated, it is worth taking the time to learn as it makes it much easier to work out logically the cause of a given set of signs and symptoms.

Symptoms and signs of heart failure

Many of the symptoms and signs of heart failure are due to reduced cardiac output, volume overload and increased venous pressures within the circulation. LVF will result in increased congestion into the pulmonary circulation and can cause further backpressure and congestion into the systemic venous circulation. RVF, on the other hand, does not cause pulmonary congestion, but does cause congestion of the systemic veins.

Because of this, right and left ventricular failure tend to present differently (Table 14.1). One or the other may be dominant and the clinical picture varies accordingly. Often there are signs of both.

The severity of the symptoms and functional capacity of patients are often described using the New York Heart Association (NYHA) classification (Table 14.2).

Dyspnoea may result from pulmonary oedema, impaired skeletal muscle function, depressed respiratory muscle function and reduced lung function. It can present in a number of ways:

• Exertional dyspnoea – as cardiac failure worsens, the level of exertion required to cause dyspnoea decreases until the patient is breathless at minimal exertion (e.g., when dressing or even when speaking).

• Orthopnoea – the increased central blood volume when the patient lies flat is often too much for the failing heart to pump, resulting in the development

Table 14.2 NYHA functional classification for heart failure.

NYHA Class	Features
Class I (mild)	No limitation of physical activity by symptoms
Class II (mild)	Symptoms with ordinary activity
Class III (moderate)	Symptoms with minimal activity
Class IV (severe)	Symptoms at rest

of pulmonary oedema. Patients who have severe LVF often sleep with several pillows to prop them up.

- Paroxysmal nocturnal dyspnoea (PND) – after being asleep for some time, the patient is awakened by severe breathlessness, which is relieved only after standing or sitting upright. It is thought that this is because of pulmonary oedema due to gradual resorption of interstitial fluid overnight and nocturnal depression of respiratory function.

Fatigue and weakness result from reduced perfusion of skeletal muscles, and nocturia is due to peripheral oedema being reabsorbed into the circulation when supine. This results in increased circulating volume, increased renal perfusion and thus increased urine output.

Cough may be:

- A nocturnal dry cough due to bronchial oedema or cardiac asthma (bronchospasm secondary to oedema).
- Productive of pink frothy sputum due to pulmonary oedema.
- Dry cough as a side effect of angiotensin-converting enzyme (ACE) inhibitor therapy.

Epigastric discomfort occurs in cases of hepatic congestion. Anorexia (due to oedema of the gut), ankle swelling (due to peripheral oedema) and shortness of breath (due to inadequate pulmonary perfusion) may occur in a patient who has predominantly right-sided heart failure.

See Fig. 14.4 and Chapter 7, for a summary of clinical examination in patients suspected of heart failure.

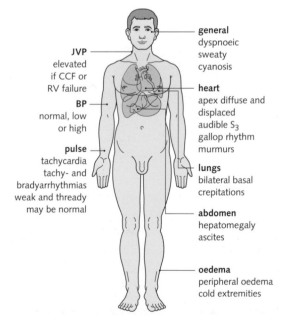

Fig. 14.4 Clinical findings in a patient who has heart failure. *BP*, Blood pressure; *CCF*, congestive cardiac failure; *JVP*, jugular venous pressure; *RV*, right ventricular.

> ### HINTS AND TIPS
>
> If a raised JVP is non-pulsatile, consider superior vena caval obstruction.

When examining the patient with heart failure, for the patient's comfort remember that:

- Dyspnoea secondary to pulmonary oedema is worse on lying flat and in severe cases the patient has to sit upright. In this situation, it may not be reasonable to ask the patient to sit at a 45-degree angle; therefore conduct the examination in the upright position.
- Take care when palpating the liver or attempting to elicit hepatojugular reflux because congestive cardiac failure can result in tender hepatomegaly.

INVESTIGATIONS

Blood tests

Electrolytes and renal function

Hypokalaemia and hyponatraemia are common findings in patients who are on diuretic therapy. There may also be renal impairment due to hypoperfusion or diuretic therapy. Hyponatraemia is common in heart failure and is due to high circulating ADH levels (dilutional hyponatraemia).

Hyperkalaemia may be seen in patients who are being treated with potassium-sparing diuretics (e.g., amiloride or spironolactone), angiotensin-converting enzyme (ACE) inhibitors (e.g., ramipril or lisinopril) or angiotensin II receptor blockers (ARBs), such as losartan or candesartan.

Full blood count

Severe anaemia may lead to heart failure. Conversely, chronic heart failure (irrespective of aetiology) frequently leads to mild anaemia. Leucocytosis may suggest infection, which may exacerbate failure.

Cardiac biomarkers in heart failure

Mild or moderate elevations in troponin are seen in patients with ongoing heart failure. It may be significantly raised if there is ongoing (or recent) ischaemia or infarction. A trend in troponin levels can be useful to assess for an acute event (in the context of history, ECG findings, etc.).

Serum natriuretic peptides may sometimes be measured. Brain natriuretic peptide (BNP) and N-terminal (NT) proBNP (a biologically inactive prohormone of BNP) are released into the bloodstream by the ventricular myocardium when excess stretch of cardiomyocytes occurs.

Levels of BNP are significantly raised in patients with heart failure and there is evidence to suggest the levels correlate with symptom severity (with a very high level indicative of poor prognosis).

BNP (and ANP) act to:

- Increase natriuresis – with loss of sodium, fluid is also lost. This helps to combat fluid overload, reducing cardiac preload.
- Vasodilate – this helps to lower TPR and therefore afterload.

The National Institute for Health and Care Excellence (NICE) guidelines on heart failure (released 2010) recommend that a BNP of less than 100 pg/mL (or NT-proBNP less than 300 pg/mL) should rule out heart failure in the acute setting. Patients with a suspected diagnosis of heart failure and a BNP of 100-400 pg/mL should be referred for specialist assessment and echocardiogram within 6 weeks. Very high levels of natriuretic peptides is correlated with poor prognosis and patients with a BNP of over 400 pg/mL (or NT-proBNP over 2000 pg/mL) should be referred for urgent assessment within 2 weeks.

The more recent European Society of Cardiology guidelines (2016) recommend that in the non-acute setting, a BNP of less than 35 pg/mL or an NT-proBNP of less than 125 pg/mL should rule out heart failure, with a threshold of a BNP of less than 100 pg/mL or NT-proBNP less than 300 pg/mL ruling out heart failure in the acute setting.

BNP and NT-proBNP have very high negative predictive values and are useful to rule-out heart failure (and identify those who do not require echocardiography and specialist assessment). However, they have poorer positive predictive values (false positives are common) and are therefore less useful in establishing a diagnosis of heart failure.

Other blood tests

A number of other blood tests may be of diagnostic use, including:

- Liver function tests – may be impaired as the result of liver congestion.
- Arterial blood gases – may show hypoxia, hypocapnoea and metabolic acidosis. Patients who are profoundly hypoxic might require artificial ventilation.
- Thyroid function tests – hypothyroidism and hyperthyroidism can both precipitate heart failure.

- Fasting lipids – may demonstrate hyperlipidaemia.
- Glucose – may diagnose co-existing diabetes or identify poor diabetic control.
- Iron studies – haemochromatosis may cause cardiomyopathy; also, iron deficiency is commonly seen in heart failure.

Electrocardiography

This may be normal or may show ischaemic or hypertensive changes. The presence of Q waves may indicate previous MI. Look for evidence of arrhythmias (such as atrial fibrillation) as these may precipitate heart failure. If arrhythmias are suspected, a 24-h ECG may be of diagnostic benefit.

Chest radiography

This may identify other causes of the patient's symptoms. Typical findings in the patient with heart failure (see Fig 14.5) include:

- Diffuse **A**lveolar oedema – classically in a bat's-wing distribution (bilateral and peri-hilar).
- Fluid in the fissures and Kerley **B** lines (interstitial oedema causing horizontal lines of fluid-filled interlobular septa at the peripheries of the lungs, usually at the bases).
- **C**ardiomegaly – seen as increased cardiothoracic ratio. This indicates ventricular hypertrophy/dilatation.
- Upper lobe venous **D**iversion (prominent veins in upper lobes).
- Pleural **E**ffusions.

These findings are easy to remember using an **ABCDE** mnemonic.

Fig. 14.5 Radiograph of the chest showing early pulmonary congestion. Note that the width of the heart shadow is greater than half the transthoracic diameter and that there are distended hila with increased lung markings. This is indicative of heart failure and pulmonary congestion. (Courtesy Newby DE, Grubb NR. *Cardiology: an illustrated colour text.* Edinburgh: Elsevier, 2005.)

Echocardiography

This is essential in heart failure; it is non-invasive and can be performed at the bedside if necessary. It can help to determine:

- Left and right ventricular dimensions and function.
- Regional wall motion abnormalities – usually indicating coronary artery disease (hypokinetic/akinetic areas may indicate ischaemia or infarction).
- Valvular structural/functional abnormalities.
- Pressure gradients across narrowed valves and estimation of pulmonary artery pressure.
- Intracardiac thrombus – may be the result of arrhythmia or previous infarction. Note transoesophageal echocardiography is more sensitive for this purpose.
- Intracardiac shunts (e.g., due to septal defect).

Cardiac catheterization

Cardiac catheterization may be of use if coronary artery disease is suspected as a cause of heart failure. Coronary revascularization (where necessary) *may* improve the pumping ability of the heart. This is generally not performed acutely unless there is objective evidence of acute ischaemia (e.g., ongoing ischaemic chest pain and new elevation in cardiac biomarkers).

Other investigations

A variety of other investigations may be of use, dependent on the clinical history and suspected aetiology of patient's presentation, including:

- Cardiac magnetic resonance imaging – can very accurately assess ventricular volume and function.

Useful for identifying myocardial scarring, infiltration and inflammation.

- Computed tomography (CT) angiography – may be useful if heart failure is precipitated by pulmonary embolus. CT coronary angiography may be used in an attempt to rule out significant coronary artery disease.
- Pulmonary function tests, urinalysis, etc. – to rule out other causes of patient's symptoms.

MANAGEMENT

Management of heart failure covers management of acute heart failure and chronic management of the patient with heart failure.

Acute left ventricular failure

Acute LVF and pulmonary oedema is very common and a medical emergency. Patients with acute LVF require rapid treatment and it is important to have good knowledge about the necessary treatments required (Table 14.3). Patients may be extremely unwell and it is therefore important to call for help at an early stage with these patients.

CLINICAL NOTE

If the patient presenting with acute heart failure is already taking β-blockers (e.g., bisoprolol), NICE recommends continuing this treatment unless the patient has a heart rate of <50 beats per minute, second or third degree atrioventricular block or shock.

Table 14.3 Algorithm for management of patient with acute left ventricular failure

Management	Notes
A. Sit the patient up.	Reduces venous return to the heart and therefore reduces accumulation of pulmonary oedema.
B. Administer high flow (15 L/min) oxygen via non-rebreathe mask.	Improvement of arterial oxygenation will reduce myocardial oxygen debt and hopefully improve myocardial function.
C. Establish peripheral intravenous access and administer IV furosemide (either as a bolus or infusion).	Furosemide acts as both a venodilator and a powerful diuretic. Its initial action as a venodilator reduces load on the heart, before diuresis occurs. Furosemide's diuretic action results in increased excretion of water and salt, reducing circulating volume. This allows resorption of fluid from the interstitial to intravascular space. Patients who are already on diuretic therapy will generally need a higher dose than that which they were prescribed pre-admission.
D. Closely monitor urine output.	Furosemide will cause diuresis and the patient will generally be unwell, making use of a bedpan difficult. A urinary catheter may be useful. It is crucial to accurately monitor fluid output to help identify oliguria and renal impairment early.
E. Consider additional treatments.	Various other treatments may be of benefit but these would generally require more intensive monitoring and potentially higher-level care (e.g., cardiac care unit, high dependency unit, intensive care unit). See below for more details.

Additional treatments

There are a number of other treatments for heart failure that may be considered in patients presenting with acute heart failure, dependent on the situation:

- Non-invasive ventilation (NIV)/continuous positive airways pressure (CPAP) –consider if the patient has severe dyspnoea and acidaemia, either at the acute presentation or as a later addition to other therapies if the patient fails to improve.
- Invasive ventilation – consider in patients who, despite other treatments, are heading towards (or develop) respiratory failure, reduced consciousness or physical exhaustion.
- Nitrate therapy – NICE recommends nitrates should not routinely be offered in acute heart failure (as they were sometimes used in the past). Intravenous nitrates may be used in certain circumstances, however, such as if there is co-existing evidence of myocardial ischaemia, severe hypertension or aortic/mitral valve regurgitation. Blood pressure should be closely monitored during nitrate infusion.
- Ultrafiltration (extracorporeal removal of fluid from the blood) – may sometimes be considered in patients with confirmed diuretic resistance.
- Inotropes or vasopressors – consider if there is acute heart failure with a potentially reversible cause of cardiogenic shock.
- Intraaortic balloon counterpulsation – especially where there is a reversible cause and cardiogenic shock.

COMMON PITFALLS

Opiates (e.g., morphine) are no longer routinely recommended to patients with acute left ventricular failure (as per NICE guidelines). There is limited evidence for benefit and some evidence of increased harm due to respiratory depression and the need for mechanical ventilation, intensive care unit admission, etc.

Acute right ventricular failure

Acute RVF is a relatively uncommon situation but may be the result of an inferior or posterior MI. If right ventricular systolic function is impaired, this results in low right ventricular stroke volume and therefore poor left ventricular filling and hypotension.

A patient who has an inferior MI and hypotension should be assessed carefully.

Hypotension after inferior MI may be secondary to the combination of RVF and relative underfilling of the right ventricle (due to nitrates, dehydration, diuretics, etc.). Provided that there is no evidence of pulmonary oedema (suggesting presence of significant left ventricular

impairment), treatment is with careful fluid challenges and central venous pressure monitoring.

Chronic management of heart failure

The general aims when treating heart failure include the following:

- Decrease preload.
- Decrease afterload by reducing both ventricular volume and blood pressure.
- Reverse or limit ventricular remodelling.
- Limit heart rate.

General measures

Patients with heart failure should restrict their intake of salt and, if they are volume overloaded, fluid restriction may also be useful. Alcohol should be avoided due to its toxic effects on the heart. Patients should also have other co-morbidities (such as hypertension, ischaemic heart disease, diabetes, etc.) effectively managed.

Pharmacological treatments

The main agents used in the treatment of heart cardiac failure are summarized in Table 14.4.

Angiotensin-converting enzyme (ACE) inhibitors

ACE inhibitors (e.g., enalapril, lisinopril and captopril) inhibit production of angiotensin II by ACE. Inhibition of Angiotensin II in heart failure limits the degree of ventricular remodelling, reduces the afterload on the heart

Table 14.4 The main pharmacological treatment options in patients with heart failure

First-line treatments	Second-line treatments	Third-line/ additional treatments
• Angiotensin-converting enzyme (ACE) inhibitors (e.g., ramipril, lisinopril). • β-Blockers (or β-adrenoreceptor antagonists) (e.g., bisoprolol, atenolol).	• Angiotensin II receptor antagonists (ARBs) if ACE inhibitor not tolerated (e.g., candesartan, valsartan). • Aldosterone antagonists (also known as mineralocorticoid receptor antagonists) (e.g., spironolactone, eplerenone).	• Digoxin. • Hydralazine and nitrates in combination (can be used as alternative first-line treatment in patients intolerant of ACE). • Ivabradine. • Sacubitril/ valsartan combination.

Diuretic therapy (e.g., furosemide, bumetanide) as required for symptomatic relief (does not give prognostic benefit).

(by removing its vasoconstrictor effect) and limits salt and water retention.

ACE inhibitors have been repeatedly demonstrated to improve survival and symptoms in heart failure. They should be offered to everyone with heart failure secondary to left ventricular systolic dysfunction whether symptomatic or not (unless not tolerated or if there is a specific contraindication). Patients taking ACE inhibitors should have regular checks of renal function and electrolytes as they may cause renal impairment and hyperkalaemia.

Around 10% of patients taking ACE inhibitors will experience a dry cough. This is caused by inhibition of the metabolism of bradykinin (another function of ACE). Cough usually appears in the first few weeks of treatment. In these cases, switch to an angiotensin II receptor blocker. Other common side effects include rashes, angioedema and loss of taste (or a metallic taste).

COMMUNICATION

A multidisciplinary team approach is the key to the modern management of patients with heart failure. Nurse specialists in heart failure can optimize drug therapy and give education and lifestyle advice, and work in conjunction with physiotherapists, dieticians, pharmacists and physicians.

Angiotensin II receptor blockers

ARBs, such as candesartan and valsartan, have the same benefits as ACE inhibitors in heart failure, but the main advantage is that these drugs do not prevent the breakdown of bradykinin, so cough does not occur as a side effect and angioedema is less common.

β-Blockers

The benefits of β-blockers in heart failure include reduction in heart rate, increasing coronary blood flow. They also decrease the metabolic demand of the myocardium. In combination with ACE inhibitors, β-blockers improve survival and reverse ventricular remodelling. β-Blockers should be offered to all patients with heart failure secondary to left ventricular systolic dysfunction (including the elderly, those with peripheral vascular disease, COPD without reversibility, etc.)

In some cases, the decreased contractility and heart rate may worsen symptoms, so they should be introduced at low doses and the dose increased slowly ('start low, go slow'). In the patient who presents with acute heart failure, β-blockers should not be started (or restarted) until their condition is stable – when they are no longer requiring intravenous diuretics, for instance.

Aldosterone antagonists

Aldosterone antagonists, such as spironolactone and eplerenone, act to reduce preload by blocking aldosterone receptors in the distal convoluted tubule of the nephron.

Aldosterone promotes sodium retention and potassium excretion; it also has a number of unfavourable extra-renal effects, including sympathetic stimulation, parasympathetic inhibition, vascular damage and impairment of arterial compliance, all of which adversely affect cardiac function. It promotes fibrosis and adverse remodelling of the heart.

Patients with severe heart failure receiving both ACE inhibitors and aldosterone antagonists have a 30% lower mortality rate than patients receiving ACE inhibitors plus a placebo. Aldosterone antagonists do, however, increase the risk of life-threatening hyperkalaemia, especially when used in combination with an ACE inhibitor, so electrolyte levels must be closely monitored.

HINTS AND TIPS

Other side effects of spironolactone include gynaecomastia and breast pain/tenderness. Eplerenone does not have the same effect.

Diuretics

Diuretics (Table 14.5) increase salt and water excretion in the kidneys. Loop diuretics, such as furosemide, are the class most widely used in heart failure to reduce circulating volume (and thus preload), reducing pulmonary congestion and peripheral oedema. Thiazide-like diuretics may also be added if loop diuretics alone are not effective in relieving symptoms. Unlike many of the other drugs used in heart failure, diuretics do not improve survival; they do, however, provide effective symptomatic relief. The exception to this statement is aldosterone antagonists, which have diuretic function but do improve prognosis.

COMMUNICATION

Communication and patient education is especially important in heart failure. The patient should be advised to monitor for acute weight changes (which may be indicative of fluid retention/loss) and advised what to do if this changes or if they deteriorate clinically. They should be aware what to do if they develop a concurrent illness (sick day rules), as ongoing treatment with certain drugs (e.g., furosemide, spironolactone and ACE inhibitors) in this setting may result in acute kidney injury and electrolyte abnormalities.

Nitrates

Glyceryl trinitrate (GTN) increases levels of cyclic guanosine monophosphate (cGMP), which acts to relax vascular

Table 14.5 Site of action (in the nephron) and adverse effects associated with commonly used diuretics

Class of diuretic	Site of action	Adverse effects
Loop diuretics (e.g., furosemide, bumetanide).	Thick ascending loop of Henle.	Electrolyte abnormalities (e.g., hypokalaemia), exacerbating of gout.
Thiazide diuretics (e.g., bendroflumethiazide, metolazone).	Distal convoluted tubule.	Hyperglycaemia, gout, electrolyte abnormalities (e.g., hypokalaemia, hyponatraemia), elevated triglycerides/low-density lipoproteins (LDL).
Potassium-sparing diuretics (e.g., spironolactone, amiloride).	Collecting duct and distal convoluted tubule.	Hyperkalaemia (use with caution with angiotensin-converting enzyme inhibitors), gynaecomastia with spironolactone.

ACE, angiotensin converting enzyme.

smooth muscle. It preferentially dilates venous vessels, thereby decreasing preload and reducing the degree of ventricular volume overload. Nitrate use in heart failure is somewhat limited to the acute setting because tolerance to its effects develops over 1 or 2 days. However, asymmetric regular dosing can be used in combination with hydralazine.

Hydralazine

Hydralazine is a potent vasodilator, predominantly of arterioles; therefore it reduces afterload, which acts to improve cardiac function. Side effects include flushing and a lupus-like syndrome. It is prescribed in combination with a nitrate medication in patients who cannot tolerate an ACE inhibitor or ARB (particularly if these medications induce renal failure), and also sometimes as an additional therapy in severe heart failure, especially where there is pulmonary hypertension.

Digoxin

Digoxin is an inhibitor of the sodium/potassium pump on the sarcolemmal and cell membranes. This adenosine triphosphate (ATP)-dependent pump plays a role in transporting calcium out of the cell. Its inhibition, therefore prevents this, resulting in increased intracellular calcium concentration, which in cardiac muscle, results in a positive inotropic effect. Digoxin also acts on the atrioventricular node to prolong the refractory period and decrease conduction velocity, thereby slowing conduction of the cardiac impulse and reducing ventricular rate – a negative chronotropic effect. The use of digoxin is recommended in patients with heart failure and atrial fibrillation to control the heart rate. It is also used in patients with heart failure (secondary to left ventricular systolic dysfunction) that is severe or worsening despite first- and second-line treatments (those mentioned previously).

Retrospective analysis showed that patients with low therapeutic digoxin levels saw a mortality benefit, whereas those with high levels saw an increase in sudden cardiac death; therefore digoxin therapy is probably best used with monitoring of drug levels.

CLINICAL NOTE

Inotropic drugs increase the contractility of the myocardium. Other than digoxin, their principal role should be restricted to the management of acute heart failure, as they are associated with increased mortality with long-term use.

Novel agents

There are a number of newer medications that are starting to be introduced in the treatment of heart failure including:

- Ivabradine – acts to reduce heart rate via inhibition of the I_f ('funny') channel. Ivabradine was initially used in the treatment of angina pectoris but has more recently entered guidelines for treatment of heart failure. The European Society of Cardiology (ESC) recommends ivabradine treatment in patients with heart failure if they have an ejection fraction of less than 35%, are in sinus rhythm at a rate of greater than 70 beats per minute and are already on treatment with a maximally tolerated dose of β-blocker, as well as an ACE inhibitor and an aldosterone antagonist.

- Sacubitril/valsartan in combination – an ARB (valsartan) in combination with sacubitril. Sacubitril acts to inhibit an enzyme called neprilysin or neutral endopeptidase; this enzyme is responsible for breakdown of several vasoactive peptides, including ATP, BNP and bradykinin. These peptides work to reduce blood volume by causing natriuresis and diuresis when the myocardium is under excessive stretch. Sacubitril therefore promotes the action of ANP and BNP and helps to reduce circulating volume. There is some recent evidence to suggest this combination may be more effective (in terms of reducing cardiovascular mortality and heart failure admissions) than an ACE inhibitor alone. However, there are concerns about long-term safety (and increased risk of symptomatic hypotension and angioedema). The ESC recommends this medication in a subset of patients as a third-line treatment; this should only be started under specialist advice.

Implantable devices

Roughly one-third of patients with heart failure have left bundle branch block. As the conduction system in these individuals is abnormal, the ventricles do not contract uniformly (there is some dyssynchrony in the ventricular contraction). In normal hearts, the effects of this are generally not noticed. However, in dilated, poorly functioning hearts it has a significant effect in reducing stroke volume and cardiac output and can lead to mitral regurgitation.

Cardiac resynchronization therapy (CRT), with a biventricular pacemaker to stimulate both the right and the left ventricle simultaneously, may be considered in certain patients. This increases cardiac output and is of benefit in patients with heart failure and broad QRS (>120 ms) complexes, in terms of significantly improving patients' quality of life, the amount of exercise they are able to perform and reducing both heart failure hospitalizations and mortality. Current NICE guidance recommends CRT in patients who are NYHA class III–IV with an ejection fraction of less than 35% and prolonged QRS duration in sinus rhythm. Some patients may also benefit from a CRT device with defibrillator function (known as a *CRT-D*) or an implantable cardioverter defibrillator (ICD), although indications are relatively complex (see **NICE guidance TA314** for further information).

Ventricular assist devices

Mechanical ventricular assist devices (VADs) are implantable devices that which take over the work of the failing ventricle(s). They are connected to an external control unit/battery. VADs can be used as a temporary solution until transplantation can be performed or in cases of cardiogenic shock that are expected to recover.

CLINICAL NOTE

Some VADs pump in a pulsatile manner (as per the natural action of the heart), whereas more recent VADs operate as continuous flow pumps. A patient with a left ventricular assist device that pumps continuously, will either have a very low intensity pulse or often no pulse at all!

Cardiac transplantation

Heart transplantation is the only definitive treatment for severe, intractable heart failure. The procedure requires lifelong immunosuppression, which puts patients at increased risk of infection. With good patient selection, the prognosis is good, with 1-year survival rates of 85%–90% and 3-year survival approaching 75%. The quality of life of the majority of patients is dramatically improved.

● Chapter Summary

- Heart failure arises when the heart is unable to maintain sufficient tissue perfusion to meet the metabolic demands of the body's tissues and is the end result of many different pathological processes.
- Heart failure occurs due to a number of adaptive changes that, as they persist and intensify, become maladaptive, accelerate disease progression and bring about the clinical syndrome of heart failure.
- The most common cause of heart failure in high-income countries is systolic failure as the result of myocardial damage, usually due to ischaemic heart disease.
- Myocardial failure can affect the left and right ventricles individually or both together. Isolated right ventricular failure is uncommon as the commonest cause of right ventricular failure is left ventricular failure.
- Left ventricular failure causes congestion into the pulmonary circulation and presenting complaints include dyspnoea (especially on exertion), orthopnoea and paroxysmal nocturnal dyspnoea.
- Right ventricular failure causes systemic venous congestion and presenting complaints include dyspnoea, ankle swelling, abdominal discomfort/lethargy and nausea.
- It is important to attempt to clarify the cause of heart failure to tailor management plans appropriately.

- Acute left ventricular failure causing pulmonary oedema is a medical emergency; treatment is with intravenous diuretics, oxygen and respiratory support as necessary. There are a number of other treatments that may be used in certain situations.
- Acute right ventricular failure is uncommon but is treated with careful fluid boluses (assuming no pulmonary oedema is present).
- The main aims in the management of chronic heart failure are to decrease preload, decrease afterload, reverse/limit ventricular remodelling and to limit heart rate – management includes optimization of comorbidities, pharmacological treatments and device therapy in certain situations.

Normal sinus rhythm is defined as a regular rhythm of normal heart rate (60–100 bpm) with every QRS complex being preceded by a P wave in a 1:1 ratio. PR interval remains constant.

Arrhythmia is a term used to describe an irregularity in the normal heartbeat or electrical conduction system of the heart. This includes:

- Bradyarrhythmias – slow heart rhythms.
- Irregular rhythms of normal rate.
- Supraventricular arrhythmias – fast heart rhythms of origin above the ventricles.
- Ventricular arrhythmias – fast heart rhythms of ventricular origin.

Cardiac arrest and resuscitation are also covered later in the chapter.

CLINICAL NOTE

Sinus arrhythmia is a normal physiological phenomenon seen in young healthy individuals where the beat-to beat heart rate varies during the respiratory cycle due to changes in vagal tone. Inspiration increases the heart rate and expiration slows it.

BRADYARRHYTHMIAS

Bradyarrhythmias are slow heart rhythms (Table 15.1). Many bradyarrhythmias are due to dysfunction in the electrical conduction pathways in the heart but bradycardia can occur in individuals without underlying heart disease.

Sinus bradycardia

Sinus bradycardia occurs when the heart is in sinus rhythm but the resting heart rate is less than 60 beats/min. This can be physiological (e.g., during sleep) and is also seen in young, fit individuals. Pathological causes include:

- Sinus node disease (especially in the elderly).
- Raised intracranial pressure (part of the 'Cushing reflex').
- Severe hypoxia.
- Hypothyroidism (myxoedema).
- Hypothermia.
- Tumours (cervical, mediastinal).
- Sepsis.
- Drugs (β-blockers, calcium channel blockers and other antiarrhythmic agents).

Patients are usually asymptomatic and no treatment is required. Occasionally, however, syncope, hypotension or dyspnoea may occur. In these circumstances, treatment

Table 15.1 Differential diagnosis of bradyarrhythmia, in order of increasing electrical dysfunction. Red denotes serious/life threatening arrhythmias that often require temporary or permanent pacemaker implantation.

Bradyarrhythmia	Features
Sinus bradycardia	Heart rate <60 beats/min.
Sinoatrial node disease and sick sinus syndrome	Bradycardia, may be associated with tachyarrhythmias and intermittently with tachy-brady syndrome.
First degree heart block	PR interval >0.20 s.
Second degree heart block- Mobitz type I	Wenckebach phenomenon - progressive prolongation of PR interval with eventual dropped beat. Generally benign and does not require intervention.
Second degree heart block- Mobitz type II	Intermittent dropped beats. No prolongation of, or unchanging, PR interval. Indicative of impending complete heart block and is an indication for permanent pacemaker implantation.
Second degree heart block - 2:1 heart block/3:1 heart block	Fixed ratio of P waves to QRS complexes e.g., 2:1, 3:1 – result of either Mobitz I or Mobitz II conduction (not always possible to differentiate for 2:1 block).
Complete heart block/Third degree heart block	Complete atrioventricular dissociation (no relationship between P waves and QRS complexes). QRS complex is often broad.
Asystole	No beats conducted, no atrial or ventricular activity.
Ventricular standstill/P wave asystole	Visible P waves but no QRS complex.

with intravenous (IV) atropine or isoprenaline, or insertion of a temporary pacing wire might be required to speed up the heart rate until the underlying condition is treated.

Sinus node disease

The sinoatrial (SA) node is the natural cardiac pacemaker. It is a crescent-shaped cluster of cells approximately 15 mm × 5 mm in size. The SA node is located just below the epicardial surface at the junction of the right atrium and the superior vena cava.

The rate at which the SA node generates impulses is determined by both vagal and sympathetic tone. The impulses are conducted via the atrial myocardium to the atrioventricular (AV) node.

Disease of the SA node may be due to:

- Age-related degeneration and fibrosis.
- Ischaemia and infarction (in 60% of patients, the SA node is supplied by the right coronary artery).
- Excessive vagal stimulation.
- Myocarditis.
- Genetic (rare).

This can result in pauses between consecutive P waves (>2 s). There are degrees of SA node conduction abnormality:

- Sinoatrial exit block – an expected P wave is absent, but the following one occurs at the expected time (i.e., the pauses are exact multiples of the basic P-P interval).
- Sinus pause or sinus arrest (Fig. 15.1) – interval between the P waves is longer than 2 s and is not a multiple of the basic P-P interval.

Tachy-brady syndrome (sick sinus syndrome)

This is a combination of sinus node disease and abnormal tachyarrhythmias. It is most commonly caused by degenerative fibrosis of the SA node in the elderly.

Management

Patients who have symptomatic or recurrent sinus pauses often require permanent pacing with a dual-chamber pacemaker (assuming rate-slowing drugs have been discontinued). Many patients with SA node disease also have more distal conduction disease, hence why dual- (rather than single-) chamber pacemakers are usually used.

Antiarrhythmic drugs may also be needed if the patient has sick sinus syndrome. Pacemaker insertion should be considered before commencing these drugs because they may make the SA node conduction defect worse. Paroxysmal atrial fibrillation (AF) often coexists and so such patients will often also need anticoagulation.

Atrioventricular block

The atrioventricular (AV) node is a complex structure that lies in the right atrial wall on the septal surface between the ostium of the coronary sinus and the septal leaflet of the tricuspid valve. In 90% of patients, the AV node is supplied by the right coronary artery. The rest are supplied via the circumflex artery.

The AV node acts so as to conduct impulses from the atria to the ventricular conductive tissue.

First-degree atrioventricular block

In this conduction disturbance (Fig 15.2), conduction time through the AV node is prolonged, but all impulses are conducted. The PR interval is longer than 0.20 s.

This condition does not require treatment in a healthy patient but should be watched because it can herald greater degrees of block (this occurs in approximately 40% of cases). This is particularly important in patients who have evidence of other conducting tissue disease, e.g., bundle branch block.

> **RED FLAG**
>
> Progressive prolongation of PR interval on serial ECGs in infective endocarditis carries a poor prognosis. This can occur secondary to the formation of a para-aortic abscess (the conducting tissue is in close proximity to the aortic valve ring) and this usually heralds rapid development of complete heart block and valve dehiscence.

Second-degree atrioventricular block

In this type of block some impulses are not conducted from the atria to the ventricles.

Figure 15.1 Sinus pause or arrest. Note the interval of more than 2 s between P waves.

First degree block (constantly prolonged PR interval)

Each QRS complex has a preceding P wave, but the PR interval is 0.36 s which is prolonged (normal is 0.12–0.20 s)

Second degree block (Mobitz type II) (PR interval constant, but some P waves have no QRS)

There is a constant, normal PR interval, but there are isolated P waves without following QRS complexes

Second degree block (Mobitz type I, Wenckebach) (PR interval increases with each beat and then results in an isolated P wave)

The PR interval progressively increases and then there is one isolated P wave without a following QRS complex; the PR interval then returns to its starting point and increases again

Third degree (complete) block (QRS complexes are independent of P waves)

There are 90 P waves/min. There is no relationship between P waves and QRS complexes

Figure 15.2 Classification of heart blocks. Note that only the large squares of the ECG are shown for clarity.

Mobitz type I heart block – Wenckebach phenomenon

Mobitz type I (also known as Wenckebach) AV block is characterized by progressive prolongation of the PR interval (see Fig. 15.2) – eventually resulting in a non-conducted P wave (dropped QRS complex). The cycle is then repeated.

This process is usually due to a reversible block in electrical conduction at the level of the AV node. Cells in the AV node become progressively fatigued until they fail to conduct an impulse.

This is a common phenomenon and can occur in any cardiac tissue, including the SA node.

Wenckebach phenomenon can occur in athletes and children and is due to high vagal tone. It is usually benign and not usually an indication for pacing.

When it occurs after an inferior myocardial infarction (MI), no treatment is required unless the patient is symptomatic. In symptomatic patients, atropine or temporary pacing may be used.

Mobitz type II heart block

In Mobitz type II AV block, the PR interval remains constant but P waves are dropped intermittently (see Fig. 15.2).

This occurs usually due to intermittent failure of the conduction system at the level of the AV node or His-Purkinje system and is often due to underlying structural damage.

It is a precursor to complete heart block and therefore requires close cardiac monitoring and insertion of a pacemaker.

Mobitz II heart block may be due to idiopathic fibrosis of the conducting system or certain inflammatory conditions but may also occur following anterior MI due to septal infarction and necrosis of the conducting system.

2:1 or 3:1 heart block

Fixed ratio heart blocks occur when the ratio of P waves to QRS complexes is fixed at 2:1 or 3:1, etc. This may be the result of either Mobitz I or Mobitz II conduction and it can often be difficult to determine the underlying pathophysiology from the ECG. There may be clues that can help, however. Often a rhythm strip or telemetry may be of use in determining the underlying disturbance as individuals with fixed ratio block may also demonstrate intermittent runs of more characteristic Mobitz I or Mobitz II conduction.

Third-degree or complete heart block

Third-degree heart block (also known as *complete heart block*) results in complete electrical dissociation of the atria from the ventricles (Fig. 15.2).

The P and QRS complexes are regular in rhythm but are completely independent and bear no temporal relationship to one another. There is a ventricular 'escape' rhythm, which usually gives rise to wide QRS complexes. Note that if the AV block is proximal ('high') the complexes may be narrow. This often occurs in congenital complete heart block.

Management depends upon the underlying cause:

- After an inferior MI, a temporary pacemaker should only be inserted in the event of haemodynamic compromise. Usually, the AV block is high (at the level of the AV node itself), temporary and the escape rate is reasonable. Most of these cases revert back to normal conduction within a few weeks and a permanent pacemaker (PPM) is rarely needed

- After an anterior MI, a PPM will be required and should be inserted promptly (unless the patient is unstable, in which case a temporary wire is inserted first, followed by a permanent system some days later). The AV block is lower, generally permanent, and the escape rate unsustainably low (the block occurs due to necrosis of the electrical conduction system).
- If the heart block is due to drugs (e.g., β-blockers) it may resolve once these are withdrawn.
- In all other patients with complete heart block, the patient should be permanently paced, whether symptomatic or not.

> **CLINICAL NOTE**
>
> Bradyarrhythmias do not usually compromise cardiac output if the rate is over 50/min and the ventricles have normal function.

Bundle branch block

Bundle branch block is an interventricular conduction disturbance. The bundle of His arises from the AV node and, at the level of the top of the muscular interventricular septum, it divides into the left and right bundle branches (Fig. 15.3), which supply the left and right ventricles, respectively. The left bundle divides again into anterior and posterior divisions (or hemifascicles).

Damage to one or more of these bundles due to ischaemia or infarction (or other conditions disturbing electrical conduction; see sinus node disease, earlier) results in a characteristic ECG picture as the ventricular depolarization pattern is altered. When conduction is blocked in one of the bundle branches, the affected areas of myocardium are stimulated later by conduction from unaffected areas of myocardium. This leads to widening and disruption of the QRS complexes (>0.12 s).

> **HINTS AND TIPS**
>
> Bundle branch block may progress to complete heart block; intermittent heart block should be suspected in patients who present with syncope and bundle branch block.

Looking at leads V1 and V6, in right bundle branch block there is:

- A second R wave (R′) in V1 and a deeper, wider S wave in V6.
- The last part of the QRS in lead V1 is positive. This is because of the delayed right ventricular depolarization.

In left bundle branch block:

- There is a Q wave with an S wave in V1.

Right bundle branch block

right bundle branch blocked here

depolarization of right ventricle delayed

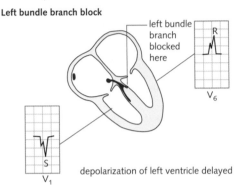

Left bundle branch block

left bundle branch blocked here

depolarization of left ventricle delayed

Figure 15.3 Left and right bundle branch blocks. Disruption of the conduction system delays activation of ventricular muscle producing a characteristic split peak in the ECG.

- There is a notched R wave in V6.
- The last part of the QRS in lead V1 is negative. This reflects the delayed depolarization of the left ventricle.

> **HINTS AND TIPS**
>
> To determine the type of bundle branch block, look at leads V1 and V6 and think of WiLLiaM MaRRoW. In LBBB, there is a W pattern in lead V1, and an M pattern in V6 (WiLLiaM). In RBBB, there is an M pattern in lead V1, and a W pattern in V6 (MaRRoW).

Asystole

This is a form of cardiac arrest with an absence of cardiac output and absence of ventricular depolarization. See the **Cardiac Arrest** section later in the chapter for more details.

Investigation of Bradyarrhythmias

Electrocardiography

This may show evidence of heart block. However, if the heart block is intermittent, the ECG may be normal.

In a patient who has unexplained syncope and an apparently normal 12-lead ECG, it is important to exclude intermittent conduction disturbances using ambulatory ECG monitoring.

Blood tests

Serum electrolytes, liver function and thyroid function tests may reveal causes of sinus bradycardia.

Chest radiography

This may reveal cardiomegaly in patients who have ischaemic cardiomyopathy or myocarditis. Pulmonary oedema may be a result of the bradycardia.

Echocardiography

This may reveal regional wall hypokinesia due to areas of ischaemia or infarction. This is especially relevant if it involves the septum.

Pacemakers

Indications for permanent pacing

A pacemaker is used to deliver electrical stimuli via leads in contact with the heart. The leads not only deliver energy, but are also able to sense spontaneous electrical activity from the heart. The aim of inserting a pacemaker is to mimic as closely as possible the normal electrical activity of the heart in a patient who has a potentially life-threatening conduction disturbance. The indications for a permanent pacemaker (PPM) are listed in Table 15.2.

Indications for temporary pacing

The following indications for temporary pacing are appropriate:

- All of those listed in Table 15.2 if there is no facility for permanent pacing immediately available.
- Symptomatic drug-induced bradyarrhythmias – a temporary wire is used until the effect of the drug has worn off, e.g., after a trial or overdose of a β-blocker.
- Heart block after inferior MI if there is haemodynamic compromise.

Table 15.2 Indications for a permanent pacemaker.

Complete atrioventricular block - should be paced whether symptomatic or not unless following inferior myocardial infarction (may recover).

Mobitz type II atrioventricular block.

Persistent atrioventricular block post anterior myocardial infarction.

Persistent atrioventricular block post inferior myocardial infarction after trial with temporary pacing wire (may recover).

Persisting symptomatic bradycardia or sinus node pauses.

Pacemaker insertion

Temporary pacing wires are inserted via a major vein (usually the right subclavian, right internal jugular or right femoral vein). The wire is advanced until it reaches the right ventricular apex and is then secured in place. The end of the wire is connected to an external pulse generator and this is then set appropriately to achieve adequate pacing.

PPM implantation is generally carried out under local anaesthetic and often conscious sedation. Insertion rarely requires general anaesthesia.

The pacemaker box is implanted in a pocket formed overlying the pectoral muscle, inferiorly to the clavicle, usually on the side of the non-dominant arm. The pacemaker lead(s) are inserted into a major vein (usually subclavian or cephalic) and advanced until secured in the appropriate region(s) of the heart muscle. The other end of the lead(s) are then attached to the pacemaker box.

Complications of pacemaker insertion

The following are recognized complications of pacemaker insertion:

- Complications of wire insertion including pneumothorax, haemorrhage, brachial plexus injury (during subclavian vein puncture), arrhythmia and infection (may progress to infective endocarditis).
- Complications of PPM box positioning (e.g., haematoma formation, infection and erosion of the box through the skin).
- Difficulties with the wire, such as wire displacement and loss of ability to pace or sense (need to reposition wire), fracture of the wire insulation (usually due to tight sutures or friction against the clavicle – need to replace wire) and perforation of the myocardium (uncommon unless after MI when the myocardium is friable – need to reposition wire).

Types of pacemaker

Pacemakers can be classified as:

- Single chamber – with a single wire into either the ventricles (most commonly) or atria (less common). A single ventricular lead might be used in AF for instance, when the atrium cannot be appropriately sensed.
- Dual chamber – with one wire into the atria and one wire into the ventricles. This more closely resembles the normal activities of the heart. The atrial contribution may be up to 25% of total cardiac output and therefore a dual chamber pacemaker should be fitted in patients in whom the atrium can be sensed and paced.
- Biventricular pacemakers – with leads into the right atrium, right ventricle and left ventricle. This is useful in the treatment of patients with heart failure and ventricular conduction abnormalities, such as left bundle branch block. This is also called *cardiac resynchronization therapy* as the pacing to the two ventricles helps to 'resynchronize' the ventricles and may improve efficiency of heart contraction.

Pacemaker syndrome

Permanent single-chamber right ventricular pacing in a patient who has intact atrial function can lead to atrial activation by retrograde conduction from the ventricle – so-called *pacemaker syndrome*. There is a cannon wave with every beat, pulmonary arterial pressure rises and cardiac output is impaired. This is managed by replacing the pacemaker with a dual-chamber device.

SUPRAVENTRICULAR TACHYARRHYTHMIAS

Supraventricular tachyarrhythmias (SVTs) are fast rhythms characterized by narrow QRS complexes (unless aberrant conduction is present). The arrhythmogenic focus is supraventricular. None of these are generally immediately life-threatening (except some situations of AF when an accessory pathway is present).

A tachycardia is defined as a rate of 100 beats/min or greater. In order of increasing atrial electrical dysfunction, these are:

- Sinus tachycardia.
- Atrial ectopics.
- Nodal ectopics.
- Atrial tachycardia.

- Junctional tachycardia and supraventricular re-entry tachycardia.
- Atrial flutter.
- Atrial fibrillation.

Sinus tachycardia

Sinus tachycardia (Fig. 15.4) is defined by:

- Heart rate of over 100 beats/min.
- Every QRS complex is preceded by a normal P wave.
- The PR interval is within normal limits and remains stable.

There are numerous physiological causes of sinus tachycardia, including:

- Fever.
- Thyrotoxicosis.
- Hypotension.
- Hypoxia.
- Any form of stress (e.g., pain, anxiety and exertion).

Occasionally, an inappropriate resting sinus tachycardia occurs. This is due to an abnormality of sinus node discharge or another atrial focus of activity located near the sinus node.

Premature atrial complexes

These are seen on the ECG as a premature P wave (may be normal or abnormal in appearance) followed by a PR interval, which may be prolonged or short, depending upon where in the atrium the impulse arises (Fig. 15.5). The QRS complex should be of normal morphology. This is often followed by a pause because the AV node is refractory and cannot conduct. In contrast to ventricular premature complexes, this pause is not fully compensatory (i.e., the next sinus beat occurs earlier than it otherwise would have done; after premature ventricular complexes the sinus beats continue on as normal).

Premature atrial complexes can be precipitated by many conditions including:

- Stress.
- Alcohol.
- Myocardial ischaemia.
- Myocardial inflammation.

Treatment is not indicated unless the patient is very symptomatic, in which case β-blockers may be of benefit.

Figure 15.4 Sinus tachycardia.

atrial ectopic

Figure 15.5 ECG illustrating an ectopic atrial beat. Note the abnormally shaped P wave and normal QRS complex. A compensatory pause follows.

Nodal and junctional ectopics

These abnormal beats arise from the AV node or the AV junctional area adjacent to it. These structures have the ability to fire autonomously but are usually suppressed as their rate of firing is slower than the SA node.

If impulses arise ectopically from these areas, the impulse is conducted to the atrium, producing a retrograde ('inverted') P wave, and also to the ventricles, where a narrow QRS complex is produced (Fig. 15.6). Depending on relative speeds of conduction, the P wave may occur before, after, or simultaneously with the QRS complex. As with atrial ectopics, treatment is not usually indicated.

Atrial tachycardia

Atrial tachycardia is a tachyarrhythmia generated in the atrial tissue. The atrial rate is usually 150–200 beats/min. Because the origin of the tachycardia is not the SA node, the P-wave morphology and axis may be different from normal (Fig. 15.7).

Causes of atrial tachycardia
The following may lead to atrial tachycardia:

- Structural heart abnormality.
- Coronary artery disease.
- Digitalis toxicity.

Investigation and diagnosis
On examination, the pulse is usually rapid and of variable intensity. The jugular venous pulse may reveal many a waves to each v wave if a degree of AV block is present.

ECG may show either 1:1 conduction or variable degrees of AV block. It is sometimes difficult to differentiate atrial tachycardia from atrial flutter. Diagnosis may be aided by enhancing

retrograde P

nodal ectopic

Figure 15.6 A nodal ectopic. The ectopic complex is similar to the normal QRS, suggesting it originates from the atrioventricular or junctional region. The P wave is retrograde and seen just after the ectopic QRS superimposed on the T wave. The ectopic beat is followed by a compensatory pause.

AV block and making the underlying atrial activity (P wave rate and morphology) easier to visualize. This may be done by:

- Valsalva manoeuvre or carotid sinus massage – increases vagal stimulation of the SA and AV node.
- Intravenous adenosine – results in transient complete AV block.

HINTS AND TIPS

Remember that atrial flutter usually has an atrial rate of 300 beats/min with a degree of AV block (e.g., 2:1, 3:1, etc.) and a 'saw-tooth' pattern. Atrial tachycardia has a slightly slower atrial rate with abnormal P waves.

Abnormal P wave superimposed on T wave

Figure 15.7 Atrial tachycardia.

Management

The underlying cause should be treated (for instance, check digoxin levels and stop the drug if appropriate).

Drugs used to treat atrial tachycardia include:

- AV blocking drugs, such as digoxin, β-blockers and calcium channel blockers (e.g., verapamil) – these slow the ventricular response rate, but do not affect the atrial tachycardia itself.
- Class IA (e.g., disopyramide), IC (e.g., flecainide) or III (e.g., amiodarone) drugs, which can be used to try to terminate the atrial tachycardia.

Electrical cardioversion is often successful.

Atrioventricular junctional tachycardia

This is a tachycardia arising from the junctional area occur when there is a focus of activity with a discharge rate faster than that of the SA node. This is abnormal and usually due to ischaemic heart disease or digitalis toxicity.

Clinical features

The following features are seen:

- Rate is usually up to 130 beats/min.
- Gradual onset.
- Terminates gradually.
- ECG shows a narrow complex tachycardia, occasionally with retrogradely conducted P waves. It is difficult to distinguish this from an AV nodal re-entry tachycardia (AVNRT).

Management

Treatment is aimed at the underlying cause:

- Antiarrhythmic agents such as digoxin, β-blockers and calcium channel antagonists may be tried.
- Electrical cardioversion may be successful.

Atrioventricular nodal re-entrant tachycardia

These tachycardias involve a re-entry circuit in or close to the AV node that allows impulses to travel round and round,

triggering the ventricles and the atria (in a retrograde manner) as they go.

Clinical features

These tachycardias display the following features:

- Rate is 150–260 beats/min.
- Usually sudden onset and offset.
- Narrow QRS complexes unless there is aberrant conduction. P waves are not always easy to see and may occur before, after, or within the QRS (Fig. 15.8).

Diagnosis

Differentiating a re-entrant tachycardia from atrial flutter or fibrillation can be difficult in some cases. The irregularly irregular rhythm of atrial fibrillation is often noticeable but this is not always the case with very fast heart rates. Diagnosis can be aided by

- Performing Valsalva manoeuvre or carotid sinus massage.
- Giving intravenous adenosine.

These procedures block the AV node and, therefore, may show underlying P waves of atrial flutter or the baseline fibrillation of AF. In re-entrant tachycardia, blocking the AV node breaks the re-entry circuit and terminates the tachycardia in most cases. Re-entry tachycardia can also be terminated by a ventricular ectopic beat.

Management

These tachycardias often terminate spontaneously.

Vagal manoeuvres, such as carotid sinus massage and the Valsalva manoeuvre, are often effective in terminating the tachycardia and patients can be taught to do these themselves.

In hospital the following treatments can be effective:

- Vagal manoeuvres.
- IV adenosine.
- AV node blocking agents (e.g., β-blockers, digoxin and calcium channel blockers).
- Direct current (DC) cardioversion if less invasive methods have been unsuccessful or if the patient is haemodynamically unstable.

In a patient with recurrent troublesome AVNRT, electrophysiological testing can locate the site of the abnormal

P wave occur after QRS complex

Figure 15.8 Atrioventricular nodal re-entry tachycardia.

circuit and this can then be ablated. This is a curative procedure. The main risk is AV node ablation resulting in complete heart block and requiring a PPM.

Wolff-Parkinson-White syndrome

In this condition, there is an abnormal connection between the atrium and the ventricle along which an impulse can travel. This is known as an accessory pathway. In Wolff–Parkinson–White syndrome the accessory pathway is known as the bundle of Kent.

The bundle of Kent

The bundle of Kent is capable of:

- Both anterograde (atria to ventricle) and retrograde (ventricle to atria) conduction.
- Conducting impulses faster than the normal His conductive tissue. If the impulse is conducted down the bundle of Kent, the ventricle is activated sooner than normal, resulting in a short PR interval. This may be referred to as 'pre-excitation'.

If, however, the impulse does not travel down the bundle of Kent, the P wave and QRS complex are normal. Therefore, it can be seen that the impulse can travel via two different routes from the atrium to the ventricle.

However, the impulse often travels both routes simultaneously; this results in a short PR interval and a slurred upstroke to the R wave (known as the delta wave of 'pre-excitation'; Fig. 15.9).

Tachycardias associated with Wolff–Parkinson–White syndrome

A number of different tachycardias may occur:

- AVNRT – the impulse is conducted from atrium to ventricle via the AV node and then back to the atrium via the accessory pathway, causing a narrow complex tachycardia.
- Similar tachycardia with conduction in opposite direction (i.e., atrium to ventricle via accessory pathway), resulting in a broad complex tachycardia due to ventricular depolarization initiating at a point away from the bundle of His.
- AF/atrial flutter – can present a risk as atrial impulses can be conducted very rapidly via the accessory pathway, giving ventricular rates of potentially 300 beats/min or greater (due to avoidance of the AV node, which usually limits conduction rate). This rapid ventricular rate can lead to ventricular fibrillation (VF).

Figure 15.9 Wolff–Parkinson–White syndrome. Note the short PR interval (0.08 s) and the slurred upstroke of the QRS complex (the delta wave). This is caused by part of the impulse travelling down the accessory pathway and causing pre-excitation (early excitation) of the ventricle (represented by the δ wave). The rest of the impulse travels via the atrioventricular node and is represented by the main QRS complex.

Clinical features

Wolff–Parkinson–White syndrome is a congenital condition. Patients present with recurrent palpitations or syncope. Sudden death is a risk due to ventricular tachyarrhythmias. The accessory pathway may cease to conduct as patients grow older, but other patients continue to have problems.

Management

Treatment of Wolff–Parkinson–White syndrome is indicated only in patients who have tachyarrhythmias. Some patients have ECG evidence of accessory pathways (short PR and delta waves), but no tachyarrhythmia, and these do not require treatment. There are a number of treatment options, including pharmacological treatments and ablation (use of radiofrequency energy to cauterize an area of myocardium).

Pharmacological treatments

The aim of drug therapy is to slow conduction in the accessory pathway as well as to slow AV nodal conduction. Drugs that do both are Vaughan Williams classification IA, IC, and III drugs.

Drugs such as digoxin and verapamil block the AV node, but do not affect the accessory pathway, so increasing the risk of rapid conduction of AF and flutter via the accessory pathway. This can sometimes result in loss of cardiac output and death.

Digoxin and verapamil **should not be used** as single agents in the treatment of tachycardias in Wolff–Parkinson–White syndrome.

Ablation therapy

This is the preferred (and hopefully curative) treatment used to abolish accessory pathways. It may be electrical or surgical:

- Electrical ablation (or radiofrequency catheter ablation) is performed after the accessory pathway has been located by electrophysiological testing.
- Surgical ablation – rare, but may be useful if electrical ablation is not successful.

Atrial flutter

Atrial flutter has the following characteristics:

- Atrial contraction rate is regular and is 250–350 beats/min (usually 300 beats/min).
- Ventricular response is rarely 1:1 (300 beats/min), but more commonly 2:1 (150 beats/min), 3:1 (100 beats/min), etc.
- Severity of the symptoms – this depends on the ventricular response rate (i.e., a rapid ventricular response is likely to cause palpitations, angina and cardiac failure).

Causes include:

- Structural heart disease (e.g., valve disease, cardiomyopathy).
- Pulmonary disease (e.g., pulmonary embolus, pneumothorax, infection).
- Toxins (including alcohol and caffeine).

Investigations and diagnosis

ECG (Fig. 15.10) may demonstrate:

- Regular 'saw-tooth' atrial flutter waves (P waves).
- Narrow QRS complexes (unless there is co-existing bundle branch block).

Figure 15.10 Atrial flutter. Note 'saw-tooth' P waves at a rate of just over 300 beats/min and the ventricular response of 4:1 (around 75 beats/min).

If diagnosis is unclear then AV nodal blocking manoeuvres (adenosine administration or vagal manoeuvres) may help to slow ventricular response and reveal underlying saw-tooth P waves.

Management

Cardioversion is the best treatment, but if not possible, then slowing of ventricular rate will provide symptomatic relief and protect against cardiac failure. Direct current cardioversion using a **synchronized** shock will rapidly and safely restore sinus rhythm in some cases.

Class IA, IC or III drugs may be useful for chemical cardioversion if DC cardioversion is unsuccessful or to maintain sinus rhythm after successful DC cardioversion.

Where cardioversion is not possible or not sustained, AV nodal blocking agents are used to slow the ventricular response rate (class II, class IV or digoxin). Note that some drugs (e.g., flecainide) may slow the flutter rate, leading to 1:1 conduction of flutter beats and a resultant *increase* in ventricular rate).

There is increased risk of thrombus formation in atrial flutter, as with AF, so anticoagulation is recommended before DC cardioversion.

If cardioversion is unsuccessful or flutter is recurrent, then ablation of the flutter circuit may be carried out. This is a relatively straightforward procedure and should be curative.

Atrial fibrillation

Atrial fibrillation is the most common sustained arrhythmia and has the following features:

- It is a common arrhythmia found in over 5% of the population over 70 years of age.
- Disorganized random electrical activity in the atria results in a lack of effective atrial contraction (and varying ventricular response).
- Stasis of blood in the atria predisposes to thrombus formation and embolic episodes.

The rhythm disturbance may be paroxysmal (transient), persistent (lasting longer than 1 week) or permanent.

Causes

Common causes include:

- Ischaemic heart disease.
- Valvular heart disease (especially mitral valve disease).
- Hypertensive heart disease.
- Pulmonary disease (e.g., embolus, infection, pneumothorax).
- Sepsis/underlying infection.
- Thyrotoxicosis.
- Alcohol excess.

Investigations and diagnosis

The ECG shows absent P waves and irregular baseline with a variable ventricular response rate (hence the irregularly irregular pulse; Fig. 15.11). Ventricular response ranges from 90 to 170 beats/min but can be faster or slower. The actual atrial rate may be from 300 to 600 beats/min. Absence of effective atrial contraction means there are no a waves in the jugular venous pressure waveform and there cannot be a fourth heart sound.

Figure 15.11 Atrial fibrillation. Note the irregular baseline and absent P waves. The rhythm is irregularly irregular.

Management

In AF, management generally involves either a rhythm control strategy (aiming to restore and maintain sinus rhythm) or rate control (controlling the ventricular response) alone (Table. 15.3). The likelihood of successful cardioversion depends upon:

- Persistence of underlying cause (e.g., a patient who has untreated mitral stenosis is unlikely to cardiovert successfully, whereas a patient who has AF secondary to sepsis and is successfully treated with antibiotics is).
- Duration of the AF (i.e., the longer the duration, the smaller the chance of cardioversion – this occurs due to atrial remodelling).

Treatment options are similar to those in atrial flutter:

- Rate control alone – usually with a β-blocker or a rate-slowing calcium channel antagonist, e.g., verapamil, or digoxin (especially in patients with heart failure).
- Synchronized DC cardioversion (often requiring higher energy than for atrial flutter) may cardiovert the patient into sinus rhythm.
- Pharmacological agents from group IC (e.g., flecainide, propafenone) (if there is no structural heart disease) or group III (e.g., amiodarone, sotalol) can be used to cardiovert or to maintain sinus rhythm after electrical cardioversion.
- Patients who have resistant AF may be treated with an AV node blocking agent to slow the electrical response (group II or IV drugs or digoxin).

Anticoagulation in atrial fibrillation

AF carries an increased risk of thromboembolism due to stasis of blood in the atria leading to thrombus formation and subsequent cerebrovascular/peripheral embolization. Benefits of anticoagulation must be balanced against the risk of haemorrhage. The CHA_2DS_2-VASc scoring system is often used to risk stratify patients' risk of stroke prior to treatment (Table 15.4).

Each additional point on the CHA_2DS_2-VASc scoring system confers additional increased risk of thrombo-

Table 15.4 The CHA_2DS_2-VASc scoring system for assessing risk of stroke in atrial fibrillation.

Congestive heart failure history	+1 point
Hypertension history	+1 point
Age ≥75	+2 points
Diabetes history	+1 point
Stroke/TIA/thromboembolism history	+2 points
Vascular disease history	+1 point
Age 65–74	+1 point
Sex **c**ategory (female)	+1 point

TIA, transient ischemic attack.

Table 15.5 Treatment recommendations for CHA_2DS_2-VASc scores.

Score	Risk	Recommendation
0 (male) or 1 (female)	Low	No anticoagulation therapy recommended.
1 (male)	Moderate	Oral anticoagulation should be considered.
2 or greater	High	Oral anticoagulation recommended.

embolic stroke. This scoring system supersedes the older $CHADS_2$ score.

Current guidelines recommend anticoagulant therapy in individuals with a CHA_2DS_2-VASc score of 2 or greater (Table 15.5). This means that females require a single additional point on the scoring system before anticoagulation would be recommended, whereas males would require 2 points for the same to apply.

However, in males with only a single risk factor for stroke (CHA_2DS_2-VASc score = 1), then anticoagulation should be *considered* but is not mandated. Oral anticoagulation has been shown in this instance to provide net benefit for prevention of stroke when compared to no anticoagulation therapy (or aspirin).

Anticoagulation in AF was traditionally with warfarin (a Vitamin K antagonist) but AF without co-existing valvular disease is increasingly treated with novel oral anticoagulants (NOACs). These medications are also sometimes called direct oral anticoagulants (DOACs) and include apixaban, rivaroxaban, dabigatran and edoxaban.

NOACs can provide adequate and predictable levels of anticoagulation easily without requirement for monitoring therapeutic levels. However, their main disadvantages are that they need to be taken consistently (half-life is shorter than with warfarin) and some NOACs have no reversal agent in the case of major bleeding (unlike warfarin).

Table 15.3 Factors to consider when deciding to treat atrial fibrillation (AF) with rhythm or rate control.

Rhythm control	Younger patients First episode of AF AF secondary to treatable cause Medications used tend to have more side effects
Rate control	Older patients Pre-existing coronary disease Contraindications to cardioversion Previous failed attempts to control rhythm

COMMON PITFALLS

Aspirin is no longer recommended for prevention of stroke in atrial fibrillation. Patients are either treated with oral anticoagulant therapy or not. Antiplatelet agents are not in current guidelines.

Sometimes the HAS-BLED scoring system may be used to quantify risk of major bleeding for patients on anticoagulation (Table 15.6).

Patients are considered high-risk for major bleeding if they score 3 points or more on the HAS-BLED scoring system. Please note that a high HAS-BLED score is not necessarily a reason to withhold anticoagulation, particularly as there is significant overlap between factors which increase bleeding risk, and those that increase stroke risk. In some patients, however, the risk of bleeding may be deemed greater than the benefits of anticoagulation.

Anticoagulation and cardioversion of atrial fibrillation

There is an increased risk of thromboembolism for a few weeks after cardioversion of AF to sinus rhythm. This is thought to be due to the formation of atrial thrombus before cardioversion and the persistence of inefficient contraction in certain parts of the atrium (e.g., left atrial appendage) for a few weeks after apparently successful cardioversion. Points to note are as follows:

Table 15.6 The HAS-BLED scoring system for assessing risk of major bleeding for patients on anticoagulation.

Hypertension: Uncontrolled; >160 mmHg systolic	+1 point
Abnormal renal function: Dialysis; transplant; Cr >200 μmol/L or >2.26 mg/dL *or* **A**bnormal liver function: Cirrhosis; bilirubin >2× normal; ALT/AST/Alk Phos >3× normal	+1 point
Stroke: Prior history of stroke	+1 point
Bleeding: Prior history of major bleeding or predisposition towards bleeding	+1 point
Labile INR: Unstable/high INRs; time in therapeutic range <60%	+1 point
Elderly: Age >65 years old	+1 point
Drug/ Alcohol usage history: ≥8 units/week *Or* **D**rugs predisposing to bleeding: Antiplatelet agents, NSAIDs	+1 point

Alk Phos, alkaline phosphatase; ALT, alanine aminotransferase; AST, aspartate aminotransferase; Cr, creatinine; INR, international normalized ratio; NSAID, nonsteroidal antiinflammatory drug.

- If the AF is of recent onset (within 48 h), it is reasonable to anticoagulate with IV heparin and cardiovert immediately.
- If the patient has a longer history, then full anticoagulation should be given (warfarin with an international normalized ratio (INR) 2–3 or NOAC treatment) for at least 4 weeks before cardioversion and continued for at least 6 months after cardioversion.
- In patients where emergency cardioversion is required (i.e., patients who have severe heart failure secondary to AF), cardioversion should be performed with heparin cover immediately.
- Transoesophageal echocardiography (TOE) is sometimes used to assess safety to proceed to cardioversion immediately in a patient who is not anticoagulated. However, TOE cannot completely exclude the presence of any thrombus and, as indicated earlier, thrombus can form after successful cardioversion.

HINTS AND TIPS

Supraventricular tachyarrhythmias may often be of concern to patients but are not generally life-threatening; the main risk is of stroke, and this is reduced effectively with the treatment strategies discussed. The only life-threatening supraventricular tachyarrhythmia is pre-excited AF in patients with an accessory pathway, as this may degenerate into ventricular fibrillation. These patients are usually treated as inpatients with radiofrequency ablation.

Investigation of supraventricular tachyarrhythmias

The following investigations are appropriate for patients presenting with an SVT.

Blood tests

Relevant blood tests include:

- Full blood count and inflammatory markers – anaemia may precipitate ischaemia. Certain arrhythmias (such as sinus tachycardia, AF) may be predisposed to by infection.
- Electrolytes – derangement of sodium, potassium or calcium may predispose to arrhythmia. Hypokalaemia predisposes to digoxin toxicity.
- Thyroid function tests – hyperthyroidism may lead to atrial tachyarrhythmias, whereas hypothyroidism

can predispose to bradyarrhythmia and sometimes ventricular tachyarrhythmias.

- Liver function tests – these tests, particularly γ-glutamyltransferase (GGT), may be abnormal in patients with a history of alcohol excess.

Electrocardiography

12-lead ECG may demonstrate:

- The arrhythmia itself.
- Ischaemic changes – usually as the result of (or contributed to by) increased cardiac oxygen demand as the result of tachycardia.
- Hypertensive changes.
- Evidence of pre-excitation (short PR interval, delta wave).

Measurement over a longer period (e.g., 24 hours, 48 hours, or longer) may be useful in demonstrating paroxysmal tachyarrhythmias.

Chest radiography

Notable features may include in some cases:

- Signs of heart failure – such as cardiomegaly or pulmonary oedema.
- Valve calcification.

Echocardiography

This may be useful because valve lesions and dilated cardiac chambers may be identified.

Electrophysiological studies

These studies involve inserting multiple electrodes into the heart via the great veins and positioning them at various intracardiac sites. Electrical activity can then be recorded from the atria, ventricles, bundle of His and so on to provide information on the type of conduction defect or rhythm disturbance.

These are useful for arrhythmias when it is difficult to identify the mechanism and also to help identify any possible focus or accessory pathway suitable for ablation. If the possible focus or an accessory pathway is identified, ablation can be attempted during the investigation.

Atrioventricular nodal blocking manoeuvres

These are used diagnostically and therapeutically:

- Diagnostically – they slow ventricular response and enable P wave morphology to be seen.
- Therapeutically – they are used to terminate arrhythmias with re-entry circuits involving the AV node. The following are appropriate:
- Valsalva manoeuvre – straining against a closed glottis.
- Carotid sinus massage.
- Adenosine administration (rapid IV injection).

Carotid sinus massage

This increases vagal tone and so prolongs AV node conduction time. The patient should be lying comfortably with the neck extended. Carotid bruits must be excluded (carotid artery massage may cause a stroke if thrombus or plaque is dislodged).

The patient should preferably be connected to a 12-lead ECG, running all leads simultaneously. The P waves might not be seen if only a few leads are running.

Initial gentle and then firm pressure is applied to the carotid pulse just below the angle of the jaw for a maximum of 5–10 s. Never do this on both sides simultaneously.

Adenosine administration

Again, the patient should be supine and connected to a 12-lead ECG continuous trace. Warn the patient that he or she may experience chest pain, flushing and dyspnoea for a few seconds after administration. Adenosine should not be administered to patients maintained on dipyridamole as it prolongs dipyridamole's action and causes prolonged complete heart block.

Establish intravenous (IV) access in a good-sized vein (antecubital fossa is ideal). Start with a 6 mg rapid IV injection; follow with a rapid normal saline flush of 20 mL. If there is no response, this may be followed by a 12 mg bolus, followed by another 12 mg bolus if necessary.

> **HINTS AND TIPS**
>
> Adenosine can precipitate bronchospasm and should be avoided in asthmatic patients. Verapamil can sometimes be used in cardioversion of asthmatics.

Adenosine activates potassium channels and hyperpolarizes the cell membrane. It causes a reduction in AV nodal conduction velocity and transient AV block as a result.

The half-life of adenosine is very short (6 s) and it can be safely used in broad complex tachycardia to differentiate ventricular tachycardia (VT) from SVT with aberrant conduction. After adenosine administration, flutter waves may be revealed or the SVT may be terminated. **Do not use verapamil for this purpose** as there is a risk of fatal myocardial depression in patients who have VT.

VENTRICULAR ARRHYTHMIAS

Ventricular arrhythmias are arrhythmias generally characterized by broad QRS complexes. The arrhythmogenic focus is within the ventricles.

Differential diagnoses of ventricular arrhythmia are:

- Ventricular ectopic beats.
- Ventricular tachycardia (VT).
- Polymorphic VT (e.g., torsades de pointes).
- Ventricular fibrillation (VF).

Except for ventricular ectopic beats, all of these may be life-threatening.

Ventricular ectopic beats

These are also known as premature ventricular complexes and have certain ECG characteristics (Fig. 15.12), including:

- They occur before the next normal beat would be due.
- They are not preceded by a P wave.
- The QRS complex is abnormal in shape and has a duration of greater than 120 ms.
- They are followed by a compensatory pause so that the RR interval between the normal beats immediately preceding and immediately following the ectopic beat is exactly twice the normal RR interval (in premature atrial complexes the RR interval is less than this).

Clinical features

It is thought that ventricular ectopics occur in over half the normal population. This prevalence increases with age. These extra beats do not in themselves imply underlying heart disease.

Most people are entirely asymptomatic; others may complain of missed or extra beats. Alternatively, others may experience thumping or heavy beats because the beat immediately following the ectopic does so after a compensatory pause during which there is a prolonged filling time, resulting in an increased stroke volume.

A number of precipitating causes are recognized, including:

- Hypokalaemia.
- Excess caffeine consumption.
- Fever.
- Underlying cardiac abnormality (e.g., myocardial ischaemia, cardiomyopathy, mitral or aortic valve disease).

Management

In a patient who has no underlying cardiac abnormality, no treatment is needed unless symptoms are severe. In this situation, a small dose of a β-blocker should suppress ectopic activity.

In the post-MI situation, there is controversy about whether ventricular ectopics are significant or need treatment. Treatment with antiarrhythmic agents increases mortality: in the CAST trial, encainide/flecainide increased the risk of death 3.6-fold. Check serum electrolytes (especially potassium and magnesium) and prescribe a β-blocker unless contraindicated.

Definition of ventricular tachyarrhythmias

A ventricular tachyarrhythmia is an abnormal rapid rhythm that originates in the ventricular myocardium or the His-Purkinje system. Ventricular tachyarrhythmias are broad complex – the QRS complex is greater than 120 ms in duration or three small squares on a standard ECG trace. Ventricular tachyarrhythmias include:

- Monomorphic VT.
- Polymorphic VT, including torsades de pointes.
- VF.

Ventricular tachycardia

VT is defined as three or more consecutive ventricular beats occurring at a rate greater than 120 beats/min (Fig. 15.13). Again, the complexes are abnormally wide; their duration is longer than 120 ms.

Clinical features

VT is often a life-threatening arrhythmia. The reduction in cardiac output caused by this arrhythmia often causes dizziness or syncope. Common precipitants include acute MI, cardiomyopathy or inherited conduction disorders. Very occasionally, patients may tolerate this rhythm well and experience only palpitations.

Figure 15.12 Ventricular ectopic beats, which are indicated by arrows.

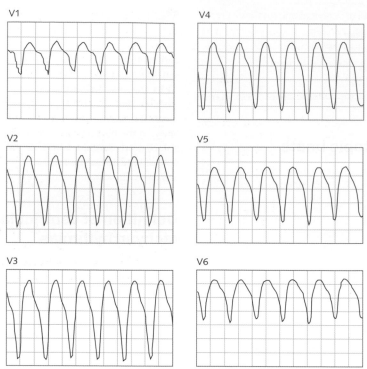

Figure 15.13 ECG illustrating ventricular tachycardia. Note the concordance shown in the chest leads. No fusion or capture beats are visible.

Table 15.7 Differences between ventricular tachycardia (VT) and supraventricular tachycardia (SVT) with bundle branch block (BBB).

Arrhythmia	VT	SVT with BBB
AV association	AV dissociation (no relationship between P waves and QRS)	P waves, if seen, are associated with the QRS
Variety of complexes	Capture beats (where a P wave is followed by a normal QRS); fusion beats (where a normal sinus beat occurs simultaneously with a ventricular beat, the resulting complex having an intermediate appearance that is a combination of the two component beats)	No capture or fusion beats
ECG pattern	May be RBBB or LBBB	Usually RBBB
Concordance	Present (the QRS complexes retain the same axis throughout the chest leads)	Absent (some QRS complexes will be positive, others will be negative)
QRS waveform	May vary from beat to beat	Constant

AV, atrioventricular; LBBB, left bundle branch block; RBBB, right bundle branch block.

Diagnosis

VT may be monomorphic (complexes on the surface ECG have the same shape) or polymorphic (beat-to-beat variations in morphology). The main differential diagnosis for VT is SVT with aberrant conduction (or bundle branch block) (Table 15.7). These arrhythmias can be difficult to differentiate. It helps if you remember the following points:

- VT is potentially fatal. If in doubt, treat as VT.

- Carotid sinus massage or adenosine may briefly block the AV node and, therefore, slow the ventricular response in SVT (it will have no effect on VT).
- **Never** use verapamil to slow the ventricular response in this situation: the negative inotropic and vasodilatory effect of this drug could have disastrous effects if the rhythm is, in fact, VT, causing rapid development of cardiogenic shock or cardiac failure.

Management

VT is very dangerous and if allowed to continue, will result in cardiac failure or death. Treatment must be prompt and depends upon the clinical scenario:

- A conscious patient with VT and no haemodynamic compromise – treatment should be with drugs (discussed later in the chapter).
- A conscious patient with both VT and haemodynamic compromise – triggered (synchronized) DC cardioversion under general anaesthetic (fast bleep the anaesthetist).
- An unconscious patient with ongoing VT and no cardiac output ('pulseless VT') – unsynchronized DC cardioversion (defibrillation) as per cardiac arrest protocol (discussed later in the chapter).

> **HINTS AND TIPS**
>
> Correct hypokalaemia promptly in all patients who have ventricular arrhythmias. Potassium can be given orally or in a dilute form via a peripheral vein. Potassium can be given more rapidly via a central line with careful monitoring of cardiac rhythm and serum potassium levels. Warning: intravenous potassium can cause ventricular fibrillation.

Polymorphic ventricular tachycardia – torsades de pointes

Polymorphic VT occurs if there are multiple ventricular arrhythmogenic foci present. This results in a broad complex tachycardia with QRS complexes varying in amplitude, axis and duration. Torsades de pointes (twisting of the points) is a specific form of polymorphic VT that occurs in the context of prolonged QT interval – the name refers to the fact that QRS complexes seem to 'twist' around the isoelectric line (Fig. 15.14).

> **HINTS AND TIPS**
>
> The QT interval corresponds to the time from depolarization to repolarization (beginning of the Q wave to end of T wave, i.e., action potential duration) and varies according to the heart rate. Therefore, a long QT interval is approximated by a corrected QT interval (QTc) of greater than 0.44s in men or 0.46s in women. QTc = QT/square root of RR interval.

Instead of correcting for heart rate, the QT interval can be plotted against heart rate on a QT nomogram (Fig. 15.15). The patient is considered to have a prolonged QT and be at risk of torsades de pointes if their QT interval–heart rate pair is plotted above the line.

Figure 15.14 Torsades de pointes. Note the irregular rhythm and twisting axis.

Figure 15.15 QT Interval Nomogram

Clinical features

The patient usually feels faint or loses consciousness as the result of a drop in cardiac output. Attacks may occur during periods of adrenergic stimulation (e.g., fear) or in some cases, in the context of bradycardia or during a compensatory pause following an ectopic beat. There are many possible causes, all of which act through a prolonged QT interval (Table 15.8).

Table 15.8 Causes of a long QT interval.

Cause	Examples
Congenital	Jervell and Lange-Nielsen syndrome (autosomal recessive, sensorineural deafness) Romano-Ward syndrome (autosomal dominant, no deafness)
Drugs (a long list!)	Class IA, IC, III antiarrhythmic agents (e.g., quinidine, flecainide, amiodarone), Tricyclic antidepressants (e.g., amitriptyline), Other antidepressants (including citalopram, venlafaxine), Antipsychotics (e.g., chlorpromazine, haloperidol, olanzapine), Antihistamines (e.g., loratadine, diphenhydramine) Macrolides (e.g., erythromycin, clarithromycin) Methadone
Electrolyte abnormalities	Hypokalaemia Hypomagnesaemia Hypocalcaemia
Others	Acute myocardial infarction Central nervous system disease Mitral valve prolapse Organophosphate pesticides

Management

Treatment of torsades de pointes differs from that of the other ventricular arrhythmias and is as follows:

- Identify and treat any precipitating factors (e.g., stop offending drugs, correct electrolyte imbalance).
- Treat with IV magnesium – this has been shown to be effective even in patients with normal serum magnesium levels.
- Atrial or ventricular pacing to maintain a heart rate of no less than 90 beats/min to prevent lengthening of the QT interval – IV isoprenaline may also be used to reduce the QT interval.
- In congenital long QT syndromes, high-dose β-blockers (β-adrenoceptor antagonists) or high left thoracic sympathectomy may be used. There is increasing use of PPMs in individuals who remain symptomatic despite maximally tolerated β-blocker dosage. ICDs are sometimes useful if episodes of torsades continue despite drug therapy.
- Torsades may degenerate into VF, which requires defibrillation. Avoid DC cardioversion in an otherwise stable patient as torsades de pointes is generally paroxysmal and often recurs following cardioversion.
- Do not use antiarrhythmic drugs.

Ventricular fibrillation

VF is irregular rapid ventricular depolarization (Fig. 15.16). There is no organized contraction of the ventricle; therefore the patient has no pulse. This arrhythmia rapidly causes loss of consciousness and cardiorespiratory arrest.

Clinical features

The most common cause of VF is acute MI. However, it is also being seen at the end-stage of many disease processes and signifies the presence of severe myocardial damage

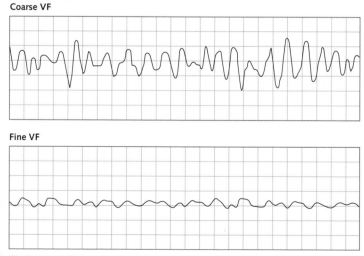

Coarse VF

Fine VF

Figure 15.16 Ventricular fibrillation (VF) can have a coarse or fine pattern.

(this is sometimes referred to as secondary VF and usually results in death despite resuscitation attempts). It may be precipitated by:

- VT, including torsades de pointes.
- Ventricular ectopic beats.
- Supraventricular arrhythmias.
- Using **unsynchronized** DC cardioversion during ventricular repolarization ('R on T' phenomenon), e.g., in an unstable patient with SVT (make sure cardioversion in these cases is **synchronized**).

Management

VF must be treated promptly with simple (non-synchronized) DC cardioversion (see the resuscitation protocol later in this chapter). It is vital to start effective chest compressions as soon as possible while the defibrillator is charging.

For secondary prevention, an ICD is indicated.

CLINICAL NOTE

Use of precordial thump is no longer recommended routinely as there is a very low success rate for cardioversion of a shockable rhythm. It should only be considered in monitored VF (or pulseless VT) arrest if used without delay while awaiting the arrival of a defibrillator.

Following defibrillation, management can be divided into pharmacological and non-pharmacological therapies. Pharmacological treatments are discussed later in this chapter (see **Antiarrhythmic drugs** sub-section).

Non-pharmacological treatments of ventricular tachyarrhythmias

Non-pharmacological treatments are used in patients who have recurrent VT or VF because:

- If successful, complete cure is achieved without the need for drugs.
- Localization of the arrhythmogenic focus is becoming possible in more cases due to increased understanding of the mechanisms of these arrhythmias.

Common methods of treatment involve electrophysiological studies and radiofrequency ablation or insertion of an ICD.

Electrophysiological studies

These studies are used mostly:

- To elucidate the mechanism of tachyarrhythmias.
- Diagnostically to evaluate the risk of sudden cardiac death in patients who have possible ventricular tachyarrhythmias.

- Diagnostically to determine conduction defects in patients who have recurrent syncope.
- Therapeutically to terminate a tachyarrhythmia by overdrive pacing or shock.
- Therapeutically to ablate potential source of recurrent tachyarrhythmia. This is intended to be a curative procedure, with the patient no longer needing antiarrhythmic agents. Note that even though these ventricular arrhythmias can sometimes be prevented, this does not in itself reduce the incidence of sudden death.

Patients who have survived a cardiac arrest will often be treated with an implantable cardioverter defibrillator (ICD) without an electrophysiological study beforehand.

Implantable cardioverter-defibrillators

ICDs are regularly used in the management of sustained or life-threatening ventricular arrhythmias. These devices are slightly larger than a PPM and are implanted in the same way. The device can sense VT and VF and can attempt to cardiovert the arrhythmia by pacing the ventricle or by delivering a DC shock.

Indications for use of ICDs are as detailed in Table 15.9.

Devices may also be recommended in patients with:

- Left ventricular systolic dysfunction with ejection fraction ≤35%.
- Co-existing broadening of the QRS interval or presence of left bundle branch block.

These patients may sometimes be treated with ICD, cardiac resynchronization therapy with pacing (CRT-P) or cardiac resynchronization therapy with defibrillator (CRT-D).

Table 15.9 Indications for implantable cardioverter-defibrillators.

Primary prevention	Secondary prevention
Familial cardiac condition with increased risk of sudden death – long QT syndrome, hypertrophic cardiomyopathy, Brugada syndrome or arrhythmogenic right ventricular dysplasia	Survivors of cardiac arrest caused by either ventricular tachycardia (VT) or ventricular fibrillation (VF)
Previous surgical repair of congenital heart disease	Spontaneous sustained VT causing significant haemodynamic compromise or syncope
	Sustained VT without syncope or cardiac arrest and left ventricular ejection fraction ≤35% but symptoms no worse than New York Heart Association class III.

The impact of an ICD on a patient's occupation and ability to drive needs to be made clear to the patient. Following ICD implantation:

- Patients are **permanently** barred from driving buses or lorries.
- If implanted due to an arrhythmia associated with incapacity, then the patient must not drive cars or motorcycles for 6 months. If not implanted for this reason, then the patient is barred for 1 month. The patient may then return to driving assuming there are no other contraindications.
- If the device delivers a shock, this has further implications upon driving cars and motorcycles. The period a patient must not drive for varies based on the context of the shock, whether there was any incapacity at the time and whether steps are taken to prevent recurrence.

- Class III – Potassium channel blockers (which inhibit repolarization, thereby prolonging the action potential and refractory period).
- Class IV – Calcium channel blockers.
- Other – Other or unknown mechanisms such as digoxin, adenosine and magnesium.

A summary of the electrophysiological actions of antiarrhythmic drugs is given in Table 15.10. The Vaughan Williams classification of antiarrhythmic drugs allows agents to be grouped according to mode of action on the myocardium and may make selection of appropriate agents for the treatment of any given arrhythmia more straightforward.

A summary of pharmacokinetics and side effects of the antiarrhythmic agents is shown in Table 15.11. These medications have a large number of interactions with other medications, particularly other antiarrhythmic agents. It is important to fully check the other medications a patient takes prior to administering an antiarrhythmic agent.

ANTIARRHYTHMIC DRUGS

Drugs used to treat tachyarrhythmias

The older Vaughan Williams classification is still sometimes used:

- Class I – Sodium channel blockers.
- Class II – β-Adrenoceptor antagonists.

HINTS AND TIPS

Antiarrhythmic agents can cause bradyarrhythmias as well as being arrhythmogenic. This can be serious and extreme caution with close monitoring is important when using antiarrhythmic agents and especially when used in combination.

Table 15.10 Electrophysiological actions of antiarrhythmic drugs.

Vaughan Williams Class	Examples	Site of Action	Sinus node rate	Atrial conduction rate	AV node refractory period	Ventricular contraction rate
IA	Quinidine, procainamide, disopyramide	Blocks fast sodium channels	No effect	Decreased	Increased	Decreased
IB	Lidocaine, mexiletine, tocainimide	Blocks fast sodium channels	No effect	No effect	Little effect	Decreased
IC	Flecainide, propafenone	Blocks fast sodium channels	Reduced	Decreased	Increased	Decreased
II	Bisoprolol, atenolol, metoprolol, sotalol	Blocks β--adrenergic receptors	Reduced	No effect	Increased	No effect
III	Amiodarone, sotalol, bretylium	Blocks potassium channels; mechanism not entirely understood	Reduced	Decreased	Increased	Decreased
IV	Verapamil, Diltiazem	Blocks slow calcium channels	Small reduction	Small reduction	Increased	No effect
Digoxin		Blocks Na$^+$/K$^+$ ATPase	No effect	Increased	Increased	Slows AV conduction
Adenosine		Slows conduction through the AV node	Reduced	Decreased	Increased	Temporarily pauses AV conduction

ATPase, adenosine triphosphatase; AV, atrioventricular.

Table 15.11 Pharmacokinetics and adverse effects of antiarrhythmic drugs.

Medication	Route of administration	Half-life	Mode of excretion	Adverse effects
Procainamide	Oral, IV or IM	3–5 h	Renal	Skin rashes, Raynaud's syndrome, hallucinations; toxicity – cardiac failure, long QT, ventricular tachyarrhythmias
Lidocaine	IV	1–2 h	Hepatic	Myocardial depression, cardiac failure, long QT; toxicity – dizziness, confusion, paraesthesia
Flecainide	Oral, IV	20 h	Renal (partly hepatic)	Myocardial depression, ventricular arrhythmias (a major problem, especially in patients with ischaemic heart disease)
Atenolol	Oral, IV	6–7 h	Renal	Myocardial depression, bronchospasm, peripheral vasoconstriction
Sotalol	Oral, IV	10–15 h	Renal	Myocardial depression, long QT, ventricular tachyarrhythmias
Amiodarone	Oral, IV	3–6 weeks	Hepatic	Pulmonary fibrosis, liver damage, peripheral neuropathy, hyper- or hypothyroidism, corneal microdeposits, photosensitivity, myocardial depression (but safe in cardiac failure), long QT.
Verapamil	Oral, IV	3–7 h	Renal	Myocardial depression, constipation
Digoxin	Oral, IV	36–48 h	Renal	Toxicity – heart block, atrial tachycardia, ventricular arrhythmia, xanthopsia
Adenosine	IV	<10 s	Rapidly broken down by enzymes in the circulatory system	Lightheadedness, sweating, nausea, 'sense of impending doom', metallic taste

Pharmacological treatments of supraventricular tachyarrhythmias

Class IA, IC and III drugs and adenosine affect conduction in the atrial and ventricular tissue; they are, therefore, useful for cardioverting many rhythms to sinus by breaking re-entry circuits or reducing the excitability of ectopic foci. Class III drugs have the added advantage of slowing atrioventricular conduction and, therefore, also slowing ventricular response.

Pharmacological treatments of ventricular tachyarrhythmias

In the acute situation, if the patient is unconscious or has no cardiac output, give prompt DC cardioversion (see **Cardiac arrest** section of this chapter).

In the acutely ill patient who has VT or VF, antiarrhythmic agents may be given after sinus rhythm has been established by DC cardioversion in an effort to stabilize the myocardium. Medications used to treat ventricular tachyarrhythmias other than torsades de pointes are mainly either class II or class III.

Amiodarone or β-blockers are commonly used, but alternative agents include flecainide and lidocaine:

- Amiodarone is a good choice in cardiac failure because it has little negative inotropic effect. If given intravenously, after the initial bolus dose, amiodarone should ideally be given centrally because it is damaging to peripheral veins. Amiodarone has a very long half-life (25 days) and oral loading takes at least 1 month. IV loading is faster.
- If there is no contraindication for β-blockers, sotalol may be considered as it has none of the long-term side effects of amiodarone. It must be used in high doses to gain the class III effect, but should be uptitrated gradually, measuring the QT interval before each dose increase.
- Flecainide is effective but avoided in patients who have suspected ischaemic heart disease because this may increase its proarrhythmic effects.

Drug treatment alone for the secondary prevention of ventricular arrhythmia has been shown to be ineffective, although β-blockers should be used where possible in patients post-MI or with heart failure. Drugs are a useful adjunct to reduce the frequency of arrhythmic events in conjunction with ICD therapy.

ALGORITHMS FOR MANAGEMENT OF ARRHYTHMIAS

Perform a comprehensive A–E assessment on all patients presenting with arrhythmia.

Many patients with arrhythmias will be stable but if patients demonstrate any of the following 'adverse features,' then urgent action is required:

- Shock (usually defined as sBP <90 mmHg).
- Syncope.
- Myocardial ischaemia.
- Heart failure.

General bradycardia algorithm

See Fig. 15.17 for an algorithm for treatment of bradycardic patients.

General tachyarrhythmia algorithm

See Fig. 15.18 for an algorithm for management of tachyarrhythmic patients.

Figure 15.17 Adult bradycardia (with pulse) algorithm. AV, atrioventricular; BP, blood pressure. (From G2015_Adult_bradycardia RESUS COUNCIL.pdf. Adult Bradycardia Algorithm Resuscitation Council (UK) Guidelines 2015, https://www.resus.org.uk/resuscitation-guidelines/peri-arrest-arrhythmias/)

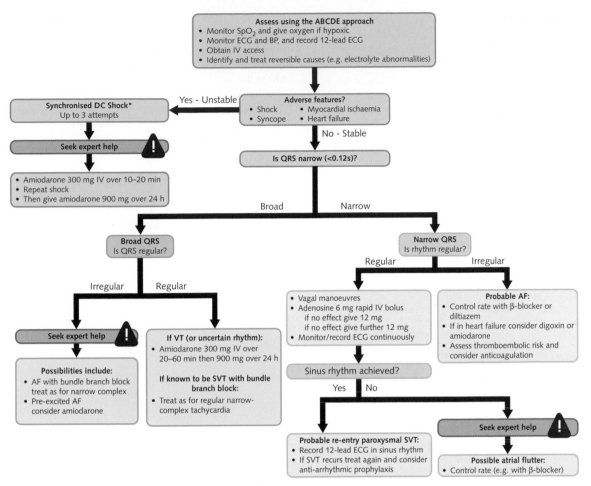

*Conscious patients require sedation or general anaesthesia for cardioversion

Figure 15.18 Adult tachycardia (with pulse) algorithm. AF, atrial fibrillation; BP, blood pressure; DC, direct current; SVT, Supraventricular tachycardia; VT, ventricular tachycardia. (From G2015_Adult_BLS Resus Council 2015.pdf. Adult Bradycardia Algorithm Resuscitation Council (UK) Guidelines 2015, https://www.resus.org.uk/resuscitation-guidelines/peri-arrest-arrhythmias/)

CARDIAC ARREST AND RESUSCITATION

Cardiac arrest occurs when there is an absence of cardiac output. Cardiopulmonary resuscitation (CPR) is the term used to describe the maintenance of adequate breathing and circulation in a patient who cannot do so for him-or herself. The aim of CPR is to restore respiration and adequate cardiac output as soon as possible to prevent death or permanent disability. CPR involves two types of protocol:

1. Basic life support (BLS) – no special equipment required.
2. Advanced life support (ALS) – requires specialist skills and equipment.

In any type of resuscitation protocol, the following three areas must be assessed and supported in order of priority:

- Airway.
- Breathing.
- Circulation.

Basic Life Support

BLS refers to the maintenance and support of airway, breathing and circulation without the aid of any specialized equipment (Fig. 15.19). This should be commenced immediately upon recognising cardiac arrest. The aim of BLS is to maintain adequate ventilation and cardiac output until the underlying problem can be reversed. There are a number of points to note:

- Open the airway if necessary, and assess if the patient is breathing (with look, listen and feel) for no more than 10 s. If trauma to the cervical spine is a possibility, the airway should be maintained without tilting the head.
- If there are two rescuers, one should go for help as soon as possible. If there is only one, the rescuer should

```
┌─────────────────────────────┐
│ Unresponsive and not breathing │
│          normally            │
└─────────────────────────────┘
              ↓
┌─────────────────────────────┐
│  Call 999 and ask for an     │
│        ambulance             │
└─────────────────────────────┘
              ↓
┌─────────────────────────────┐
│    30 Chest compressions     │
└─────────────────────────────┘
              ↓
┌─────────────────────────────┐
│      2 Rescue breaths        │
└─────────────────────────────┘
              ↓
┌─────────────────────────────┐
│     Continue CPR 30:2        │
└─────────────────────────────┘
              ↓
┌─────────────────────────────┐
│   As soon as AED arrives     │
│   switch it on and follow    │
│       instructions           │
└─────────────────────────────┘
```

Figure 15.19 Adult basic life support algorithm (Resuscitation Council 2015 Guidelines). AED, automated external defibrillator; CPR, cardiopulmonary resuscitation. (From G2015_Adult_BLS Resus Council 2015.pdf. Adult Bradycardia Algorithm Resuscitation Council (UK) Guidelines 2015, https://www.resus.org.uk/resuscitation-guidelines/peri-arrest-arrhythmias/)

shout for help and, if necessary, very quickly (i.e., taking seconds) go to obtain help after establishing that the patient is not breathing. If, however, the patient is a child, then 1 min of CPR should be given before the rescuer goes for help – in these situations the collapse is likely to be due to respiratory arrest and rescue breaths, if given early, will improve prognosis.

- Chest compressions are performed by placing the heel of the hand over the lower half of the sternum. Enough pressure should be applied to depress the sternum 5–6 cm and no more.
- The rescuer should be vertically above the patient's chest and the arms should be kept straight. The rate of compressions should be 100–120/min. After each compression the pressure should be released and the chest wall allowed to rise back up. The sequence is 30 compressions followed by 2 rescue breaths.
- Each rescue breath is given by mouth-to-mouth inflation, ensuring there is a good seal and the nose is occluded. Blow steadily for 1 minute. The rescuer should watch the chest wall of the patient to ensure that it rises and falls with each breath. It is important to allow the chest wall to fall back completely before taking the next breath.

Use of automated external defibrillators

Automated external defibrillators (AEDs) are increasingly prevalent in public places and can be used with minimal or no training. They allow for early defibrillation, often long before the arrival of professional help. AEDs provide full instructions to the user throughout the defibrillation process.

AEDs are useful in areas with high densities of people (e.g., airports, railway stations, stadiums, etc.) but also in remote areas in which, if an arrest occurred, response would be significantly delayed.

Recovery position

This position should be adopted if an unresponsive patient is both breathing and has a pulse whilst the rescuer goes for help. It has several important functions (Fig. 15.20), including keeping the patient's airway straight, allowing the tongue to fall forward and not obstruct the airway, and minimising risk of aspiration of gastric contents.

Airway straight with no obstruction from tongue – minimises risk of aspiration

hand under cheek keeps head tilted back

lower arm not under body

upper leg, hip and knee are at right angles

Manoeuvres
Remove patient's glasses (if worn).
Kneel beside patient and make sure their legs are straight.
Place patient's near-side arm at right angles to their body, elbow bent with palm up.
Bring patient's far-side arm across the chest and hold back of their hand against the cheek on near-side.
With other hand, grasp far-side leg above the knee and pull it up, keeping the foot on the ground.
Keeping their hand against the cheek, pull on the far-side leg to roll the patient towards you.
Adjust the upper leg so the hip and knee are both at right angles.
Tilt the head back to ensure airway remains open.
If necessary, adjust hand under the cheek to keep head tilted.
Re-assess breathing regularly.

Figure 15.20 The recovery position.

Advanced life support

The Resuscitation Council's current adult ALS guidelines were most recently updated in 2015 (Fig. 15.21). This guideline has two main arms, based on dividing cardiac arrest patients into two main groups:

1. Those with shockable rhythms - VF/ pulseless VT (pVT).
2. Those with non-shockable rhythms – asystole/ pulseless electrical activity (PEA).

Points to note
For optimum efficacy of ALS:

- Ensure BLS is commenced immediately and, once a cardiac monitor is available, that defibrillation is administered immediately if shockable rhythm is present. Minimize interruptions to CPR.
- Ensure the airway is protected throughout – ideally this should be with insertion of a cuffed endotracheal (ET) tube, preferably by an anaesthetist. This minimizes the

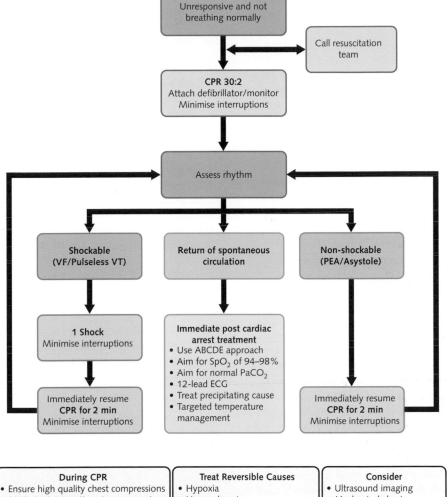

Figure 15.21 Adult advance life support algorithm (2015 guidelines). CPR, cardiopulmonary resuscitation; PEA, pulseless electrical activity VF, ventricular fibrillation; VT, ventricular tachycardia. (From G2015_Adult_BLS Resus Council 2015.pdf. Adult Bradycardia Algorithm Resuscitation Council (UK) Guidelines 2015, https://www.resus.org.uk/resuscitation-guidelines/peri-arrest-arrhythmias/)

risk of aspiration of gastric contents and can increase the efficacy of ventilation. If an ET tube can be placed, then ventilate the patient at a constant rate of 10 breaths/min and continue chest compressions at a rate of 100–120 compressions/min without pauses for ventilation.

- The defibrillator pads should be placed to allow optimum energy delivery to the myocardium – the right pad should be below the clavicle in the mid-clavicular line and the left pad should be on the lower rib cage on the anterior axillary line.

'Shockable rhythms' arm of the advanced life support algorithm

In the event of pVT or VF, one DC shock should be administered as soon as the rhythm is identified and it is safe to deliver the shock. Generally, an energy setting of at least 150 J should be used in the first instance when using a bi-phasic defibrillator. Following delivery of the shock, CPR should be resumed immediately. Rhythm and pulse is assessed following a further 2 minute cycle of CPR. A further shock may be delivered at this time if indicated. Adrenaline is given at a dose of 1 mg intravenously after the third shock is delivered, and then every 3–5 minutes (generally every two rhythm checks). Amiodarone (300 mg IV) should be given after the third shock. Look for reversible causes of cardiopulmonary arrest.

'Non-shockable rhythms' arm of the advanced life support algorithm

This arm of the ALS algorithm includes asystole, PEA and profound bradyarrhythmias. Prognosis is generally poorer for patients with non-shockable rhythms. Defibrillation is not indicated unless the rhythm check shows change to VF/pVT. Adrenaline should be given intravenously at a dose of 1 mg as soon as IV access is achieved. This may be repeated every 3–5 minutes. Look for reversible causes of cardiac arrest.

Reversible causes – '4 Hs and 4 Ts'

A number of reversible causes for cardiac arrest have been identified and these are sometimes referred to as the *4 Hs and 4 Ts*. Attempts should be made to rule these out or treat as appropriate during all cardiac arrests:

- **H**ypoxia – ensure maximal possible inspired oxygen is delivered during CPR and that ventilation is adequate. Ensure the chest is rising and falling and that there are bilateral breath sounds.
- **H**ypovolaemia – attempt to stop any obvious haemorrhage and restore circulating volume with fluids and/or blood products.
- **H**ypo-/hyperkalaemia, hypoglycaemia or other metabolic disorders – patient history may suggest presence of a metabolic abnormality; ABG and blood glucose may allow for rapid diagnosis/treatment.
- **H**ypothermia – may be suggested by the history e.g., cardiac arrest associated with drowning.

- **T**hrombosis (coronary or pulmonary) – if pulmonary embolus is suspected, consider giving thrombolysis if there are no contraindications. If thrombolysis is given, consider performing CPR for at least 60–90 minutes before resuscitation efforts are terminated.
- **T**ension pneumothorax – suspect in trauma cases or after insertion of a central line; it is also seen spontaneously in fit young men and in patients with asthma or COPD. Look for unilateral absence of chest movements and breath sounds. Treat it with a large-bore cannula into the pleural space at the second intercostal space in the mid-clavicular line, followed by the insertion of a chest drain.
- **T**oxins – may be suggested by the history, may occur due to prescribed medications, over-the-counter medications or recreational drugs. Use a toxicology database (e.g., Toxbase) for specific guidelines.
- **T**amponade (cardiac) – suspect in trauma cases and post-thoracotomy patients. Tamponade can be confirmed by ultrasound imaging. It needs rapid insertion of a pericardial drain.

In-Hospital cardiac arrest

When a cardiac arrest occurs in hospital, a call is put out to the arrest team. Most hospitals in the UK have a standard number (2222), which is a direct line to the switchboard operator. The caller should state in a clear voice, 'Cardiac arrest, ward X'. The switchboard operator will then repeat the information back to the caller before alerting the arrest team. Generally, the arrest team comprises at least an anaesthetist, a medical registrar, a senior house officer and an FY1, as well as a porter who can take urgent blood samples to the laboratory. The anaesthetist or registrar usually leads the resuscitation effort.

Many hospitals now use audit forms to analyse the response to each cardiac arrest call. These forms collect information on the condition of the patient on arrival, events during the arrest and whether it was successful or not. The results of audit sheets are used as part of ongoing quality improvement and to direct further training of the arrest team.

ETHICS

'Do Not attempt Resuscitation' or 'DNR' orders are written by senior members of staff when it is thought that death is expected, resuscitation under the circumstances would be futile, or the patient's quality of life would subsequently be very poor. These are difficult decisions to make, and a sound knowledge of ethical principles and medical law is essential. The principles of beneficence and non-maleficence are particularly important here; CPR should not be carried out if felt not to be in the best interests of the patient. Even if CPR is a valid treatment option, the patient may exert their autonomy and refuse resuscitation in advance.

● **Chapter Summary**

- Arrhythmia is a term used to describe an irregularity in the normal heartbeat. Many patients with arrhythmia may be asymptomatic, whereas others can be critically unwell.
- Certain patients with bradycardia (such as patients with complete heart block) warrant pacemaker insertion.
- Patients with atrial fibrillation are at increased risk of stroke – it is important to balance stroke risk against the increased bleeding risk of anticoagulation.
- Familiarity with the indications (and contra-indications) of antiarrhythmic agents is vitally important – some can cause profound instability if given in an inappropriate setting.
- Arrhythmia and the presence of myocardial ischaemia (either in the form of chest pain or on the ECG) syncope, shock (systolic blood pressure <90 mmHg) or signs of heart failure indicate the arrhythmia is 'unstable'. These patients require urgent intervention.
- If the patient has a pulse but warrants defibrillation, then remember to use synchronized DC cardioversion. In ventricular fibrillation or pulseless ventricular tachycardia, proceed with unsynchronized defibrillation immediately.
- For cardiac arrest and resuscitation, follow the BLS and ALS algorithms.
- Rapid recognition of arrest with early CPR, early defibrillation and prompt post-resuscitation care improves arrest outcomes.

Valvular disease can manifest as either stenosis or regurgitation, or sometimes both simultaneously. Stenosis is a narrowing or obstruction to normal flow through the valve. In regurgitation, the valve fails in its function to prevent backflow of blood and is 'leaky'. This can also be described as an incompetent or insufficient valve.

Valvular disease can be caused by:

1. Direct damage to the valve leaflets (usually the case in stenosis).
2. Damage to the valve ring (the annulus).
3. Damage to the supporting structures (papillary muscles, chordae tendineae).

The most commonly affected valves are the aortic and mitral valves. This is due to the high pressures to which they are exposed (compared to those in the right side of the heart). Multiple valves may be diseased. Any valvular abnormality will predispose to infective endocarditis (IE).

See Chapter 10 for a summary of causes of valvular disease (and other murmurs) and clinical findings on examination.

HINTS AND TIPS

Valve lesions are a common short-case question both in finals and in membership examinations.

RHEUMATIC HEART DISEASE

Rheumatic fever is now rare in the developed world due to improved sanitation, reduced overcrowding, effective antibiotic therapy and a reduction in the virulence of β-haemolytic streptococcus. It is still a major problem in the developing world, where it is the most common cause of acquired valvular disease. Acute rheumatic fever most frequently affects children aged 5–15 years.

Acute rheumatic fever is an inflammatory disease caused by an autoimmune reaction initiated by infection with group A β-haemolytic streptococcal pharyngitis 2–3 weeks earlier. Antibodies directed against bacterial cell membrane antigens cross-react with the patient's own proteins (in a type II hypersensitivity reaction). It may cause multi-organ disease, affecting the heart, skin, joints and central nervous system.

Rheumatic heart disease is a consequence of rheumatic fever that may have occurred many years previously. The acute process can leave the valves scarred and deformed,

and progressive fibrosis can occur causing chronic rheumatic heart disease. It is more common in females.

Clinical features

The patient may not recall a preceding sore throat. Diagnosis of rheumatic fever is based on the revised Jones criteria.

Major criteria:

1. Carditis – involves all three layers (pancarditis), see later.
2. Arthritis – a migrating polyarthritis affecting the large joints.
3. Sydenham's chorea – occurs months after the initial disease and is characterized by rapid, involuntary purposeless movements of the face and limbs due to inflammation of the caudate nucleus, also known as *St Vitus' dance*.
4. Erythema marginatum – seen mainly on the trunk; the shape of the lesions change with time and the asymptomatic rash spreads outwards with raised red circular edges and a centre which clears.
5. Subcutaneous nodules – pea-sized, firm, painless, subcutaneous nodules on the extensor surfaces (overlying joints, on the scalp and over vertebrae).

Minor criteria are:

1. Fever.
2. Raised erythrocyte sedimentation rate (ESR) or C-reactive protein (CRP).
3. Prolonged PR interval (only if carditis is not a major criteria).
4. Arthralgia.
5. Previous rheumatic fever.

Diagnosis requires two major criteria, or one major and two minor criteria, plus evidence of preceding streptococcal infection (e.g., increased antistreptolysin O (ASO) titres). Evidence of streptococcal infection is not required if there is isolated pancarditis or chorea, and if all other causes of these are excluded. If diagnosing recurrent rheumatic fever, only evidence of previous streptococcal infection and 2 minor criteria are required.

Carditis predominantly affects the valves (valvulitis) but can affect the endocardium, myocardium and pericardium concomitantly (pancarditis). It is usually asymptomatic even though a murmur or echocardiographic evidence may be found. The patient may present with breathlessness, chest pain or palpitations. Signs may include a new murmur, or features of pericarditis or heart failure.

Aschoff nodules (granulomatous lesions with a central necrotic area) are pathognomonic of rheumatic fever, and initially have an inflammatory infiltrate that is eventually replaced by fibrous tissue. Commonly, rheumatic fever affects the mitral valve (65%) or the mitral and aortic valves (25%). In the long-term, progression can lead to commissural fusion (fusing of valve leaflets), shortening/thickening of the chordae and cusp fibrosis. The most common chronic sequelae are mitral stenosis (MS) with or without regurgitation, although other valves may be affected.

Investigations

Blood tests are expected to reveal raised inflammatory markers (ESR and CRP) and leucocytosis.

Evidence of streptococcal infection should be looked for. Throat swab should be taken for culture (although often too late for positive results when rheumatic fever presents) and may be used for the rapid streptococcal antigen detection test (RADT) if available. Blood tests 2 weeks apart may demonstrate rising antibodies, e.g., ASO titres.

First degree atrioventricular (AV) block may be seen on the ECG, although this is not a specific finding despite being a minor criterion. Features of pericarditis or other non-specific ST or T wave changes may be seen.

A chest X-ray may demonstrate cardiomegaly or evidence of heart failure.

An echocardiogram may demonstrate valvular abnormalities, cardiac enlargement and pericardial effusion in acute rheumatic fever. The so-called fish-mouth or button-hole mitral valve deformity can be seen on echocardiogram in MS secondary to chronic rheumatic heart disease.

Management

Treatment with high-dose penicillin (benzylpenicillin, single intramuscular injection or phenoxymethylpenicillin, 10-day oral course) is started immediately to eradicate the causative organism.

Antiinflammatory agents are given to suppress the autoimmune response and to relieve arthritis. Aspirin is effective, and although in children there is a small risk of Reye's syndrome, it is still sometimes used in preference to nonsteroidal antiinflammatory drugs at small doses. Corticosteroids are used if there is any carditis.

Bed rest reduces cardiac workload and reduces joint pain. Cardiac failure is treated with supportive therapy, although sometimes the rheumatic fever causes severe mitral regurgitation (MR) which does not respond to medical treatment and requires valve replacement.

Long-term antibiotics (usually penicillin) are recommended for a minimum of 5 years (or until the patient is 21) to prevent recurrent rheumatic fever. Long-term follow-up is needed to identify any valve disease.

> **HINTS AND TIPS**
>
> Acute rheumatic fever is not common in the developed world, but there are still many elderly people suffering the after-effects of a childhood infection. It is also important to recognize and treat acute rheumatic fever promptly.

AORTIC STENOSIS

This is the most common valvular disease in the developed world. The most common form of aortic stenosis (AS) is valvular AS from degenerative calcification; however, AS may also occur at the sub- or supravalvular level in congenital disease (Table. 16.1).

> **CLINICAL NOTE**
>
> Congenitally bicuspid valves are one of the most common congenital cardiac abnormalities; however, most do not cause any problems until later in life. On average, patients with bicuspid valves develop aortic stenosis 10 years earlier than those with normal valves. It is also associated with aortic aneurysm and dissection.

Table 16.1 Causes of aortic stenosis

Site of aortic stenosis (AS)	Causes
Valvular AS	Degenerative calcification of normal tricuspid valve or congenitally abnormal valve (tends to occur at a younger age) Rheumatic fever Congenital, males > females (malformed valve can be uni-, bi- or tricuspid)
Subvalvular AS	Fibromuscular ring Hypertrophic cardiomyopathy
Supravalvular AS	Associated with hypercalcaemia in Williams syndrome – a syndrome associated with elfin facies, intellectual disability, affable 'cocktail party' personality, strabismus, hypervitaminosis D and hypercalcaemia; autosomal dominant inheritance although mostly arises de novo.

Pathophysiology

In adults, left ventricular outflow obstruction usually develops over a number of years. The stenosis increases afterload on the left ventricle (LV), increasing the force required to eject blood into the aorta. This causes left ventricular hypertrophy (LVH) and increase in myocardial oxygen demand. More vigorous and prolonged contraction aims to overcome the obstruction and maintain an adequate cardiac output, but as systole is prolonged, diastole is shortened. Coronary artery flow occurs during diastole; therefore, myocardial blood supply from the coronary arteries is reduced. If myocardial perfusion is outstripped by demand, angina occurs even in the presence of normal coronary arteries. Inadequate tissue perfusion (e.g., of the brain) may cause syncope. Reduction in cardiac output and pulmonary oedema can result in breathlessness.

Clinical features

Although patients are often asymptomatic, there is a classic triad of symptoms:

1. Angina – see earlier.
2. Dizziness and syncope – especially on exertion.
3. Dyspnoea – initially exertional due to the inability to increase cardiac output adequately. May lead to orthopnoea and paroxysmal nocturnal dyspnoea as the LV fails.

Sudden death and systemic emboli may occur but these are rare.

HINTS AND TIPS

Patients who have aortic stenosis may present with angina, but an exercise test is usually contraindicated in patients who have severe aortic stenosis, as exertion can cause syncope or sudden death. It is therefore crucial to examine every patient carefully before recommending an exercise ECG.

Examination

The following findings are common in valvular AS (Fig. 16.1):

1. Slow rising, low volume pulse – best felt at the carotid pulse.
2. Narrow pulse pressure.
3. Heaving apex beat – rarely displaced.
4. Ejection systolic murmur heard loudest over the aortic area, may radiate to the carotids and be accompanied by a palpable thrill.
5. Quiet or absent aortic component of the second heart sound (A_2).
6. Signs of left ventricular failure (LVF).

Investigations

Electrocardiography

This usually shows sinus rhythm and a picture of LVH with strain – a tall R wave in lead V5–V6, with a deep S wave in lead V1 and T wave inversion in the lateral leads.

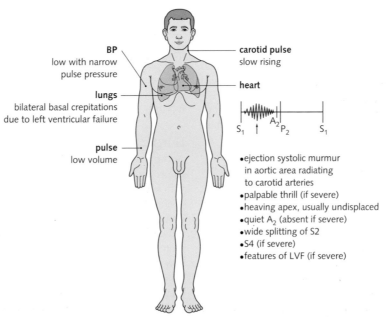

Fig. 16.1 Possible clinical findings in aortic stenosis. A_2, aortic component of second heart sound; LVF, left ventricular failure; P_2, pulmonary component of second heart sound; S_1, first heart sound; S_2, second heart sound.

Chest radiography

The cardiac shadow is often of normal size in LVH but can be enlarged if there is co-existent aortic regurgitation (AR) or LVF. The valve may be calcified and, therefore, visible. The aorta is often enlarged due to turbulent blood flow. There may also be evidence of pulmonary oedema in LVF.

Echocardiography

This is the standard method to assess and follow up AS. It will show the valve in great detail, including the number of cusps and their mobility, and the presence of calcification. Doppler echocardiography allows blood flow velocity to be measured and the calculation of the effective orifice area and aortic valve gradient, which are all measures of AS severity. It will also demonstrate resultant LVH or LVF. Aortic size can be measured, and co-existent AR or mitral valve disease may be seen.

Cardiac catheterization

This may provide information on the valve gradient and LV function, although echocardiography is sufficient in the vast majority. The main indication is assessment of coronary arteries prior to surgical valve replacement, to identify patients who may benefit from concurrent bypass grafting.

Management

Medical management

Prognosis is good if the patient is asymptomatic. Patients with asymptomatic severe AS may be followed up with intermittent echocardiography as the patient may attribute gradual decrease in exercise tolerance to age. Patients should be educated to look out for warning symptoms, such as chest pain, syncope and breathlessness. As soon as mild symptoms are present, survival becomes poor unless left ventricular outflow tract obstruction is promptly relieved either surgically or percutaneously. The average time between symptom onset and death is 5 years with angina, 3 years with syncope and 2 years with heart failure. Valve replacement may prevent LVF or sudden death.

Medication use is limited. Diuretics can be helpful to remove abnormal fluid accumulation in heart failure, but use cautiously – hypovolaemia will overcome the compensatory raised end-diastolic LV pressure and reduce cardiac output. The positive inotropic effects of digoxin also have some theoretical benefits and can be used in patients with AS and heart failure. Many antianginal drugs and angiotensin-converting enzyme (ACE) inhibitors are avoided in AS because they theoretically might:

1. Have a negative inotropic effect and result in acute pulmonary oedema (if LV function is impaired).
2. Cause vasodilatation, resulting in worsening of the gradient across the aortic valve, and inability to produce a compensatory increase in cardiac output.

Fig. 16.2 Example of a transcatheter heart valve (Sapien 3). (Courtesy Prof. D Newby.)

However, there is interest in the potential protective effects of ACE inhibitor therapy, especially longer acting agents without acute falls in blood pressure.

Transcatheter aortic valve implantation (TAVI)

In recent years, balloon-expandable valves have been developed that can be deployed either through percutaneous catheters or using a trocar through the apex of the heart (Fig. 16.2). This has become a valuable treatment in those that are at very high surgical risk due to co-morbidities, and, as technologies develop further, may replace some traditional surgery in the future.

Balloon aortic valvuloplasty (BAV)

This procedure stretches the stenotic valve with a balloon inserted via a percutaneous catheter. It is not a long-term solution and is associated with significant risks; therefore it is only used as a palliative measure or bridge to surgery.

Surgical management

Aortic valve replacement (AVR) is still the treatment of choice and should be considered without delay in all patients with symptomatic severe AS. Most centres have experience operating on very old patients (e.g., in their 80s) with improved quality of life and survival. AVR is usually performed using a median sternotomy incision and requires cardiopulmonary bypass. In some young patients, a Ross procedure may be performed. In this case, the patient's own pulmonary valve is moved to the aortic position. A porcine or cadaveric graft is then implanted into the pulmonary position; this replacement will last much longer than if inserted into the aortic position as it is not exposed to systolic pressures.

Aortic valvotomy is performed to repair congenital AS in children.

AORTIC REGURGITATION

AR may be due to an abnormality of the valve cusps themselves and/or dilatation of the aortic root and therefore the valve ring (Table 16.2).

Pathophysiology

The regurgitation of blood back into the LV after each systole results in an increased end-diastolic volume and an increased stroke volume. The LV works harder and becomes hypertrophied and dilated. The aorta may also dilate with increased stroke volumes, worsening AR. As AR progresses, the LV may no longer be able to compensate, resulting in LVF and pulmonary congestion. The LV backpressure may also cause pulmonary hypertension and right ventricular failure (RVF) but this is uncommon.

If onset is acute (e.g., ruptured valve with IE), these compensatory structural changes cannot take place and the increase in LV pressure causes premature closure of the mitral valve and prevents diastolic filling.

Clinical features

Moderate and mild AR is usually asymptomatic. Patients often have an increased awareness of their heartbeat due to increased stroke volume years before any other symptom. Dyspnoea is the main presenting symptom and develops insidiously in chronic severe AR, with accompanying features of LVF, such as orthopnoea and paroxysmal nocturnal dyspnoea. Angina can develop as hypertrophy increases demand and abnormally low diastolic blood pressure decreases coronary flow.

Table 16.2 Causes of aortic regurgitation

Site of disease	Cause
Valve disease	Infective endocarditis Rheumatic fever Congenital – e.g., prolapse with ventricular septal defect Rheumatoid arthritis Systemic lupus erythematosus
Aortic root disease	Osteogenesis imperfecta Type A aortic dissection Aortic root aneurysm Trauma Takayasu arteritis Reiter syndrome Psoriatic arthritis Syphilis
Both	Degenerative Hypertension Connective tissue disease (e.g., Marfan syndrome) Bicuspid aortic valve Ankylosing spondylitis

Acute severe AR may present with profound hypotension due to cardiogenic shock, weakness and breathlessness.

Examination

Characteristic findings in chronic AR (Fig. 16.3) are:

1. Collapsing high-volume pulse.
2. Wide pulse pressure.
3. Downward and laterally displaced apex, which has a thrusting nature.
4. Murmur best heard with the diaphragm at the lower left sternal edge with the patient sitting forward and in full expiration. It is a soft, high-pitched, early diastolic murmur, sometimes difficult to hear – be sure to listen for it properly with the diaphragm of the stethoscope.
5. Increased flow across the aortic valve in significant AR frequently produces an ejection systolic murmur even without AS, which is often louder than the early diastolic murmur.
6. Third heart sound due to rapid ventricular filling.
7. A number of eponymous signs (see Chapter 10).
8. Austin Flint murmur – heard when the regurgitant jet causes vibration of the anterior mitral valve leaflet. The murmur is similar to that of MS, but with no opening snap.
9. May include signs of LVF, see Chapter 14.

CLINICAL NOTE

Also known as a *water hammer pulse*, the collapsing pulse is due to the increased stroke volume and the rapid run-off of blood back into the left ventricle after systole. It is accentuated at the radial pulse by lifting the arm rapidly – use the base of your fingers across the patient's radial artery at the wrist to best appreciate the tapping quality of the collapsing pulse. Remember to check whether the patient has any shoulder pain first! The abrupt expansion and collapse can be better felt at the carotid pulse (Corrigan's sign).

In acute AR, the patient may appear very unwell, with cyanosis, hypotension, and pulmonary congestion. Prominently, tachycardia occurs to compensate for the inability of the heart to dilate and hypertrophy quickly. This usually leads to shortening of the murmur, and most of the other peripheral signs are also less evident.

Investigations

Electrocardiography

In early AR, the ECG is normal. As chronic AR progresses, there may be left axis deviation, then LVH with strain pattern.

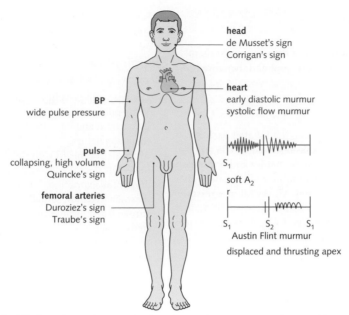

Figure 16.3 Possible clinical findings in aortic regurgitation. A_2, aortic component of second heart sound; S_1, first heart sound; S_2, second heart sound.

Chest radiography

The LV does not have time to enlarge in acute AR but may be markedly enlarged in chronic AR. Marked aortic root enlargement may suggest this as the cause for AR. If there is LVF, there may be evidence of pulmonary oedema.

Echocardiography

The structure of the aortic valve can be evaluated and fluttering of the anterior mitral valve leaflet is frequently seen as the regurgitant jet hits the leaflet from above. Doppler echo demonstrates the size of the regurgitant jet as a measure of severity. Left ventricular size and function can be assessed. Aortic root size can be assessed, although sometimes this will require additional evaluation. Transthoracic echo is usually sufficient, although sometimes transoesophageal echo may provide more detailed information.

Cardiac catheterization

This enables assessment of aortic root size, severity of AR, left ventricular function and co-existent coronary artery disease.

Cardiac magnetic resonance imaging (MRI)

Cardiac MRI can accurately assess AR severity, flow reversal in the aorta, and LV volume and mass. It is helpful when echocardiography has not provided optimal views.

Management

Medical management

Treatment for an underlying cause (e.g., IE) may be required. Isolated systolic hypertension can increase regurgitant volume and therefore should be treated – vasodilators (e.g., ACE inhibitors, nifedipine) are preferred. The use of diuretics and ACE inhibitors is valuable to treat cardiac failure in these patients.

Prognosis for asymptomatic patients is generally good in chronic AR. Once symptoms develop, prognosis is poor without valve replacement (average time from symptom onset to death is 4 years with angina, 2 years with LVF). Irreversible dilatation and significant LV systolic impairment can occur in some patients before symptoms occur; therefore follow-up is valuable. It is important to make the diagnosis and surgically treat this condition before the LV dilatation and failure becomes irreversible. Patients with severe AR should be educated to look out for symptoms and are followed up with intermittent echocardiography.

Surgical management

AVR is considered promptly in chronic AR if the patient is symptomatic, if there is significant progressive LVF or if there are signs of progressive LV dilatation (end systolic diameter >55 mm). The aortic root may also need to be replaced if it is grossly dilated. Concurrent coronary artery bypass graft may also be required. In a small proportion of cases, aortic valve repair rather than replacement may be possible.

In acute AR, urgent AVR is recommended – in the case of IE in haemodynamically stable patients, this may be deferred for 5 to 7 days for intensive antibiotic treatment.

MITRAL STENOSIS

MS is almost always caused by rheumatic fever. Other causes are rare:

1. Calcification of the mitral valve annulus in old age.
2. Congenital.
3. Malignant – lung carcinoid (systemic carcinoid causes right-sided valve disease).
4. Systemic lupus erythematosus.
5. Rheumatoid arthritis.
6. Other conditions may mimic MS by causing obstruction of inflow to the LV. These include left atrial (LA) myxoma, LA thrombus, large vegetations (IE) and hypertrophic cardiomyopathy.

Pathophysiology

Rheumatic fever causes thickening of the cusps and fusion of the cusps and commissures, which then become immobile and stenosed in a fish-mouth configuration. An immobile valve cannot close properly and is often regurgitant as well.

The stenosis limits passive diastolic filling of the LV, increasing the contribution of atrial systole. It also increases LA pressure, producing atrial distension (often causing atrial fibrillation (AF)) and increasing pulmonary venous pressure. In turn, this can cause pulmonary hypertension and right heart failure (Fig. 16.4). This may occur over decades.

Tachycardia shortens diastole (LV filling time) and increases LA pressure. In AF, loss of coordinated LA contraction (upon which the heart has become dependent) reduces cardiac output by ~20%. Both tachycardia and AF are poorly tolerated and may precipitate the onset of pulmonary oedema in previously asymptomatic patients.

Clinical features

The main presenting features of MS are exertional dyspnoea and fatigue:

1. Dyspnoea – this may be due to pulmonary oedema or pulmonary hypertension. Patients who have MS are more susceptible to chest infections, which may cause dyspnoea.
2. Fatigue – due to reduced cardiac output.
3. Ankle swelling – if right heart failure develops.
4. Palpitations – AF is common in MS (due to LA enlargement) and may cause palpitations, often accompanied by a sudden deterioration in dyspnoea.
5. Haemoptysis – this can be frank blood (bronchial vein or alveolar capillary rupture) or frothy pink sputum (pulmonary oedema).
6. Chest pain – thought to be due to severe pulmonary hypertension.
7. Systemic emboli (higher risk with AF) – the dilated left atrium predisposes to thrombus formation and thromboembolism, e.g., stroke, acute limb ischaemia, renal emboli causing hypertension.

Rare symptoms secondary to LA enlargement include:

1. Hoarseness due to stretching of the recurrent laryngeal nerve.
2. Dysphagia due to oesophageal compression.
3. Left lung collapse due to compression of the left main bronchus.

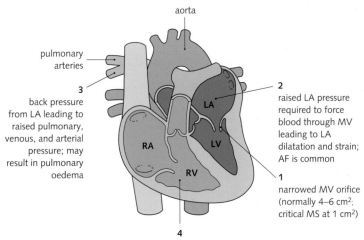

aorta

pulmonary arteries

3 back pressure from LA leading to raised pulmonary, venous, and arterial pressure; may result in pulmonary oedema

LA

RA

LV

RV

2 raised LA pressure required to force blood through MV leading to LA dilatation and strain; AF is common

1 narrowed MV orifice (normally 4–6 cm^2; critical MS at 1 cm^2)

4 back pressure from pulmonary artery causes RV strain and hypertrophy and eventually RV failure with raised JVP, ascites, hepatomegaly, and peripheral oedema; dilatation of RV may lead to dilatation of tricuspid valve ring and TR

Fig. 16.4 Pathophysiology of mitral stenosis. AF, atrial fibrillation; LA, left atrium; LV, left ventricle; JVP, jugular venous pressure; MV, mitral valve; RA, right atrium; RV, right ventricle; TR, tricuspid regurgitation.

Examination

Clinical findings (Fig. 16.5) include:

1. Loud first heart sound (S_1) due to slow diastolic filling.
2. Tapping apex beat (palpable S_1) that is not displaced.
3. Opening snap after the second heart sound (S_2). Both the opening snap and loud S_1 may be absent if the valve is heavily calcified.
4. Low rumbling mid-diastolic murmur following the opening snap – heard loudest with the bell at the apex with the patient lying on their left side and in full expiration. Pre-systolic accentuation of the murmur if the patient is in sinus rhythm (absent in AF). Severity is related to the duration, not the intensity, of the murmur.
5. Pulse may be irregularly irregular signifying AF, which becomes common as the disease progresses and with older age.
6. A common presentation is with pulmonary oedema (bibasal crepitations, possible effusions).
7. As the pulmonary vascular resistance rises, if the patient is still in sinus rhythm, prominent a waves in the jugular venous pressure (JVP) are seen. Pulmonary hypertension in MS can cause mitral facies (malar flush), a loud palpable pulmonary component of the second heart sound (P_2), a Graham Steell murmur (pulmonary regurgitation early diastolic murmur) and a parasternal heave due to right ventricular hypertrophy. Right ventricular dilatation can cause tricuspid regurgitation (TR) with a pansystolic murmur and giant v waves in the JVP.
8. If RVF develops, signs include a raised JVP, peripheral oedema, ascites and hepatomegaly.

Investigations

Electrocardiography

AF may be seen. P mitrale may be shown in LA enlargement (only in sinus rhythm) – the P wave in lead II is abnormally long (>0.12 s) and may have a bifid 'M' shape. There may also be evidence of right ventricular hypertrophy (right axis deviation, tall R wave in V1 or deep S wave in V6 >7 mm).

Chest radiography

This may show evidence of an enlarged left atrium (the normal concave upper left heart border can be straightened or convex, the left atrium can indent the right lung to cause the double density sign at the right heart border and the carina can be splayed with a horizontal left main bronchus). The mitral valve itself may be calcified and visible. There may be prominent pulmonary vessels or frank pulmonary oedema.

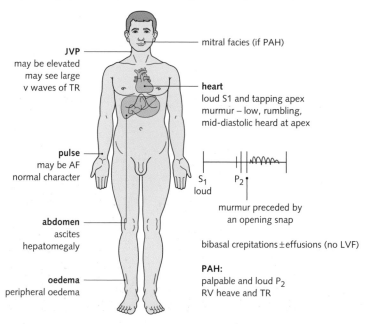

Fig. 16.5 Possible clinical findings in mitral stenosis. AF, atrial fibrillation; JVP, jugular venous pressure; LVF, left ventricular failure; P_2, pulmonary component of second heart sound; PAH, pulmonary arterial hypertension; RV, right ventricular; RVF, right ventricular failure; S_1, first heart sound; SR, sinus rhythm; TR, tricuspid regurgitation.

Echocardiography

This is the most accurate investigation to assess MS (Fig. 16.6). The mitral valve structure and mobility can be visualized and the cross-sectional area measured. This can also be estimated using Doppler as a measure of severity. Left ventricular function, LA size, pulmonary hypertension and right ventricular complications can be evaluated. Transoesophageal echocardiography (TOE) can be helpful sometimes to identify LA thrombus.

Cardiac catheterization

This is performed on most patients before valve replacement to exclude any coexistent coronary artery disease and evaluate any MR or pulmonary hypertension that may be present.

Management

Medical management

Medical treatment of MS may consist of antibiotic prophylaxis, management of AF and heart failure, and follow-up.

If MS is due to rheumatic heart disease, antibiotics are given to prevent worsening of MS from recurrent rheumatic fever.

AF management is similar to management due to any other cause of AF (see Chapter 15):

1. Digoxin, small dose of β-blocker or rate-limiting calcium channel antagonist – helpful for ventricular rate control in AF, as prolonging diastole allows the LV more time to fill. A β-blocker may be lifesaving in pregnancy (MS is often previously undiagnosed).
2. Direct current (DC) cardioversion – may be successful in AF of recent onset, although rhythm control can be difficult to achieve in MS. Only attempt it if confident that onset was within 48 hours or the patient has been fully anticoagulated for at least 4 weeks to reduce the risk of embolization.
3. Anticoagulation – recommended in all patients who have AF or previous embolic complications; aim for international normalized ratio (INR) between 2 and 3.

Diuretics are useful to treat pulmonary and peripheral oedema.

Prognosis is good in asymptomatic MS; follow-up is helpful to determine optimal timing of intervention. In patients with symptomatic severe MS (poor outcomes if stenosis is not relieved) or pulmonary hypertension, consider intervention.

Mitral valvuloplasty

Mitral balloon valvuloplasty is the intervention of choice if suitable. A balloon is passed across the mitral valve and inflated, separating the commissures of the stenosed valve. This procedure is carried out percutaneously and only requires a local anaesthetic and light sedation. The following features make a patient unsuitable for this procedure:

1. Marked MR.
2. LA thrombus (must have TOE to exclude) or history of systemic emboli.
3. Calcified or thickened rigid mitral valve leaflets or sub-valvular apparatus.

Complications include embolization, cardiac perforation and MR requiring valve replacement.

Surgical management

This is indicated in patients who have severe MS (mitral valve area $\leq 1\,\text{cm}^2$) with significant symptoms (New York Heart Association class III or IV), severe pulmonary hypertension (pulmonary artery systolic pressure >60 mmHg) or persistent LA thrombus. Note that restenosis may occur after percutaneous valvuloplasty or surgical valvotomy and

Fig. 16.6 (A) Normal echocardiogram of the parasternal long axis view (diastolic frame) (Ao, aorta; AV, aortic valve; IVS, intraventricular septum; LA, left atrium; LV, left ventricle; MV, mitral valve; PW, posterior LV wall; RV, right ventricle). (B) Echocardiogram of mitral stenosis (long axis). The mitral valve (MV) leaflets are densely thickened and the left atrium (LA) is severely dilated. (Courtesy Dr A Timmis and Dr S Brecker.)

patients should be followed up. In carefully selected patients, this does not occur for many years; early restenosis within 5 years may occur in those who have thickened or rigid valves.

Open mitral valvotomy

Open mitral valvotomy is performed under general anaesthetic using a median sternotomy incision and requires cardiopulmonary bypass. Any thrombus in the left atrium or LA appendage is removed, the mitral valve commissures are carefully separated under direct vision, and fused chordae tendineae can be split. It is used when balloon valvuloplasty is not suitable, e.g., in mitral valves that are too calcified or distorted, co-existent mild MR amenable to surgical repair, presence of LA thrombus, previous failed balloon valvuloplasty and co-existent disease of other heart valves.

Closed mitral valvotomy

This has now been superseded by mitral valvuloplasty. It does not require cardiopulmonary bypass; access is gained through a submammary incision (curved under the left breast) with a dilator passed into the LV apex to separate the valves. It is worth knowing this because patients in finals examinations may have this scar.

Mitral valve replacement (MVR)

MVR can be used for calcified or very rigid valves that cannot be split with valvuloplasty or valvotomy without causing significant regurgitation, or if there is already significant co-existent MR which is not amenable to repair.

MITRAL REGURGITATION

MR can occur if any of the following components of the mitral valve apparatus are abnormal: (Table 16.3):

1. Mitral valve annulus.
2. Mitral valve leaflets.
3. Chordae tendineae.
4. Papillary muscles.

The most common causes are mitral valve prolapse (MVP), ventricular and annular dilatation, rheumatic heart disease, IE and ischaemic damage to the chordae tendineae or papillary muscles.

Pathophysiology

In chronic MR, to accommodate the increased volume of blood flowing back into the left atrium during systole, LA dilatation occurs over time, which often causes AF. Regurgitant flow also increases back-pressure in the pulmonary veins, causing the development of pulmonary hypertension, which may eventually lead to RVF. The LV also becomes gradually dilated as it compensates for chronic volume overload, which can then further worsen MR and lead to LVF. Therefore, untreated severe MR may result in

Table 16.3 Causes of mitral regurgitation

Site of pathology	Cause
Mitral annulus	Senile calcification LV dilatation and annular enlargement – IHD, dilated cardiomyopathy IE (abscess formation)
Mitral valve leaflets	IE (vegetations preventing leaflet closure or causing perforation) Chronic rheumatic heart disease MVP Congenital malformation Connective tissue disorders – Marfan syndrome, Ehlers-Danlos syndrome, osteogenesis imperfecta, pseudoxanthoma elasticum Systemic lupus erythematosus (Libman-Sacks lesion)
Chordae tendineae	Idiopathic rupture Myxomatous degeneration (MVP, connective tissue disorders) Acute rheumatic fever IE
Papillary muscle	Myocardial infarction Infiltration – amyloidosis, sarcoidosis Myocarditis

IE, infective endocarditis; IHD, ischaemic heart disease; LV, left ventricular; MVP, mitral valve prolapse.

biventricular failure. MS on the other hand does not cause LVF.

In acute MR, the left atrium does not have time to dilate to accommodate the increased volume, and the pressure increase is transmitted directly to the pulmonary veins, resulting in pulmonary oedema.

Clinical features

These vary depending upon whether the MR is chronic or acute:

1. Chronic MR develops slowly, allowing the heart to compensate, and usually presents with a history of fatigue and reduced exercise tolerance (primarily decreased cardiac output); dyspnoea can be due to eventual LVF. Palpitations can occur due to awareness of increased stroke volume, or due to development of AF. Peripheral oedema may occur with development of pulmonary hypertension.
2. Acute MR presents with severe dyspnoea due to acute pulmonary oedema, or cardiogenic shock.

Acute MR can be rapidly fatal. Look for this in patients following myocardial infarction (MI) (papillary muscle rupture or dysfunction occurs in the first 7 days after MI) and in patients who have IE.

Examination

Features that may be seen (Fig. 16.7) include:

1. Irregularly irregular pulse – AF is common, especially in chronic MR.
2. Displaced thrusting apex – downward and lateral displacement as the LV dilates – eventually LVF may result. Note that in MS, the apex is not displaced as the LV is protected by the stenosed mitral valve.
3. Soft S_1 – quiet if mitral valve leaflets malfunctioning.
4. Pansystolic murmur – best heard at the apex, may radiate to the axilla. May obliterate the second heart sound. Note that murmur intensity is not an indicator of MR severity.
5. May have a mid-systolic click and late systolic murmur in mitral valve prolapse (MVP).
6. Signs of LVF – i.e., bilateral basal inspiratory crepitations, basal dullness due to effusions. S_3 is less useful as it is often present without LVF due to the increased flow volume and rapid LV filling in MR.
7. Signs of RVF (more common in acute MR, or if pulmonary hypertension and RVF develop) - elevated JVP, peripheral oedema, ascites and congestive hepatomegaly.
8. Loud P_2 and right ventricular heave – may be present if developed pulmonary hypertension.

Investigations

Electrocardiography

There may be P mitrale or AF, and LVH. Evidence of right ventricular hypertrophy may be present in late stages.

Chest radiography

Cardiothoracic ratio may be increased due to left ventricular enlargement. Left atrial enlargement, pulmonary venous congestion or overt pulmonary oedema may be seen. The mitral valve can be visible if it is calcified.

Echocardiography

The mitral valve leaflets (including vegetations) and supporting structures (e.g., ruptured chordae tendineae) can be clearly visualized. The regurgitant jet is seen and severity quantified using colour Doppler. The left atrium and LV may be enlarged and left ventricular dysfunction may be seen in severe MR. Pulmonary artery pressures can be estimated. Suitability for mitral valve repair is better evaluated with TOE.

Cardiac catheterization

Most patients have minimal MR on echocardiography and do not require catheterization. This is performed to further assess the severity of the MR, measure pulmonary hypertension and to exclude other valve lesions and coronary artery disease in the assessment for valve replacement.

Management

Medical management

Vasodilators (e.g., ACE inhibitors) are valuable in hypertension or congestive cardiac failure to prevent increased afterload worsening MR. If left ventricular function is impaired, other standard management (e.g., β-blockers, diuretics) is helpful. Management of AF is important with rate-limiting medicines and anticoagulation.

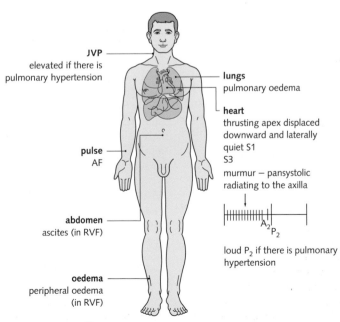

Fig. 16.7 Possible clinical findings in mitral regurgitation. A_2, aortic component of second heart sound; AF, atrial fibrillation; P_2, pulmonary component of second heart sound; RVF, right ventricular failure; S1, first heart sound; S3, third heart sound.

Percutaneous mitral valve repair

In the last few years, percutaneous devices have been developed to reduce MR by drawing in the mitral valve ring or clipping together the centre of the two mitral valve leaflets. This is only considered in patients who are not suitable for surgery.

Cardiac resynchronization therapy (CRT)

In functional MR (dilated annulus secondary to e.g., dilated or ischaemic cardiomyopathy), CRT with dual ventricular pacing may improve leaflet coaptation and reduce the severity of MR and is indicated in patients with significantly reduced left ventricular ejection fraction and left bundle branch block (see Chapter 14).

Surgical intervention

Patients are considered for surgery if there is symptomatic severe MR, or if there is progressive cardiac enlargement or deterioration of left ventricular function. Surgery may be considered if AF or pulmonary hypertension have developed in asymptomatic patients, as these are associated with worse prognosis. If possible, it is important to act before irreversible left ventricular damage and severe pulmonary hypertension have occurred.

In acute MR, in addition to aggressive medical therapy, surgery is indicated if there is acute LVF; without it the patient is unlikely to survive.

Mitral valve repair

This may take the form of mitral annuloplasty, repair of a ruptured chorda or repair of a mitral valve leaflet. These procedures are performed on patients who have mobile non-calcified and non-thickened valves. Both repair and replacement of the mitral valve require a median sternotomy incision and cardiopulmonary bypass.

Mitral valve replacement

This is only performed if mitral valve repair is not possible and the higher operative risks are deemed necessary. Replacement may paradoxically worsen left ventricular function by preventing reduction of afterload through MR or interrupting the continuity of the annulus with the chordae tendineae and the papillary muscles.

Mitral valve prolapse

MVP is also known as floppy mitral valve or click-murmur syndrome. Important points include:

1. This is common (2%–3% of the population), with a female preponderance.
2. The mitral valve may billow minimally into the left atrium with a click but no regurgitation, or may cause varying degrees of MR.
3. Most cases are idiopathic, but it is seen more frequently in connective tissue disorders e.g., Marfan syndrome.
4. Most patients are asymptomatic, and are diagnosed incidentally on examination. Infrequently, some patients present with fatigue, atypical chest pain, palpitations, infective endocarditis or embolic phenomena.
5. Examination reveals a mid-systolic click at the apex. If there is regurgitation, this may be followed by a systolic murmur of MR. The murmur may be best heard at the left sternal edge or round the patient's back.
6. Most patients require no further treatment other than reassurance as it generally follows a benign course. However, it is one of the commonest causes of MR, which can become severe as the chordae tendineae elongates. Rarely, rupture can cause acute severe MR. It is a common predisposing condition to IE.

TRICUSPID DISEASE

Tricuspid stenosis

Tricuspid stenosis (TS) is rare. It is almost always due to rheumatic fever; even so, it only affects a small proportion of those with rheumatic fever – the mitral and aortic valves are usually also affected. Infrequently, it can be due to carcinoid syndrome or congenital tricuspid atresia.

Clinical features

The most prominent symptoms are usually related to concurrent left-sided valvular disease. However, if TS is severe, this may prevent enough forward flow to cause breathlessness; conspicuously little orthopnoea or paroxysmal nocturnal dyspnoea should raise suspicion of severe TS. Fatigue may be present due to reduced cardiac output. Systemic congestion (hepatic congestion, ascites and peripheral oedema) may be pronounced; severe generalized oedema is known as anasarca.

The most obvious examination findings are those of venous congestion. The JVP is raised with large a waves (if the patient is in sinus rhythm) and slow y descent. There may be hepatomegaly, ascites and peripheral oedema. A soft mid-diastolic murmur at the lower left sternal edge may be heard, although this can be difficult to differentiate from the murmur of MS. Lack of the parasternal heave of right ventricular hypertrophy may be helpful.

Management

The mainstay of management in severe TS is surgery; this may be either valve replacement or valvotomy. Concurrent operation on other valves might be necessary. Balloon valvuloplasty is very rarely used. Medical management with salt restriction and diuretics may help with systemic congestion.

Tricuspid Regurgitation

Most cases of TR are due to dilatation of the tricuspid annulus resulting from dilatation of the right ventricle. This may be due to any cause of RVF or pulmonary hypertension including cor pulmonale (see Table 10.1).

Occasionally, the tricuspid valve is affected by IE (usually in intravenous drug abusers). Rheumatic disease can cause TR uncommonly. Rarer causes include congenital malformations, including Ebstein anomaly and carcinoid syndrome.

CLINICAL NOTE

Ebstein anomaly is a congenital malformation and is caused by downward displacement of the tricuspid valve into the body of the right ventricle. The valve is regurgitant and malformed. The condition is associated with other structural cardiac abnormalities and there is a high incidence of both supraventricular and ventricular tachyarrhythmias.

Clinical features

The symptoms and signs are due to the backpressure effects of the regurgitant jet into the right atrium.

The most common features are fatigue due to reduced cardiac output, and symptoms of RVF, including discomfort secondary to hepatic congestion, ascites or peripheral oedema. Patients usually present with symptoms of the disease causing the underlying RVF; the TR is often an incidental finding.

Examination

The regurgitant jet is transmitted to the venous system causing a 'giant' v wave in the jugular venous waveform (Fig. 16.8). There are signs of RVF with systemic venous congestion, and there may be pulsatile hepatomegaly. AF is common. There may be signs corresponding to the cause in functional TR.

Management

TR due to right ventricular overload can improve with treatment of the cause. The mainstay of management is medical, with diuretics and ACE inhibitors to treat the fluid overload (which is due to LVF in most cases). Isolated RVF is less common; in this case, use caution with diuretics as they may adversely reduce left ventricular preload and consequently cardiac output. Instead, cautious fluid challenges may be helpful (see Chapter 14). Annuloplasty in functional dilatation or tricuspid valve replacement may be considered in very severe cases. In IE, the excision of the infected valve without immediate replacement is usually well tolerated if there is no concurrent pulmonary hypertension and avoids infection of the prosthetic valve; the valve is replaced when the infection is controlled.

PULMONARY DISEASE

Pulmonary stenosis

Pulmonary stenosis (PS) is usually a congenital malformation, e.g., tetralogy of Fallot, Noonan syndrome, congenital

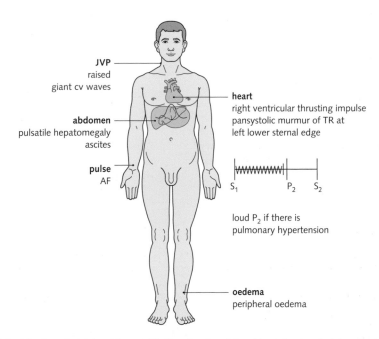

Fig. 16.8 Possible clinical findings in tricuspid regurgitation. Look out for signs of an underlying cause of right-heart failure such as mitral valve disease or pulmonary disease. AF, atrial fibrillation; JVP, jugular venous pressure; P_2, pulmonary component of second heart sound; S_1, first heart sound; S_2, second heart sound.

rubella syndrome. Rarely, PS can be caused by carcinoid syndrome or rheumatic heart disease.

Clinical features

If mild, PS is asymptomatic. If it is severe, there may be features of RVF (systemic venous congestion). If PS occurs in a neonate, there may be cyanosis due to right-to-left shunting. In neonates and infants, PS may present with failure to thrive, or diagnosed as an incidental murmur at neonatal check. In older children and adults, there may be a right ventricular equivalent of AS symptoms (exertional fatigue, exertional lightheadedness and angina).

Possible signs on examination include an ejection systolic murmur in the pulmonary area, an ejection click preceding the murmur and wide splitting of second heart sound or quiet P2. In severe PS, there may be a prominent a wave in the JVP, right ventricular heave and features of RVF.

Management

Balloon valvuloplasty is the mainstay of treatment, with surgical valvotomy less frequently used.

Pulmonary regurgitation

Pulmonary regurgitation (PR) is most frequently due to dilatation of the valve ring or pulmonary artery. This can be secondary to pulmonary hypertension due to left-sided heart disease, for instance in MS (Graham Steell murmur), primary pulmonary hypertension or Eisenmenger syndrome. Marfan syndrome can also cause dilatation. The valves can be affected by disease, such as IE, rheumatic fever, carcinoid syndrome and tetralogy of Fallot (or previous surgical correction).

Clinical features

Frequently, the clinical features of the underlying disease causing PR are the main issue, and the murmur of PR is found incidentally without causing much problem. If isolated, PR is frequently asymptomatic, although in severe cases, it may cause RVF. In association with pulmonary hypertension, it can exacerbate RVF, and pulmonary septic emboli may be seen if PR is due to IE.

Possible signs include a low-pitched early diastolic murmur in the pulmonary and tricuspid area, which may also be accompanied by an ejection systolic flow murmur due to increased RV stroke volume. In severe PR, the murmur is high-pitched due to the forceful jet and best heard at the left parasternal edge (i.e., similar to that in AR but with signs of severe pulmonary hypertension, wide splitting of S2, RV heave and RVF).

Management

Treat any underlying disease. PR is usually benign and mostly does not require treatment. Valve replacement may be considered in PR caused by surgical correction of tetralogy of Fallot.

ASSESSING THE SEVERITY OF A VALVE LESION

Once a valve lesion has been diagnosed, it is important to evaluate its severity. This is judged in most cases by clinical and echocardiographic means; angiography is occasionally also helpful. The more common left-sided valvular lesions are discussed here (Table. 16.4).

Table 16.4 Severity markers for valve disease

Valve disease	Features
AS	Presence of AS symptoms. Slow-rising pulse and narrow pulse pressure, obscured or absent A_2, paradoxical splitting of S2, S4, associated thrill, generally a louder/harsher or later peaking murmur (NB: if severe AS complicated by LVF, murmur may be very quiet or disappear, may only have signs of severe LVF and low CO). Severe AS (jet velocity >4 m/s, aortic valve area <1.0 cm², mean gradient >40 mmHg) and poor LV function on echo or cardiac catheterization.
AR	Symptoms and signs of LVF (may be one the only signs in acute AR). Collapsing pulse and wide pulse pressure, eponymous signs, S3, increased decrescendo murmur duration, Austin Flint murmur. Size of regurgitation jet and LV enlargement/dysfunction on echo or cardiac catheterization.
MS	Symptoms of pulmonary congestion or RVF. OS earlier and closer to S2 (OS/loud S1 may be lost in severe MS), soft S1, increased murmur duration (quieter if reduced CO), mitral facies, signs of pulmonary congestion, signs of pulmonary hypertension and RVF, Graham Steell murmur, signs of TR. Severe MS (valve area <1.0 cm², mean gradient >10 mmHg) or significant pulmonary HTN (pulmonary artery systolic pressure >50 mmHg) on echo or cardiac catheterization.
MR	Symptoms and signs of LVF, pulmonary HTN or RVF. Size of regurgitant jet, LA enlargement, LV enlargement/dysfunction or evidence of pulmonary HTN on echo and cardiac catheterization

A_2, aortic second heart sound; AR, aortic regurgitation; AS, aortic stenosis; CO, cardiac output; echo, echocardiography; HTN, hypertension; LA, left atrial; LV, left ventricular; LVF, left ventricular failure; MR, mitral regurgitation; MS, mitral stenosis; OS, opening snap; RVF, right ventricular failure; S1, first heart sound; S2, second heart sound; S3, third heart sound; S4, fourth heart sound; TR, tricuspid regurgitation.

PROSTHETIC HEART VALVES

Examples of mechanical and biological heart valves are shown in Fig 16.9 and Table 16.5. Aim to be familiar with mechanical valve sounds as they commonly pop up in exams. Mechanical valves impart a metallic quality to the first (mitral) or second (aortic) heart sound, and both opening and closing clicks can be heard. Some patients may have both types of valve. Biological valves produce normal heart sounds. All patients with prosthetic aortic valves (even tissue valves) will have a systolic flow murmur. Patients with mitral valves may have a quiet pansystolic murmur due to turbulent blood flow in the LV, but loud pansystolic murmurs require investigation. Diastolic murmurs are generally a worrying sign and require investigation for endocarditis, valve thrombosis, paravalvular leak or valve failure. A short, quiet diastolic murmur in a mitral prosthesis may be innocent but it is better to investigate if there is any doubt.

> **RED FLAG**
>
> Remember to investigate urgently for valvular dysfunction if a patient with a prosthetic valve develops unexplained heart failure.

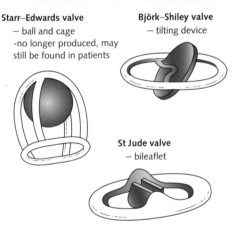

Starr–Edwards valve
— ball and cage
-no longer produced, may still be found in patients

Björk–Shiley valve
— tilting device

St Jude valve
— bileaflet

Fig. 16.9 Types of mechanical heart valve.

Table 16.5 Types of biological heart valve

Type of valve	Features
Xenograft	Manufactured from porcine valve or bovine pericardium and mounted on a frame (on chest X-ray, only the mounting ring can be seen)
Homograft	Cadaveric valve graft, does not require prosthetic mounting ring. A subtype is an autograft (from the same patient), e.g., a pulmonary valve transplanted into the aortic position.

All patients must be anticoagulated for life with mechanical valves. The target INR varies between 2.5 and 3.5, depending on the type of valve, the position of the valve and other patient risk factors for thromboembolism. Lower target INRs are used when thromboembolic risk is lower, e.g., the St Jude valve is less thrombogenic than the Starr-Edwards valve, and aortic valves are less thrombogenic than mitral or tricuspid valves. Targets vary with local, national and international guidelines. Anticoagulation is not required with bioprosthetic valves, unless there is another indication, e.g., co-existent AF (common in mitral disease).

Bileaflet valves are currently the most widely used mechanical valve due to their superior haemodynamic characteristics and lower risk of thromboembolism.

Mechanical valves last longer than bioprosthetic valves. Bioprosthetic valves may last an average of 10 years, but failure may occur in as early as 4–5 years or as late as 20 years. Mechanical valves have been shown to usually last more than 25 years.

In general, older patients (e.g., over 65) are suitable for bioprosthetic valves as the valves are likely to last the patient's lifetime. Younger patients should be considered for mechanical valves (even though this will entail the risks of lifelong anticoagulation), as the mortality for repeat valve replacement is much higher. However, some younger patients may choose bioprosthetic valves for lifestyle reasons, accepting the risk of tissue valve deterioration and the likely need for a future second valve replacement. Increasingly, patients with bioprosthetic valve failure are being treated with a 'valve-in-valve' procedure where a TAVI valve is inserted into the bioprosthetic valve.

In MS, mechanical valves are used frequently, as MS tends to present at a younger age and often the patient is in AF for which they will already require long-term anticoagulation. Bioprosthetic valves are generally preferred in the tricuspid position, as mechanical valves in this position have a much higher risk of thromboembolism.

Although guidelines have changed to state that antibiotic prophylaxis against IE is not required in native valve disease, it should still be considered in those with prosthetic valves, especially during procedures with a high risk of bacteraemia, as the outcome of IE in prosthetic valves is much worse.

INFECTIVE ENDOCARDITIS

IE is an infection of the endocardium. This usually involves the heart valves (native or prosthetic), but it can affect the chordae tendineae, the surface of the cardiac chamber or blood vessel, and indwelling cardiac devices (e.g., pacemakers leads).

The development of IE depends on a number of factors:

1. Presence of anatomical abnormalities in the heart surface.
2. Haemodynamic abnormalities within the heart.

3. Presence of bacteraemia.
4. Host immune response.
5. Virulence of the organism.

Transient bacteraemia is a common occurrence, e.g., associated with activities such as brushing teeth and chewing, as well as both dental and non-dental procedures. Despite this, IE is rare; therefore the endothelium of a healthy individual with normal cardiac anatomy is well protected.

IE occurs more commonly at sites of endothelial injury, for example on valves that have been previously damaged or are congenitally abnormal, or any area damaged by a high-pressure jet through a narrow orifice (e.g., ventricular septal defect). The resultant inflammation and platelet and fibrin aggregation at the site is easier for bacteria to adhere to; the infecting organism becomes incorporated into the site to form a vegetation. This causes further destruction of the valve(s), and often leads to valvular regurgitation (either perforation of the valve leaflets or vegetations and adhesions impeding valve closure). These vegetations can also throw off emboli to other organs, causing ischaemia or infection.

There is a mortality of up to 20% even with treatment. This is largely due to the potentially fatal complications:

1. Local destructive effects – valve regurgitation (occasionally stenosis with large vegetations), paravalvular abscess or fistulae, prosthetic valve dehiscence, arrhythmia, pericarditis and myocardial rupture. These can cause congestive cardiac failure and cardiogenic shock, sometimes rapidly.
2. Embolization of infected or non-infected fragments (may be clinically silent) – left-sided IE can result in mycotic (infected) aneurysm, stroke or cerebral abscesses, digital infarcts, renal/hepatic/splenic abscesses, renal/splenic infarcts (hepatic infarcts are rare because the liver is supplied by the hepatic artery and the hepatic portal system), MI from coronary emboli, and ischaemic bowel. Right-sided IE can lead to septic pulmonary emboli.
3. Type III autoimmune reaction to the organism – resulting in the deposition of immune (antibody-antigen) complexes and a subsequent inflammatory response. A diffuse or focal glomerulonephritis or arthritis may occur.

HINTS AND TIPS

If you remember these three classes of complications, it is easy to fit symptoms and signs into each category. Classifying signs according to the pathophysiology shows that you have a full understanding of the disease process and will impress examiners.

Previously, endocarditis was classified by onset as acute or subacute; now it is classified according to the valves involved, whether native or prosthetic, whether community or healthcare-acquired, and the causative organism.

Diagnostic criteria

The modified Duke criteria are used in the diagnosis of IE (Table 16.6).

COMMON PITFALLS

The modified Duke criteria does not require either of the major criteria to be met, as infective endocarditis can be culture-negative and vegetations are not always visualized. Conversely, not all endocarditis is infective (termed *marantic endocarditis*), and can occur with systemic lupus erythematosus, other connective tissue diseases and malignancy.

In injection drug users, microorganisms are introduced via the intravenous route or from injection-related soft tissue infections. They are included in the minor criteria because their risk of IE is several times higher than in patients with predisposing heart conditions, such as rheumatic heart disease or prosthetic valves.

Epidemiology

IE is an evolving disease. Traditionally, the main predisposing condition was rheumatic heart disease; however, the incidence of rheumatic fever in developed countries has dropped significantly because of improved social conditions and antibiotic therapy. Now, incidence in the UK is increasing due to an increase in the following:

1. Increased number of prosthetic valve insertions, pacemakers and long lines.
2. Increased number of patients who have congenital heart disease surviving to adulthood.
3. Increasing elderly population.
4. Increasing injection drug abuse.
5. Antibiotic resistance.

With this change in the population affected by IE, the organisms are also changing. *Staphylococci* have overtaken *Streptococci* as the most common cause, due to increased healthcare-associated infection and injection drug abuse. Coagulase-negative staphylococci, which used to be uncommon, are now the most common organisms seen on prosthetic valves (Table. 16.7).

There are a number of conditions that put people at increased risk of developing IE (see clinical note box below). Previously, such patients were routinely given

Table 16.6 Modified Duke criteria for the diagnosis of infective endocarditis (IE)

Criteria	Description
Major	
1	Positive **blood culture** – one of:
	1 – Typical IE microorganism from 2 separate blood cultures: • Viridans streptococci, *Streptococcus gallolyticus (Strep. bovis)*, or HACEK* group, or • *Staphylococcus aureus* or community-acquired enterococci, in the absence of a primary focus,
	2 – Persistently positive blood cultures with microorganism consistent with IE, defined as: • 2 positive cultures drawn >12 h apart • All of 3 or majority of 4 separate cultures (first and last samples drawn > 1 h apart)
	3 – Single positive blood culture for *Coxiella burnetii* or anti–phase I IgG antibody titre >1:800
2	Evidence of **endocardial involvement** – one of:
	1 – Positive echocardiogram: vegetation, abscess, pseudoaneurysm, intracardiac fistula, valvular perforation or aneurysm, or new partial dehiscence of a prosthetic valve
	2 – New valvular regurgitation (worsening or changing of pre-existing murmur not sufficient)
Minor	
1	**Predisposition:** predisposing heart condition or injection drug use
2	**Fever** ≥ 38.0°C (100.4°F)
3	**Vascular phenomena:** major arterial emboli, septic pulmonary infarcts, mycotic aneurysm, intracranial haemorrhage, conjunctival haemorrhages, Janeway lesions
4	**Immunological phenomena:** glomerulonephritis, Osler nodes, Roth's spots, rheumatoid factor
5	**Microbiological evidence:** positive blood culture but does not meet a major criterion as noted above, or serological evidence of active infection with an organism consistent with IE.
Clinical diagnosis of infective endocarditis (IE) is based on:	

Definite IE:
• Two major criteria, or
• One major and three minor criteria, or
• Five minor criteria.

Possible IE:
• One major and one minor criteria, or
• Three minor criteria.

*HACEK group: *Haemophilus spp., Aggregatibacter spp.* [previously known as *Actinobacillus spp.*], *Cardiobacterium spp., Eikenella corrodens, Kingella spp.*

antibiotic prophylaxis before a variety of procedures anticipated to cause bacteraemia. Since 2008, the National Institute for Health and Care Excellence (NICE) no longer recommends routine antibiotic prophylaxis and recommends that infections are treated promptly in those at risk. NICE recommends patients receive prophylactic antibiotics (chosen to cover common organisms that cause endocarditis) only when they undergo gastrointestinal or genitourinary procedures where there is already suspected infection. This change was made due to lack of evidence of benefit (there is no association between these procedures and the development of IE) and a known risk of harm (including anaphylaxis and the development of antibiotic resistance). The new guidelines have caused controversy, and antibiotics may still be considered in patients at the highest risk.

CLINICAL NOTE

Conditions predisposing to infective endocarditis: (**Bold denotes highest risk group**):

• Acquired valvular heart disease.
• **Prosthetic valve.**
• Congenital heart disease (**especially cyanotic heart disease with residual defect, within 6 months of complete repair with prosthetic material, or residual defect at the site of repair with prosthetic material**).
• Hypertrophic cardiomyopathy.
• **Previous infective endocarditis.**

Table 16.7 Common causative organisms in infective endocarditis

Organism	Comments
Staphylococcus aureus	Acute; highly invasive, can cause rapid destruction of previously normal valves, abscesses, septic emboli and high mortality; common in patients with indwelling lines, skin and soft tissue infections, post-operatively and in injection drug users; has overtaken streptococci to become the most common cause.
Viridans streptococci [α-haemolytic] (e.g., S. *mutans*, S. *mitis*, S. *sanguinis*, S. *anginosus* group, S. *gallolyticus*)	Subacute; common with brushing teeth, poor dentition, and after dental procedures, tonsillectomy or bronchoscopy as they are upper respiratory commensals; predominantly found on rheumatic heart valves or congenitally abnormal valves, although can be found in other situations. S. *gallolyticus* (formerly S. *bovis*) and *Streptococcus anginosus* group (formerly S. *milleri*) are found in the gastrointestinal tract and are associated with colorectal malignancies, and patients should be considered for colonoscopy.
Coagulase-negative staphylococci (e.g., S. *epidermidis*, S. *lugdunensis*)	S. *epidermidis* (a skin commensal) is the most common cause within 2 months of prosthetic valve replacement (the high-risk period), may be introduced from a wound infection; after the early period, the risk is much lower and the above organisms are more common. S. *epidermidis* can also be found on native valves. S. *lugdunensis* is more invasive. May be mistaken for a contaminant.
Enterococci (*E. faecalis, E. faecium*)	May be acute but more often subacute; third most common cause after staphylococci and streptococci; usually in patients with gastrointestinal or urinary tract infections or surgery; can cause endocarditis in any situation.
HACEK group (fastidious gram-negative bacteria)	These fastidious slow-growing organisms are commensals of the upper respiratory tract and require prolonged culture to be detected. May be resistant to penicillin.
Coxiella burnetii (Q fever)	Subacute; usually a history of contact with farm animals; can be associated with a purpuric rash, pneumonia or hepatitis.
Other gram-negative bacteria (e.g., *Chlamydia, Brucella, Bartonella*), diphtheroids	These are less common causes of endocarditis. Brucellosis is associated with contact with farm animals. *Bartonella* may be from cats (cat scratch fever) or infected lice (trench fever). Diphtheroids (*Corynebacterium spp.*) are gram-positive bacilli and an important cause in prosthetic valves.
Fungi (*Candida, Aspergillus, Histoplasma*)	More common in immunocompromised patients, those with indwelling catheters, prosthetic valves and injection drug users (*Candida* from contaminated lemon juice used to dissolve heroin); invasive and can affect normal valves; associated with abscesses, emboli and high mortality. There may be concurrent bacterial infection.

Note that infective endocarditis may be polymicrobial (involve multiple organisms), and a significant number of cases are culture negative (grow no organism).

Clinical features

History

The duration of the symptoms is variable, from a few days to several months. This tends to reflect the virulence of the organism – *Staphylococcus aureus* causes rapid valvular destruction and presents early whereas a *Staphylococcus epidermidis* infection of a prosthetic valve may take a few months to present. Previous antibiotics (partially treated endocarditis) also causes a subacute picture, and symptoms and signs vary by site of infection. Common symptoms are:

1. Fever.
2. Sweats.
3. Anorexia and weight loss.
4. General malaise.

Other symptoms may relate to cardiac complications, embolic events and vasculitic phenomena:

1. Valve dysfunction and heart failure in severe cases.
2. Stroke (may be the presenting complaint).
3. Other systemic emboli (symptoms depending on site) – bear in mind IE if the source of emboli is unknown.
4. Septic pulmonary emboli from tricuspid IE (pleuritic chest pain, breathlessness, cough and haemoptysis).
5. Myalgia and arthralgia (relatively common).

COMMON PITFALLS

Given symptoms are frequently non-specific, the diagnosis of IE can be easily missed unless there is a high index of suspicion. Early treatment reduces the risks of severe complications, such as stroke and rapid valve destruction (with heart failure or cardiogenic shock) and therefore lowers mortality. Until proven otherwise, any patient with a fever and a new murmur should be investigated and potentially treated for endocarditis.

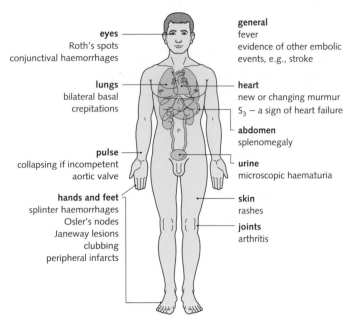

eyes
Roth's spots
conjunctival haemorrhages

general
fever
evidence of other embolic
events, e.g., stroke

lungs
bilateral basal
crepitations

heart
new or changing murmur
S_3 – a sign of heart failure

abdomen
splenomegaly

pulse
collapsing if incompetent
aortic valve

urine
microscopic haematuria

hands and feet
splinter haemorrhages
Osler's nodes
Janeway lesions
clubbing
peripheral infarcts

skin
rashes

joints
arthritis

Fig. 16.10 Possible clinical findings in infective endocarditis.

For clues about the causative organism, enquire about:

1. Any history of rheumatic fever, other valvular disease (e.g., MVP), valve replacement or indwelling cardiac devices or lines.
2. A detailed history of any dental work, operations, or infections.
3. Any history of intravenous drug abuse.
4. Occupation, and any pets or environmental contacts.

It is also important to find out about any drug allergies – this may affect the choice of long-term intravenous antibiotics that may be required. Ensure you clarify the nature of drug allergies, as ruling out penicillins unnecessarily may result in prolonged drug combinations particularly toxic to the kidneys, e.g., vancomycin and gentamicin.

Examination

A thorough examination of all systems is vital (Fig. 16.10). Aim to identify the multiple components of the modified Duke criteria, and cardiac complications not included in the criteria (e.g., heart failure), as well as look for other possible sources of infection or fever.

The following signs are characteristic of IE (see Chapter 10 for more details):

1. Clubbing – (see Chapter 5) seen with chronic subacute endocarditis. Other causes include cyanotic congenital heart disease, suppurative lung disease, lung cancer and inflammatory bowel disease.
2. Splinter haemorrhages – infrequently found in IE (~10%), although the most common cause of these is trauma in most patients.

> **COMMON PITFALLS**
>
> Some findings (e.g., finger clubbing, splenomegaly) take a few weeks to develop, and do not occur with a short history of illness (i.e., acute endocarditis). Although some of these signs (e.g., Osler nodes, Roth's spots) are famously associated with IE, they are rare, and none of the characteristic findings in IE are pathognomonic. However, the diagnosis is suggested by the constellation of signs and symptoms.

3. Osler nodes – painful raised papules on the pulps of digits (infrequent). They occur due to immune complex deposition with vasculitic changes.
4. Janeway lesions – non-tender erythematous flat lesions on the palms or soles (rare). They represent peripheral microabscesses from emboli.
5. Pulse – collapsing pulse may be found in AR with IE. Occasionally, bradycardia (due to complete heart block) may be present if there is an aortic root abscess complicating aortic valve endocarditis.
6. Murmur – usually that of a regurgitant valve, although large vegetations may cause stenosis and, of course, a flow murmur is possible in sepsis of any origin. It is important to perform regular cardiac auscultation because the murmur may change due to progressive valve damage; this may signify imminent

valve failure, and a repeat echocardiogram may be necessary to evaluate any progression.

7. Congestive cardiac failure – remember to look for this complication. In IE, this is most commonly due to valve disruption or rupture of chordae tendineae.
8. Splenomegaly – a common finding in subacute endocarditis.
9. Rash – a vasculitic (purpuric) rash may be found.
10. Roth's spots (retinal haemorrhages with a pale centre) and subconjunctival or buccal haemorrhages.
11. Examine for neurological features carefully – there may be a cerebral infarct from emboli, a haemorrhagic stroke from a mycotic aneurysm or multiple cerebral abscesses. Confusion is common.
12. There may be evidence of other peripheral emboli, such as digital or nailfold infarcts, or abdominal tenderness from splenic or mesenteric infarcts.
13. Inflamed joints – although joint pain is common, a truly swollen hot joint is uncommon; if it occurs, it should be considered as a possible septic arthritis and source of IE until excluded.
14. Look for poor dentition, which may be the source of bacteraemia.

> ### HINTS AND TIPS
>
> Remember to listen for prosthetic valve sounds – this is a risk factor for endocarditis, infection is notoriously difficult to eradicate, patients will often require cardiac surgery to remove infected material, and prosthetic valve infective endocarditis has a higher mortality rate than that in native valves. Working closely with microbiologists and cardiothoracic surgeons is crucial.

Investigations

As expected with the modified Duke criteria, blood cultures and echocardiography are central to the diagnosis and management of IE.

Blood tests

Blood cultures
These are the most important of all the investigations, as it is crucial to identify the causative organism and its sensitivities to guide the prolonged antibiotic therapy required. Positive blood cultures are usually obtained in around 95% cases of bacterial endocarditis if taken before antibiotic therapy.

In contrast to most other infections, *three to six sets* of (aerobic and anaerobic) cultures should be performed to increase the chances of isolating the cause. If possible, at least three sets should be taken with the first and last at least 1 h apart *before* commencing antibiotic therapy. If the patient is very ill and there is a high index of suspicion of IE, it is appropriate to start antibiotics after one or two sets have been obtained, otherwise it is preferable to establish the microbial cause first.

> ### HINTS AND TIPS
>
> When taking blood cultures, strict aseptic technique, multiple venepuncture sites and avoiding indwelling lines are crucial to reduce the risk of contamination. Clean the skin thoroughly with a 2% chlorhexidine swab and allow to dry, and do not re-palpate. Take the blood and then inject it into the culture bottles using new needles, or if available, use direct attachments from the needle onto swabbed culture bottles. Maintain aseptic technique throughout.

Full blood count
Anaemia of chronic disease is common (~90%) in patients who have a subacute presentation. Other findings can include:

1. Leucocytosis – a sign of inflammation (usually a neutrophilia).
2. Thrombophilia – may be seen as part of the acute phase response.
3. Thrombocytopenia – may occasionally be an indication of disseminated intravascular coagulopathy, a severe disorder with a high mortality rate.

Inflammatory markers
ESR and CRP are raised (>90%). CRP is particularly valuable as an acute marker of disease activity, and repeated measurements every few days provide information on the patient's response to treatment.

Renal function
This may be impaired due to infarction or immune complex-mediated glomerulonephritis, or due to reduced renal perfusion in cardiac failure. This should be monitored during treatment as aminoglycoside (gentamicin) and glycopeptide (vancomycin) antibiotics and disease progression may all cause renal impairment.

Liver function tests
These may be deranged due to septic microemboli.

Serological tests
These may be considered for *Coxiella, Brucella, Bartonella, Legionella,* and *Chlamydia* if there is possible exposure and blood cultures remain negative.

Urinalysis

Microscopic haematuria is commonly present in the majority (~90%) of patients with IE; therefore, if you suspect this diagnosis, always perform a bedside urine dipstick (quick, easy and cheap). Formal urine microscopy may also reveal casts in associated immune-complex glomerulonephritis.

Electrocardiography

In aortic abscess formation, development of AV block may be seen – regular ECGs are helpful in patients with IE at the aortic valve due to this risk. Embolization to the coronary arteries may cause MI with ECG changes.

Chest radiography

This may show signs of pulmonary oedema, or evidence of pulmonary abscesses from septic emboli in right-sided IE.

Echocardiography

Echocardiography (echo) may demonstrate vegetations and their size, valvular regurgitation and its severity, paravalvular leak with prosthetic valves, and complications such as abscesses or systolic dysfunction. Repeat echo is helpful to assess progression or development of complications. Transthoracic echo is not as sensitive for IE as transoesophageal echo (which is over 90% sensitive).

Echo may help confirm the diagnosis, but even if vegetations are not detected, IE cannot be excluded if the clinical picture is suggestive as echo is not 100% sensitive. It is also not 100% specific – oscillating masses thought to be vegetations may be non-infective in origin.

Management

There are two main aims in the management of IE:

1. To treat the infection effectively, with the minimum of antimicrobial-related complications, surgery if required, and source control.
2. To diagnose and treat complications of the endocarditis (i.e., congestive cardiac failure, severe valvular regurgitation, peripheral abscesses, renal failure, etc.).

Treatment of infection

If IE is suspected and the patient is unwell, empirical intravenous antibiotic therapy is started as soon as the blood cultures have been taken. The choice of agent can then be modified once the organism is known. Most commonly, therapy will consist of antibiotics, although antifungals may be required. Surgery may be required. Any identifiable source of infection should be controlled to prevent recurrent bacteraemia. The patient requires a thorough dental examination, and for example, a tooth with an apical abscess should be extracted.

Choice of antibiotic regimen

Antibiotics not only treat infection but also reduce risk of complications, such as embolization of vegetations. Always discuss the choice of antibiotic regimen with the microbiologist as soon as possible. Choice of empirical therapy depends on whether the valve affected is native or prosthetic, most likely organisms (likely route of infection), local epidemiology (including resistance), any prior antibiotic therapy and patient allergies.

Penicillin-based antibiotics are effective against Gram-positive cocci (usually benzylpenicillin for streptococci, flucloxacillin for staphylococci, ampicillin or amoxicillin for enterococci as they are resistant to benzylpenicillin). Bactericidal regimens are more effective to eradicate infection, as bacteriostatic therapy inhibits microbial growth, but allows resurgence of infection once antibiotics are stopped. Aminoglycosides (e.g., gentamicin) are typically combined with the above penicillins for synergistic activity to achieve bactericidal action. A reasonable first-line regimen may be amoxicillin, flucloxacillin and gentamicin in native valve infections before the organism is known.

In empirical treatment for prosthetic valves or if Methicillin-resistant *Staphylococcus aureus* is found, vancomycin is generally used instead of penicillin and rifampicin may be added.

When the organism and its sensitivity is known, discuss the most suitable ongoing agents and duration with the microbiologist. Sensitivity of the organisms to antibiotics may be reported with the minimum inhibitory concentration; if it is not satisfactory an antimicrobial may be added or switched.

Duration of antibiotic therapy

The avascular nature of the valves protects the microorganism from host defences, and formation of a biofilm on prosthetic material can further prevent clearance using antimicrobials. Antibiotic tolerance (bacteriostatic rather than bactericidal action) is another problem. This is why prolonged antibiotic courses are required to fully eradicate infection, and prevent serious complications.

Required duration of therapy depends on the:

- Presence of a prosthetic valve (always at least 6 weeks).
- Causative organism and its sensitivity to the antibiotics used.
- Size of the vegetation(s).
- Presence of complications.
- Clinical response to therapy.

Most bacterial infections require 4–6 weeks of intravenous therapy. As little as 2 weeks may be sufficient if response is swift with small vegetations on native valves without any complications and the organism is suitable. In some situations, it may be possible to switch to oral antibiotics. Remember, the patient must be closely monitored after changing to oral or finishing therapy. If there is any evidence of recurrent disease activity, intravenous therapy should be recommended.

Surgery

Although operative intervention in active IE carries a significant morbidity and mortality rate, surgery is required to control infection or prevent worsening heart failure or thromboembolism in a significant number of cases already at high risk of IE-related mortality. This is especially the case in endocarditis associated with prosthetic valves or those caused by *Staphylococcus aureus* or fungi. The difficult decision regarding whether to undertake surgery and the timing of surgery is made in collaboration with cardiothoracic surgeons, after consideration of high-risk IE features and co-morbidities.

Surgery may involve drainage of abscesses or debridement of infected material, repair or valve replacement; indications are listed in the box below. The patient should complete a full course of intravenous antibiotic treatment postoperatively.

Management of complications

CLINICAL NOTE

Indications for surgery in infective endocarditis:

- Heart failure.
- Uncontrolled infection (or abscess/fistula).
- Large left-sided vegetations with systemic embolization or high embolic risk.

There are numerous complications, as listed earlier. Treatment of these may require input from other teams, e.g., stroke, renal etc.

Congestive cardiac failure should be treated with diuretics and ACE inhibitors (see Chapter 14). If cardiac failure remains severe despite medical treatment, a valve repair or replacement may be required.

Conduction defects are uncommon and may be temporary (related to inflammation); therefore pacemakers for high-grade AV block are not always required. See Chapter 15 for detailed management.

The use of antithrombotic therapy can be controversial as there is limited evidence, and it may theoretically prevent thromboembolic complications but increase the risk of haemorrhage from mycotic aneurysms. Indications in IE patients are the same as in other patients. If there are thromboembolic complications, such as pulmonary embolus or deep vein thrombosis, anticoagulation is used as it is normally. Patients with metal prosthetic valves should remain on anticoagulation, although it is often preferable to change from warfarin to heparin as this is more easily reversed. Patients with ischaemic stroke are not anticoagulated because of the risk of haemorrhage into the infarct which can worsen the outcome.

Monitoring of patients who have infective endocarditis

To follow the course of infection and identify new complications early, this should include:

1. Daily history and examination – this is the most important. Look for signs of worsening valvular incompetence, cardiac failure, new splinter haemorrhages, Roth's spots, Osler nodes and so on, all of which are suggestive of ongoing active disease.
2. Temperature chart – an increase in temperature after the patient has been apyrexial for some time can represent reactivation of the infection and blood cultures (as well as other samples of possible infection) should be sent immediately, with reconsideration of possible sources (e.g., endocarditis, abscess formation, thromboembolism of vegetation, other infections, reaction to drugs, etc.).
3. Blood tests – monitor infection with full blood count and CRP. Renal function and liver function may deteriorate due to disease activity or as a side effect of medications. Antibiotic levels (e.g., gentamicin, vancomycin) will need to be closely monitored, and doses should be adjusted for renal function.
4. ECG – in some cases this may be required daily to look for lengthening of the PR interval; highest risk is in left-sided IE. If an abscess develops around the aortic root or in the septum, this can affect the AV node and may lead to complete heart block.
5. Echocardiography – this may be required as frequently as weekly to monitor response, or urgently if there is clinical deterioration. This will assess vegetation size, abscess formation, severity of valvular regurgitation and left ventricular function.

HINTS AND TIPS

Close monitoring is crucial in patients with IE, to identify and treat new complications early. Indications for surgery may develop, and deterioration may lead to severe morbidity and mortality.

● **Chapter Summary**

- Echocardiography is key to the diagnosis and management for all valvular diseases.
- Rheumatic fever is an important cause of valvular disease in the developing world, although there are still numerous affected patients in the developed world. It is caused by an autoimmune reaction to group A β-haemolytic streptococci.
- Diagnosis of rheumatic fever is made according to the revised Jones criteria. Treatment is with antibiotics and antiinflammatory drugs.
- Left-sided valvular diseases and tricuspid regurgitation are the most common valvular abnormalities; knowing the causes, clinical signs, severity markers, complications and management options is essential for exams.
- Patients with valvular disease may benefit from follow-up, as the timing for possible valve replacement or repair is critical.
- Development of heart failure in valvular disease is usually a sign of decompensation and the need to consider further intervention in addition to medical management.
- Prosthetic valves can be metallic or bioprosthetic; metallic valves require lifelong anticoagulation.
- Infective endocarditis is a serious infection with a high mortality rate.
- Diagnosis of infective endocarditis is made using the modified Duke criteria; multiple minor criteria may be fulfilled with careful examination of the patient.
- Taking multiple blood cultures at an early stage is crucial to the subsequent management of infective endocarditis.
- Remember to conduct urinalysis in suspected infective endocarditis, as microscopic haematuria is found commonly due to immune-complex glomerulonephritis and may provide an early part of the puzzle in a frequently non-specific presentation (but bear in mind other causes). This is much more common than the famous but rare signs, e.g., Osler nodes and Janeway lesions.
- Treatment of infective endocarditis involves prolonged antibiotics with infectious diseases input, source control (if identified), surgery (if any of the 3 indications are met) and multidisciplinary management of any complications.

Diseases of the myocardium and pericardium 17

DISEASES OF THE MYOCARDIUM

Myocardial damage can be caused by a number of processes. Ischaemia/infarction, arrhythmia, valvular disease and hypertension can all cause myocardial damage and have been discussed elsewhere. There are also a number of conditions that cause intrinsic damage to the myocardium. These include myocarditis and cardiomyopathy.

Myocarditis

Myocarditis is inflammation of the myocardium and may be either acute or chronic in nature. It can present in a similar way to myocardial infarction (MI). Substantial damage to the myocardium may result in dilated cardiomyopathy (DCM).

There are numerous causes of different aetiology (Table 17.1).

Clinical features

The clinical course is very variable. Many patients present with chest pain with features that often overlap with pericarditis. Patients with evidence of myocarditis may be asymptomatic and only recognized following identification of ECG changes. Other patients may present with severe heart failure, arrhythmia or even sudden cardiac death.

Table 17.1 Causes of myocarditis.

Aetiology	Examples/Comment
Idiopathic	No specific cause is found in many cases of myocarditis.
Viral infections	Numerous causes – including Coxsackie virus, echovirus, human immunodeficiency virus (HIV).
Bacterial infection	Numerous causes – including *Staphylococcus*, tuberculosis, diphtheria.
Other infections	Various fungal, parasitic, protozoal causes.
Immunological	Including systemic lupus erythematosus, sarcoidosis, rheumatoid arthritis, Kawasaki disease, scleroderma.
Toxins	Numerous causes including ethanol, cocaine, doxorubicin, cyclophosphamide, heavy metal poisoning (such as lead, iron, cadmium), arsenic, various insect bites/ stings.
Other	Radiotherapy, electric shock.

Symptomatic patients may complain of:

- Lethargy/malaise.
- Chest pain – may be the result of either pericarditis or myocardial damage.
- Fever.
- Breathlessness.
- Palpitations.
- Ankle swelling.

Examination may be unremarkable. There may be clinical evidence of heart failure or arrhythmia.

Investigation

The following investigations may be appropriate:

- Blood tests – inflammatory markers such as erythrocyte sedimentation rate (ESR) and C-reactive protein (CRP) may be raised. Full blood count, urea and electrolytes, liver function tests, troponin (often elevated). The magnitude and pattern of troponin release is very important.
- Electrocardiography – may show non-specific ST segment changes, T wave changes or abnormalities of conduction (such as bundle branch block).
- Chest X-ray – may be normal. There may be signs of cardiac failure or co-existing pericarditis (e.g., pericardial effusion).
- Echocardiogram – may identify left ventricular dysfunction, ventricular wall motion abnormalities or altered myocardial image texture. Useful for serial monitoring of cardiac function.
- Cardiac magnetic resonance imaging (MRI) – is particularly helpful to differentiate between myocarditis and MI. Certain sequences are used to look for oedema of the myocardium.
- Myocardial biopsy – is rarely performed. Histological analysis may identify inflammatory infiltrates with significant numbers of lymphocytes and macrophages.

Management

Management is focused on treatment of the underlying cause if possible. Patients who develop florid myocarditis and marked impairment of left ventricular function may require cardiovascular support in an intensive care or high dependency setting.

Treatments are generally supportive (administration of oxygen, intravenous fluids, etc.) but management may also include:

- Treatment of heart failure if present.
- Treatment of arrhythmia if present.

- Restriction of physical activity – sometimes for a number of months, to reduce strain on the heart.
- β-Blocker therapy ± angiotensin-converting enzyme (ACE) inhibitor therapy.

Cardiomyopathy

Cardiomyopathy is heart muscle disease, often of unknown cause. Ischaemic cardiomyopathy is heart failure due to underlying coronary artery disease; this is discussed elsewhere. There are several types (Fig. 17.1):

- DCM.
- Hypertrophic cardiomyopathy (HCM).
- Restrictive cardiomyopathy.
- Arrhythmogenic right-ventricular cardiomyopathy (ARVC).
- Others, including Takotsubo cardiomyopathy and left ventricular non-compaction cardiomyopathy (LVNC).

Dilated Cardiomyopathy

DCM is the most common type of cardiomyopathy and results in dilated ventricles and poor systolic function.

The coronary arteries are often normal. Often DCM is a result of a combination of different factors, with causes including:

- Idiopathic – in many cases no obvious cause is identified.
- Genetics (familial DCM) – usually autosomal dominant but not exclusively.
- Alcohol excess.
- Thyrotoxicosis.
- Autoimmune disease – including rheumatoid arthritis and systemic lupus erythematosus.
- Viral infection – numerous infective agents including adenovirus, parvovirus, echovirus, Coxsackievirus, and human immunodeficiency virus (HIV).
- Drugs and toxins (e.g., cocaine, doxorubicin, cyclophosphamide, trastuzumab (herceptin), lead).
- Infiltrative conditions – haemochromatosis, amyloidosis, sarcoidosis, etc.
- Untreated hypertension.
- Tachycardia cardiomyopathy – chronic tachyarrhythmia causing heart failure.

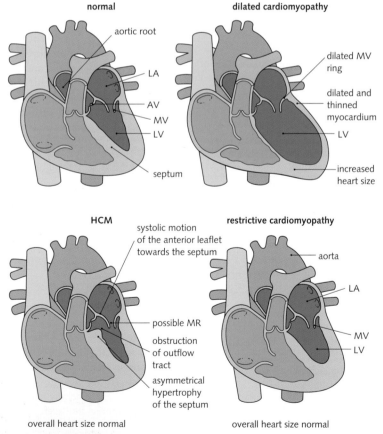

Fig. 17.1 Different types of cardiomyopathy. AV, aortic valve; HCM, hypertrophic cardiomyopathy; LA, left atrium; LV, left ventricle; MR, mitral regurgitation; MV, mitral valve.

Clinical features

Progressive biventricular cardiac failure leads to:

- Fatigue.
- Dyspnoea.
- Peripheral oedema.
- Ascites.

Other complications secondary to the progressive dilatation of the ventricles include:

- Mural thrombus with systemic or pulmonary embolization.
- Dilatation of the tricuspid and mitral valve rings leading to functional valve regurgitation.
- Atrial fibrillation (AF).
- Ventricular tachyarrhythmias and sudden death.

Investigation

Investigations to aid diagnosis include:

- Chest radiography – may show cardiomegaly, signs of pulmonary oedema (upper lobe blood diversion or interstitial shadowing) or pulmonary effusions.
- Electrocardiography – may show tachycardia, poor R wave progression across chest leads, aberrancy of conduction (e.g., bundle branch block).
- Echocardiography – may identify dilated ventricles or regurgitant valves. Occasionally, intracardiac thrombus may be seen (this is easier to identify on transoesophageal echocardiography than transthoracic echocardiography).
- Cardiac catheterization – it is important to exclude coronary artery disease (the most common cause of ventricular dysfunction).
- MRI – this is an excellent non-invasive tool for assessment of patients with cardiomyopathy, and late enhancement with gadolinium can provide useful information about the aetiology and prognosis.
- Blood tests – thyroid function tests, calcium (sarcoidosis), ferritin and iron binding studies (haemachromatosis), creatine kinase (to look for primary muscle diseases), a full blood count (anaemia) and autoimmune screen. Viral titres may be useful.

Management

Management of DCM follows four basic steps (the same applies for any other case of cardiac failure):

1. Search for and treat any underlying cause (e.g., abstinence from alcohol).
2. Treat cardiac failure (diuretics, ACE inhibitors and β-blockers).
3. Treat any arrhythmias (β-blockers, digoxin or amiodarone for AF, or amiodarone for ventricular arrhythmias).
4. Consider anticoagulation to prevent mural thrombi.

After optimization of medical therapy, device therapy should be considered. Cardiac transplantation may also be a treatment option.

Hypertrophic cardiomyopathy

HCM is characterized by hypertrophy of the ventricles. The pattern of hypertrophy is variable but tends to preferentially affect the interventricular septum.

HCM may be diagnosed following detection of left ventricular wall thickness of ≥15 mm, or ≥13 mm if the patient is a known gene carrier or has a known first-degree relative with HCM.

The majority of mutations resulting in HCM are autosomal dominant and affect genes encoding sarcomere proteins.

The myocytes of the left ventricle are abnormally thick when examined microscopically and their layout is disorganized ('myocardial disarray'). This makes left ventricular filling more difficult than normal and grossly disordered.

This condition was previously known as hypertrophic obstructive cardiomyopathy (HOCM). Dynamic left ventricular outflow tract obstruction occurs in around 25% of cases, most commonly due to systolic anterior motion of the mitral valve into the thickened septum, but sometimes the cavity can become occluded. As this only happens in a minority of patients the term HOCM is now only used if there is evidence of obstruction (and HCM otherwise).

HINTS AND TIPS

It is important to realise that the management of HCM involves alleviation of symptoms in some patients, but risk assessment for sudden death is vital in everyone. Certain mutations are particularly associated with sudden death, so genetic testing can sometimes help.

Clinical features

There are four main symptoms:

1. Angina (even in the absence of coronary artery disease) – due to the increased oxygen demands of the hypertrophied muscle.
2. Palpitations – there is an increased incidence of AF and ventricular arrhythmias in this condition.
3. Syncope and sudden death – which may be due to left ventricular outflow tract obstruction by the hypertrophied septum or due to a ventricular arrhythmia. Syncope may often result from inappropriate vasodilatation on exercise.
4. Dyspnoea – due to the stiff left ventricle, which leads to a reduced cardiac output and to pulmonary venous congestion.

Signs (Fig. 17.2) on examination to watch for are:

- Jerky peripheral pulse – the second rise palpable in the pulse is due to the rise in left ventricular pressure as the left ventricle attempts to overcome the outflow tract obstruction.

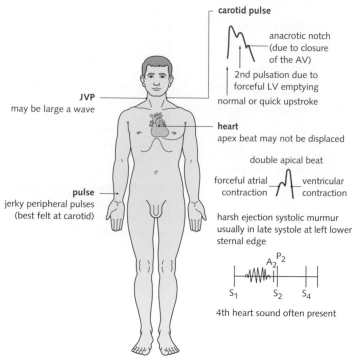

Fig. 17.2 Important clinical signs in hypertrophic cardiomyopathy. AV, aortic valve; JVP, jugular venous pressure; LV, left ventricle.

- Double apical beat – the stiff left ventricle causes raised left ventricular end-diastolic pressure. The atrial contraction is, therefore, very forceful to fill the left ventricle. It is this atrial impulse that can be felt in addition to the left ventricular contraction that gives this classical sign.
- Systolic thrill – felt at the left lower sternal edge.
- Systolic murmur – crescendo and decrescendo in nature, and best heard between the apex and the left lower sternal edge.

It can be difficult to differentiate between HCM and aortic stenosis (AS) on examination. Use the following features to help:

- Pulse character – slow rising in severe AS, jerky or with a normal upstroke in HCM.
- Second heart sound – reduced in intensity in significant AS.
- Thrill and murmur – found in the second right intercostal space in AS and at the left lower sternal edge in HCM.
- Variation of the murmur with Valsalva manoeuvre or with standing from squatting – the murmur of HCM (but not AS) is increased because the volume of the left ventricle is reduced by these manoeuvres and, therefore, the outflow gradient worsens.

HINTS AND TIPS

Remember that the outflow obstruction of aortic stenosis is fixed and is present throughout systole, whereas the obstruction of HCM is often absent at the start of systole and worsens as the ventricle empties.

Investigation

Investigation of HCM involves:

- Electrocardiography - this is usually abnormal (most common abnormalities are T wave and ST segment abnormalities). Signs of left ventricular hypertrophy may also be present. Q waves due to the hypertrophied septum may mimic old MI.
- Continuous ambulatory electrocardiography – presence of non-sustained ventricular tachycardia (VT) is common and is a risk factor for sudden death. Sustained VT is relatively uncommon.
- Echocardiography – may be used to confirm the diagnosis and assess the degree of left ventricular outflow tract obstruction. There may be evidence of unexplained hypertrophy or abnormal systolic

anterior motion of the anterior leaflet of the mitral valve.

- Exercise testing – lack of the normal rise (or a fall) in blood pressure on exercise is a risk factor for sudden death in HCM. All patients with HCM should have an exercise test to look for this, and it should be repeated periodically.
- MRI– fibrosis is associated with a worse prognosis.

Prognosis
For the majority of patients, HCM carries a relatively benign prognosis. Approximately 90% will be asymptomatic at diagnosis and most will remain so long-term.

Patients who present with symptoms generally experience slow progression of symptoms over time.

Children who are diagnosed when they are under 14 years of age have a poor prognosis and a high incidence of sudden death.

Adults have a better prognosis, but they also have a higher sudden cardiac death rate than the general population.

CLINICAL NOTE

Features that increase the risk of sudden cardiac death are:
- Genetic – first-degree relative with sudden cardiac death at a young age, certain high-risk genetic mutations.
- Clinical – non-sustained VT or history of syncope or previous arrest.
- Haemodynamic – exercise-related fall in blood pressure or presence of obstruction.
- Structural – extreme LV hypertrophy (≥30 mm)
ICDs are often recommended in patients with 2 or more risk factors.

Another outcome is progressive cardiac failure with cardiac dilatation. This carries a poor prognosis and a high mortality rate after symptoms of heart failure develop. Risk factors for cardiac failure in HCM patients include young age at diagnosis, severe symptoms, large left ventricular cavity and family history of advanced cardiac failure.

AF is common (seen in roughly 20% of adult patients) and often tolerated poorly. The presence of AF is a poor prognostic marker due to the increased risk of death from heart failure.

Pharmacological treatments
As with AS, vasodilators should be avoided because they worsen the gradient across the obstruction. Therefore, patients who have HCM should not receive nitrates.

β-Blockers (β-adrenoceptor antagonists) are used because their negative inotropic effect acts to decrease the contractility of the hypertrophied septum and reduces the

outflow tract obstruction. Disopyramide may be used in combination or alone to treat obstruction – it is a negative inotrope that reduces myocardial contractility and as a result reduces resting pressure gradients and improves symptoms. Verapamil or diltiazem may be given in symptomatic HCM in the absence of obstruction. Antiarrhythmic agents are important in patients with documented arrhythmias. Amiodarone or sotalol may be used for AF (along with anticoagulation).

COMMUNICATION

Patients should be advised that first-degree relatives should be screened with a transthoracic echocardiogram and undergo gene testing in cases of dilated or hypertrophic cardiomyopathy as these are often hereditary.

Non-pharmacological treatments
These include:

- Device therapy – dual chamber pacing to reduce the outflow gradient may be considered in selected patients. An implantable cardioverter defibrillator (ICD) should be considered in patients at high risk of sudden cardiac death.
- Percutaneous treatment (alcohol septal ablation) – alcohol can be injected down the septal branch of the left anterior descending coronary artery, causing necrosis of the myocardial tissue that gives rise to the obstruction.
- Surgery – a myomectomy is performed on the abnormal septum. This is the treatment of choice if other cardiac structural abnormalities need surgical correction.
- Cardiac transplant – may be necessary in patients with advanced heart failure.

Restrictive cardiomyopathy
Restrictive cardiomyopathy is an uncommon cause of cardiomyopathy in developed countries where most cases of restrictive cardiomyopathy are a variant of HCM – first-degree relatives may have classical HCM.

In this condition, the ventricular walls are excessively stiff and impede ventricular filling; therefore, end-diastolic pressure is increased. The systolic function of the ventricle is often normal.

Presentation is identical to that of constrictive pericarditis, but the two must be differentiated because pericardial constriction can be treated with surgery.

Possible causes of restrictive cardiomyopathy include:

- Idiopathic – no particular cause identified.
- Infiltrative diseases – such as amyloidosis (most common cause), sarcoidosis and haemochromatosis.

- Numerous other rare conditions including scleroderma, glycogen storage diseases, endomyocardial fibrosis, hypereosinophilic syndrome, etc.

Clinical features

The main features are:

- Dyspnoea and fatigue due to poor cardiac output.
- Peripheral oedema and ascites.
- Elevated jugular venous pressure (JVP) with a positive Kussmaul sign (increase in JVP during inspiration).

Management

There is no specific treatment and the condition usually progresses towards death relatively quickly; most patients do not survive beyond 10 years after diagnosis. Treatment focuses on management of causative conditions (if identified) and heart failure treatments.

Arrhythmogenic right-ventricular cardiomyopathy

ARVC is a rare condition characterized by fibrofatty replacement of the myocardium, particularly in the right ventricular free wall. The main problem that this causes is heart rhythm disturbance, ranging from ectopic beats to sustained ventricular arrhythmias, and even sudden cardiac death. There may also be impairment of right ventricular function.

Patients present with palpitation, syncope, heart failure or sudden death. Characteristic features are often seen on cardiac MRI.

There is no curative treatment, so management is aimed at preventing complications. This includes the use of ACE inhibitors and diuretics for the treatment of heart failure, antiarrhythmic agents and consideration of ICD implantation in patients at high risk of sudden cardiac death.

Takotsubo cardiomyopathy

'Takotsubo' cardiomyopathy is named after a type of Japanese octopus pot, which resembles the characteristic shape of the left ventricle in this condition (Figs 17.3

Fig. 17.4 Takotsubo cardiomyopathy seen during angiography. Note how the contrast demonstrates the unusual shape of the left ventricle.

and 17.4). Typically, the apex dilates ('ballooning'), with the rest of the ventricle spared, though mid- and basal versions have been described.

The cardiomyopathy frequently presents after a stressful event, most commonly in a post-menopausal woman, and patients may complain of chest pain or shortness of breath, with ischaemic ECG changes. After the initial presentation (which may be life-threatening) the prognosis is usually good, with full resolution of the cardiomyopathy in weeks or months. A small proportion die acutely of arrhythmia (generally torsades de pointes due to QT prolongation) or cardiogenic shock. The disease may recur.

Left ventricular non-compaction cardiomyopathy

LVNC cardiomyopathy is a rare condition caused by abnormal development of the left ventricular myocardium. This condition is characterized by prominent left ventricular trabeculae and deep intertrabecular recesses.

Symptoms are variable and, when they occur, are generally due to non-compaction impacting upon left ventricular systolic function or due to arrhythmia (and potentially sudden cardiac death).

This is a relatively newly identified condition and prognosis is therefore unclear at present. There are no specific targeted treatments.

DISEASES OF THE PERICARDIUM

The pericardium forms a strong protective sac around the heart. It is composed of an outer fibrous and an inner serosal

Takotsubo cardiomyopathy

aortic root

apical dilatation of left ventricle

Fig. 17.3 Takotsubo cardiomyopathy. Sudden weakening of the myocardium results in ballooning of the left ventricular apex to take on a shape resembling a Japanese octopus pot.

layer with approximately 50 mL of pericardial fluid between these in the healthy state. The main clinical conditions affecting the pericardium and the pericardial space are:

- Pericarditis – inflammation of the pericardium.
- Pericardial effusion – increased fluid in the pericardial space.

Pericarditis

Acute pericarditis is more common (history of less than 6 weeks) but pericarditis can in some cases be chronic and have a clinical course that runs over many months. There is a wide differential for patients presenting with pericarditis (Table 17.2).

Clinical features

History

The chest pain of acute pericarditis is usually central or left-sided pain that is sharp in nature and classically relieved by sitting forwards. Aggravating factors include lying supine, coughing or swallowing.

Dyspnoea may be caused by the pain of deep inspiration or the haemodynamic effects of an associated pericardial effusion.

Examination

The patient may have a fever and tachycardia.

A pericardial friction rub may be heard on auscultation of the heart. This is a high-pitched scratching sound (heard best with the diaphragm). It characteristically varies with time and may appear and disappear from one examination to the next. It occurs in both systole and diastole.

Investigation

Blood tests

A number of blood tests may be helpful:

- Full blood count, ESR and CRP – may provide evidence of active inflammation and also clues as to the underlying cause.
- Urea, creatinine and electrolytes.
- Cardiac biomarkers (e.g., troponin) – may be elevated, suggesting that the inflammatory process involves the myocardium (myopericarditis).
- Blood cultures.
- Antibodies for HIV, Coxsackie virus, Epstein-Barr virus.
- Autoantibody titres (e.g., antinuclear antibodies and rheumatoid factor).
- Antistreptolysin titres.

Electrocardiography

Superficial myocardial injury caused by pericarditis characteristically results in four stages of ECG changes (Table 17.3), although all four are only present in approximately 50% of patients. Some patients may be left with permanent ECG changes.

Other Investigations

Other investigations may be appropriate:

- Chest X-ray – may demonstrate enlargement of cardiac shadow. An enlarged, globular or 'flask-shaped' cardiac shadow can be a sign of large volume pericardial effusion. Pleural effusions can sometimes be seen.
- Echocardiography – useful if suspicion of pericardial effusion. May be normal in acute uncomplicated pericarditis.

Table 17.2 Causes of pericarditis.

Aetiology	Examples/Comment
Idiopathic	No specific cause is found in many cases of pericarditis.
Viral infections	Numerous causes – including Coxsackie virus, echovirus, Epstein-Barr virus, human immunodeficiency virus (HIV).
Bacterial infection	Numerous causes – including *Staphylococcus*, tuberculosis.
Fungal infections	Especially in immunosuppressed patients – including aspergillosis, histoplasmosis.
Rheumatological	Including systemic lupus erythematosus, sarcoidosis, rheumatoid arthritis.
Neoplastic	Both primary (e.g., sarcoma) and metastatic.
Pharmacological	Numerous causes – including hydralazine, procainamide.
Other	Variety of causes – including uraemia, mediastinal radiotherapy, myocardial infarction (acutely), post-myocardial infarction or peri-cardiotomy (weeks later, i.e., Dressler syndrome).

Table 17.3 ECG changes seen in pericarditis. Not all changes may be seen in every patient and time course may vary.

First few hours to 2 weeks	Widespread concave ST segment elevation (often present in all leads, except aVR and V1). PR segment depression is more specific for acute pericarditis.
1 to 3 weeks	Subsequently, the ST segments return to normal and T wave flattening occurs.
3 to several weeks	T waves later may become inverted.
Several weeks to months	Finally, all of the changes resolve and the ECG trace returns to normal

- Computed tomography (CT)/MRI – can be useful if diagnosis is unclear. Cross-sectional imaging techniques may demonstrate pericardial thickening >5 mm or presence of pericardial fluid.
- Pericardial fluid analysis – if large effusion present and pericardiocentesis carried out. Fluid can be sent for biochemical, microbiological and pathological analysis.
- Pericardial biopsy – rarely carried out but may be useful in recurrent or chronic pericarditis.

> **HINTS AND TIPS**
>
> A dissecting thoracic aortic aneurysm may occasionally present as acute pericarditis or a pericardial effusion. Therefore, be careful to look for a widened mediastinum on the chest radiograph and, if clinically suspicious, a computed tomography scan of the chest or trans-oesophageal echo (TOE) should be performed to avoid missing this diagnosis.

Management

Treat any identifiable underlying cause. Most cases of pericarditis are viral or idiopathic. The main aims of management are, therefore, analgesia and bed rest. Nonsteroidal antiinflammatory agents are the most effective for this condition. Colchicine may be useful and occasionally a short course of oral corticosteroids is required.

A pericardial effusion may be present. If large or causing tamponade, this can be drained. Analysis of the effusion may provide clues about the underlying cause of the pericarditis. Recurrence is rare but, if it does recur, colchicine or steroids will generally abort the episode.

Dressler Syndrome

Dressler syndrome is a syndrome of fever, pericarditis and pleurisy occurring generally 3 to 8 weeks after a cardiac operation or MI. It can occur only if the pericardium has been exposed to the blood. Antibodies form against the pericardial antigens and then attack the pericardium in a type III autoimmune reaction.

Patients present with fever, malaise and chest pain. They exhibit the classic signs of acute pericarditis; they may also have arthritis. Pericardial effusions are frequently seen, but cardiac tamponade is uncommon.

Chest radiography may show pleural effusions. Echocardiography may reveal a pericardial effusion.

Initial management consists of aspirin or nonsteroidal antiinflammatory agents; corticosteroids may be added if the symptoms persist.

Chronic pericarditis

Any cause of acute pericarditis can persist and lead on to chronic pericarditis. Some diseases, however, may result in chronic pericarditis more commonly, including:

- Viral infection.
- Tuberculosis.
- Mediastinal radiotherapy.
- Mediastinal malignancy.
- Cardiac surgery.
- Auto-immune disease.

There are two main types of chronic pericarditis:

- Constrictive pericarditis.
- Effusive-constrictive pericarditis.

Constrictive pericarditis

Constrictive pericarditis occurs when the pericardium becomes fibrosed and thickened and eventually restricts the filling of the heart during diastole. Restricted filling of all four chambers of the heart results in low-output failure. Initially, the right-sided component is more marked, resulting in a high venous pressure and hepatic congestion. Later, left ventricular failure becomes apparent with dyspnoea and orthopnoea.

On examination, the signs of right and left ventricular failure are evident, but the ventricles are not enlarged. The most important feature in the examination of such a patient is the JVP, which is elevated. Kussmaul sign – an increase in the JVP during inspiration – may be evident. Another important feature of the JVP is a rapid x and y descent (quite difficult sign), the presence of which excludes cardiac tamponade. The heart sounds are often soft. AF is common.

Investigation of constrictive pericarditis is as follows:

- Blood tests – as for acute pericarditis.
- Chest radiography – heart size may be normal. There may be signs of a neoplasm or tuberculosis. Pleural effusions are not uncommon. Tuberculous pericarditis may be associated with visible calcification.
- Chest CT often raises the diagnosis with extensive pericardial calcification or thickening.
- Other imaging – echocardiography shows good left ventricular function.
- Cardiac catheterization – usually diagnostic, showing the classic pattern of raised and equal left and right end-diastolic pressures with normal left ventricular function on the ventriculogram.

The only definitive management is with pericardiectomy (surgical removal of part or the whole of the pericardium). Antituberculous therapy may be required if the underlying cause is tuberculosis and should be continued for 1 year.

Effusive-constrictive pericarditis

This is a rare variant of chronic pericarditis characterized by the presence of both pericardial effusion and pericardial constriction. It is not uncommon for these patients to present with evidence of cardiac tamponade or increased ventricular filling pressures.

Patients may present with a variety of symptoms, including dyspnoea on exertion, chest pain (or discomfort), syncope, light-headedness, palpitations, cough, lethargy, etc. Many patients will be asymptomatic until pericardial effusion is very large.

Patients may require treatment with repeated pericardiocentesis or pericardiectomy.

Pericardial Effusions

A pericardial effusion is an accumulation of fluid in the pericardial space.

Causes

Pericardial effusion can be caused by a number of different pathologies. Any cause of acute pericarditis may cause an effusion. Pericardial effusions may be classified based on the nature of the fluid in the pericardial space (Table 17.4).

Clinical features

Clinical features depend on the rate and volume of fluid accumulation.

A pericardial effusion may remain asymptomatic, even if very large, if it accumulates gradually (due to the pericardium having time to stretch). As much as 2 L of fluid can be accommodated without an increase in intrapericardial pressure if it accumulates slowly.

Cardiac tamponade describes the condition where a pericardial effusion increases the intrapericardial pressure such that it leads to haemodynamic compromise.

As little as 100 mL of fluid (or blood) can cause tamponade if it accumulates suddenly.

History

The only symptoms produced by a large chronic effusion may be a dull ache in the chest or dysphagia from compression of the oesophagus.

If cardiac tamponade is present, however, the patient may complain of dyspnoea, lightheadedness, abdominal swelling (due to ascites) and peripheral oedema.

Examination

The classic signs of cardiac tamponade are described by Beck's triad and include:

- Hypotension – due to low end-diastolic volume (and therefore stroke volume). If severe, then shock may be present.
- Muffled heart sounds.
- Raised JVP.

Other signs to examine for include:

- Pulse – tachycardia with low volume pulse.
- Pulsus paradoxus – exaggerated reduction of the blood pressure of >10 mmHg during inspiration. This in combination with a pericardial effusion is diagnostic of cardiac tamponade.
- Kussmaul's sign – a paradoxical rise in JVP during inspiration (raised intrapericardial pressure impairs right ventricular filling and results in impaired venous return to the heart).

CLINICAL NOTE

Pulsus paradoxus occurs due to increased venous return during inspiration filling the right heart and restricting left-ventricular filling (because the pericardium forms a rigid sac with limited space within). This results in a reduction in stroke volume occurring during inspiration and consequently, a drop in blood pressure.

Investigation

Investigation of pericardial effusions include:

- Electrocardiography – small voltage complexes with variable axis may be seen (electrical alternans is caused by the movement of the heart within the fluid).
- Chest radiography – the heart may appear large and globular.
- Echocardiography – reveals the pericardial effusion. Right ventricular diastolic collapse is a classical sign of tamponade.

Management

The pericardial effusion should be drained if it is causing haemodynamic compromise or may be drained to aid diagnosis. If the patient is in cardiogenic shock due to tamponade, then emergency needle aspiration (pericardiocentesis) should be performed, followed by formal drainage once the patient has been resuscitated. Aspirated fluid should be sent for biochemical, microbiological and pathological analysis.

Long-term treatment depends upon the underlying cause; a surgical pericardial 'window' may be required if effusion is recurrent.

Type of effusion	Examples
Transudate (<30 g/L protein)	Congestive cardiac failure, hypoalbuminaemia.
Exudate (>30 g/L protein)	Infection (viral, bacterial or fungal), immediately post-myocardial infarction and Dressler syndrome, malignancy (e.g., local invasion from lung tumour), systemic lupus erythematosus
Haemorrhagic (known as haemopericardium)	Malignancy, uraemia, aortic dissection, chest trauma, ventricular wall rupture, following cardiac surgery.

Table 17.4 Causes of pericardial effusions.

COMMUNICATION

Following drainage of pericardial effusion and prior to discharge from hospital, patients should be made aware of the symptoms they may experience should the effusion re-accumulate and to seek medical help should these symptoms occur.

Chapter Summary

- Cardiomyopathies are rare and presentation can be very variable – some patients may be symptomatic while others present with sudden cardiac death.
- Risk of sudden cardiac death is important to assess in patients with cardiomyopathy – some patients may warrant insertion of implantable cardioverter defibrillators (ICDs) if there is a high risk of arrhythmia.
- Genetic testing/counselling is important with inherited forms of cardiomyopathy.
- Myocarditis and pericarditis have numerous causes; treatment generally consists of supportive treatments and attempting to treat the underlying cause.
- Pericardial effusion can be acute or chronic – small volumes of pericardial fluid can cause tamponade if accumulation is rapid, whereas large volumes (up to 2L) may be relatively asymptomatic if accumulation is slow.
- The classic signs of cardiac tamponade are described by Beck's triad – hypotension, muffled heart sounds and raised jugular venous pressure.
- Cardiac tamponade is an emergency and warrants urgent needle aspiration (pericardiocentesis), followed by formal drainage of effusion.

Congenital heart disease

Congenital heart disease refers to cardiac lesions present from birth.

The embryological development of the heart is a complex process involving many coordinated steps. Defects arise if the process does not occur correctly. Congenital heart defects have an incidence of 6–8 per 1000 live-born infants. They may present in the first year of life, during childhood or remain asymptomatic for life.

There are a number of different congenital abnormalities, listed below in descending order of incidence:

- Ventricular septal defect (VSD).
- Atrial septal defect (ASD).
- Patent ductus arteriosus (PDA).
- Pulmonary stenosis.
- Coarctation of the aorta.
- Aortic stenosis.
- Tetralogy of Fallot.
- Transposition of the great arteries.
- Other congenital heart disease – e.g., pulmonary atresia, hypoplastic left heart or severe Ebstein anomaly with ASD.

CAUSES OF CONGENITAL HEART DISEASE

There are many different genetic and environmental factors that affect fetal cardiac development. Genetic associations with congenital heart disease include:

- Trisomy 21 – atrioventricular septal defect, ASD, VSD, PDA and tetralogy of Fallot.
- Turner syndrome (XO) – coarctation of the aorta, bicuspid aortic valve, partial anomalous venous drainage and aortic dilatation.
- Other chromosomal abnormalities, such as Patau syndrome (trisomy 13) and Edwards' syndrome (trisomy 18).
- A number of rare single gene mutations have been associated with specific defects, e.g., mutations in a gene coding for alpha-myosin heavy chain (a cardiac muscle protein) are associated with ASDs.

Maternal infection or exposure of the fetus to drugs or toxins may result in a number of congenital defects:

- Maternal rubella – in addition to cataracts, deafness and microcephaly, this can cause PDA, ASD and pulmonary valvular and/or arterial stenosis.
- Maternal alcohol use – may result in fetal alcohol syndrome which can cause a number of cardiac defects (especially septal defects), as well as microcephaly, micrognathia, microphthalmia and growth retardation.
- Maternal systemic lupus erythematosus – associated with fetal complete heart block (due to transplacental passage of anti-Ro and anti-La antibodies).
- Numerous other toxins/medications – e.g., thalidomide, lithium, etc.

CLINICAL NOTE

Patients with congenital heart disease may have other congenital abnormalities. The VACTERL association, for instance, describes the recognized association of the following conditions with one another:

- **V**ertebral abnormalities.
- **A**norectal malformations.
- **C**ardiac defects.
- **T**racheo-oesophageal fistula.
- **O**esophageal atresia.
- **R**enal anomalies.
- **L**imb anomalies.

SHUNTS IN CONGENITAL HEART DISEASE

When considering congenital disorders of the heart, it is important to visualize the pressure changes that occur in the cardiac cycle to work out which shunting mechanism and murmur occurs with each defect; this will for the most part allow you to understand the symptoms and signs that arise.

A left-to-right shunt results in oxygenated blood going from the left side of the heart to the right side of the heart, therefore will not cause cyanosis at birth. For example, in a VSD, the left ventricular pressure is greater than the right (due to its larger muscle mass), therefore blood will flow from left to right. This can result in increased flow and pressure in the right side of the heart and eventually pulmonary hypertension and right ventricular hypertrophy.

A right-to left shunt results in deoxygenated blood going from the right side of the heart to the left side of the heart. This commonly results in cyanosis early in life but also can result in paradoxical emboli – the situation where a venous thromboembolus (e.g., embolus from a deep vein thrombosis) can enter the arterial circulation and cause a stroke or other arterial thrombosis.

COMPLICATIONS OF CONGENITAL HEART DISEASE

Before discussing individual lesions, it is important to have a grasp of the significance of congenital heart disease. Lesions have effects depending upon their size and location. These include:

- Central cyanosis – defined as the presence of more than 5 g/dL of deoxyhaemoglobin in arterial blood. Central cyanosis can be caused by congenital heart disease due to the shunting of venous blood straight into the arterial circulation, bypassing the lungs.

This type of cyanosis does not, therefore, respond to increasing the concentration of inspired oxygen.

- Congestive cardiac failure – this occurs due to the inability of the heart to maintain sufficient tissue perfusion as a result of the cardiac lesion. This may occur in infancy (e.g., due to a large VSD or transposition of the great arteries), or in adulthood in less severe conditions.
- Pulmonary hypertension and Eisenmenger syndrome – discussed in detail later.
- Infective endocarditis – congenital heart disease may result in lesions prone to bacterial colonization. Appropriate antibiotic prophylaxis is occasionally considered where appropriate to prevent this – it is not needed with some lesions, e.g., ASD.
- Paradoxical emboli – venous emboli entering the arterial circulation via a right-to-left shunt.
- Aortic dilatation/dissection – certain defects such as bicuspid aortic valves may put patients at increased risk of aneurysm or dissection of the aortic root or ascending aorta.
- Sudden death – this may be due to arrhythmias (more common in these disorders) or outflow tract obstruction as seen in aortic stenosis.

HINTS AND TIPS

NOTES ON CYANOSIS:
- Central cyanosis is cyanosis of the mucous membranes of the lips and tongue. Patients with central cyanosis will generally also be peripherally cyanosed, however peripheries are generally normal temperature unless there is associated poor peripheral circulation.
- Peripheral cyanosis is cyanosis of the peripheries (hands, feet, etc.). Pure peripheral cyanosis will cause cold, blue hands and feet but no cyanosis centrally.

Pulmonary hypertension

This develops over time as a result of an abnormal increase in pulmonary blood flow due to a left-to-right shunt. This increased flow results in changes to the pulmonary vessels, with smooth muscle hypertrophy and obliterative changes. The pulmonary vascular resistance increases causing pulmonary hypertension.

The patient becomes increasingly dyspnoeic with the progression of pulmonary hypertension. Signs on examination include:

- Dominant a wave in the jugular venous pulse.
- Palpable and loud pulmonary component of second heart sound.

- Ejection systolic murmur in pulmonary area due to increased flow.
- Right ventricular heave.
- Tricuspid regurgitation if the right ventricle dilates.

Echocardiography allows assessment of the pulmonary pressures. This is vital because the shunt should be corrected before significant pulmonary hypertension develops.

Eisenmenger syndrome

Eventually, as pulmonary hypertension progresses, pulmonary pressure exceeds systemic pressure causing reversal of a left-to-right shunt, resulting in a syndrome of cyanotic heart disease called Eisenmenger syndrome (Fig. 18.1).

Dyspnoea is usually relatively mild considering the profound hypoxia these patients have (oxygen saturations of 50% are not uncommon). There is no treatment at this late stage, save for combined heart and lung transplantation; therefore it is important to intervene early, before pulmonary hypertension and Eisenmenger syndrome develop.

> **HINTS AND TIPS**
>
> Cyanosis caused by pulmonary disease or cardiac failure improves on increasing inspired oxygen. Cyanosis caused by a right-to-left shunt bypassing the lungs does not improve on increasing inspired oxygen.

Complications include:

- Clubbing – develops in the fingers and toes (can be just in toes when Eisenmenger syndrome occurs with a PDA).
- Polycythaemia and hyperviscosity – with resulting complications of stroke and venous thrombosis. Regular venesection or anticoagulation may be necessary.
- Cerebral abscesses – especially in children.
- Paradoxical emboli – emboli from venous thrombosis may pass across the shunt and give rise to systemic infarcts.

These clinical features are also seen in patients who have cyanotic congenital heart disease (i.e., where the lesion results in a right-to-left shunt from the outset).

> **COMMUNICATION**
>
> Female patients with congenital heart disease should be counselled regarding the potential risks of becoming pregnant and, in appropriate cases, be referred to a specialist at a stage when they are considering starting a family.

LEFT-TO-RIGHT SHUNTS

Left-to-right shunts do not cause cyanosis at birth because all the blood is passing through the pulmonary circulation and being oxygenated. Cyanosis may result eventually if shunt reversal occurs (see **Eisenmenger syndrome**).

Atrial septal defect

An ASD is an abnormal opening in the wall between the right and left atria (Fig. 18.2). Blood moves from the left atrium to the right atrium due to the pressure gradient. ASDs are common, accounting for roughly 10% of congenital heart disease. However, ASDs are often not diagnosed early because they can be difficult to detect clinically.

There are three main types of ASD based on the location of the defect in the atrial septum (Fig. 18.3):

1. Septum primum (also called ostium primum ASD) – this defect lies adjacent to the atrioventricular valves and these are often also abnormal and incompetent.
2. Septum secundum (also called ostium secundum ASD) – the most common form of ASD, it is mid-septal in location.
3. Sinus venosus ASD – this rarer type of ASD lies high in the septum and may be associated with anomalous pulmonary venous drainage (where one of the pulmonary veins drains into the right atrium instead of the left).

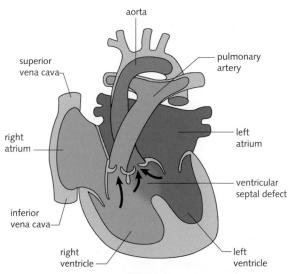

Fig. 18.1 Eisenmenger syndrome with ventricular septal defect. Patients initially will have a left-to-right shunt with ventricular septal defect; this has reversed due to pulmonary hypertension (and now flows from right to left). Less blood now reaches the pulmonary trunk and the patient becomes cyanosed. (Courtesy Lissauer T, Clayden G. *Illustrated textbook of paediatrics,* 2nd edn. London: Mosby, 2001.)

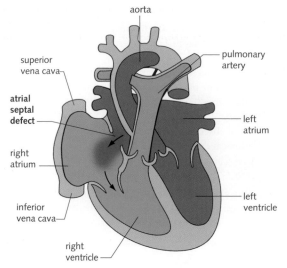

Fig. 18.2 Atrial septal defect. Note the flow of blood from the higher-pressure left atrium to the lower-pressure right atrium. (Courtesy Lissauer T, Clayden G. *Illustrated textbook of paediatrics,* 2nd edn. London: Mosby, 2001.)

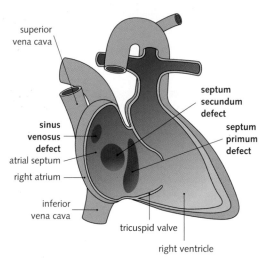

Fig. 18.3 Location of the three main types of atrial septal defect. The heart is viewed from the right side. The right atrial and ventricular walls have been omitted to reveal the septum.

The magnitude of the left-to-right shunt seen in ASD depends upon the size of the defect and also the relative pressures on the left and right sides of the heart.

History

In early life, patients are usually asymptomatic. In adult life, however, symptoms of dyspnoea, fatigue and recurrent chest infections can occur. As time goes by, the increased pulmonary blood flow can result in pulmonary hypertension and eventually reversal of the shunt and

Eisenmenger syndrome. Supraventricular arrhythmias may develop later.

Examination

The findings on examination of a patient who has an ASD (Fig. 18.4) depend upon the following factors:

- Size of the ASD.
- Presence of pulmonary hypertension.
- Presence of shunt reversal.

The second heart sound is widely split because closure of the pulmonary valve is delayed due to increased pulmonary blood flow. The splitting is fixed in relation to respiration because the communication between the atria prevents the normal pressure differential between right and left sides that occurs during respiration.

The increased pulmonary blood flow causes a mid-systolic pulmonary flow murmur.

If pulmonary hypertension has developed, there is reduction of the left-to-right shunt and the pulmonary flow murmur disappears; instead, there is a loud pulmonary component to the second heart sound because the increased pressure causes the pulmonary valve to slam shut.

Patients may later develop Eisenmenger syndrome.

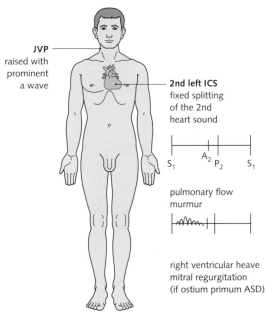

Fig. 18.4 Possible physical findings in a patient with an atrial septal defect (ASD). If the ASD is large and there is pulmonary hypertension, check for loud P_2 at the second left intercostal space (ICS) and for prominent right ventricular heave. If there is shunt reversal, you may find clubbing, central cyanosis and signs of congestive cardiac failure. A_2, aortic component of second heart sound; JVP, jugular venous pressure; P_2, pulmonary component of second heart sound; S_1, first heart sound.

Investigation

Investigation includes:

- Electrocardiography – patients with ostium secundum ASD usually have right axis deviation. Those who have an ostium primum defect usually have left axis deviation.
- Chest radiography – the pulmonary artery may appear dilated with prominent branches. There may be enlargement of the right atrium seen at the right heart border and enlargement of the right ventricle causes rounding of the left heart border.
- Echocardiography – the right side of the heart and the pulmonary artery may be dilated. The ASD may be directly visualized and a jet of blood may be seen passing through it. Associated mitral or tricuspid valve incompetence may be seen.
- Cardiac catheterization – The ASD can be demonstrated by passing a catheter across it. Oxygen saturations can be measured at locations throughout the right side of the heart and this can be used to calculate the size of the shunt, which helps determine whether operative correction is required.
- Magnetic resonance imaging (MRI) – offers excellent image quality and haemodynamic data without the use of ionising radiation.

Management

If there are signs of congestive cardiac failure, diuretics and angiotensin-converting enzyme (ACE) inhibitors may be of benefit.

The primary aim in these patients is to diagnose and evaluate severity of the ASD early, and repair the defect (if necessary) before pulmonary hypertension occurs. Once the patient has developed pulmonary hypertension, repair does not stop its deterioration. All ASDs with pulmonary to systemic flow ratios exceeding 1.5:1 should be repaired. Operative closure requires cardiopulmonary bypass and involves a median sternotomy scar.

Most ASDs are amenable to percutaneous closure, dependent on location and size. A device with two deformable discs connected by a narrow waist is inserted across the septal defect – this is introduced via a catheter inserted into the femoral vein and advanced up to the heart.

Patent foramen ovale

Around 25% of the population have a patent foramen ovale (PFO), which is a remnant of the fetal circulation that allows blood to bypass the lungs. In the remaining 75%, the foramen ovale closes with the increase in left atrial pressure that occurs during the neonate's first breaths. If present, a PFO may allow blood to cross (shunt) to the left atrium at all times, or sometimes only during Valsalva.

If a patient with venous thromboembolism has a PFO, then there is theoretically a risk of embolus crossing from the right atrium to the left atrium (as with an ASD or VSD) and potentially causing an arterial embolism, e.g., an ischaemic stroke if the embolus travels to the brain.

Stroke of unknown aetiology in a young patient with a PFO may be an indication to undergo percutaneous device closure to prevent further paradoxical emboli, although the evidence is not clear on the benefits of such a strategy. It has also been suggested that PFO might be associated with migraine, though trials of closure have had mixed results.

Ventricular septal defect

A VSD is a failure of fusion of the interventricular septum (Fig. 18.5). Blood shunts through a hole in the interventricular septum down the pressure gradient from the left ventricle to the right ventricle.

The ventricular septum is made up of two main components:

1. The membranous septum – situated high in the septum and relatively small. This is the most common site for a VSD.
2. The muscular septum – this is lower and defects here may be multiple.

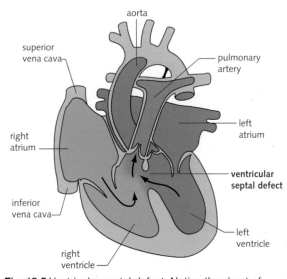

Fig. 18.5 Ventricular septal defect. Notice the shunt of blood from the left ventricle to the right ventricle. This results in oxygenated blood from the left ventricle re-entering the pulmonary circulation. (Courtesy Lissauer T, Clayden G. *Illustrated textbook of paediatrics,* 2nd edn. London: Mosby, 2001.)

History

In the neonate, a small VSD will be asymptomatic but a large VSD may result in the development of left ventricular failure (LVF). The signs of LVF in a neonate are as follows:

- Failure to thrive, feeding difficulties and sweating on feeding.
- Tachypnoea and intercostal recession.
- Hepatomegaly.

The adult who has a VSD may be asymptomatic or may present with dyspnoea due to pulmonary hypertension or Eisenmenger syndrome.

Examination

The findings on examination of a patient who has a VSD (Fig. 18.6) vary according to the following criteria:

1. Size of the VSD – a small VSD causes a loud pansystolic murmur that radiates to the apex and axilla. A very large VSD causes a less loud pansystolic murmur but may be associated with signs of left ventricular and right ventricular hypertrophy.
2. Presence of pulmonary hypertension.
3. Presence of shunt reversal.

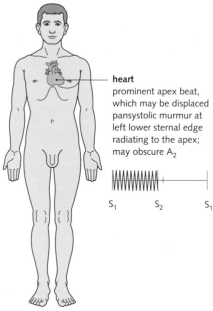

heart
prominent apex beat, which may be displaced pansystolic murmur at left lower sternal edge radiating to the apex; may obscure A_2

S_1 S_2 S_1

Fig. 18.6 Possible physical findings in a patient with a ventricular septal defect (VSD). If the VSD is large, the apex is displaced and pulmonary hypertension can develop. This results in a loud P_2 (pulmonary component of second heart sound) and right ventricular heave. Eisenmenger syndrome might also develop, with clubbing, cyanosis and disappearance of the pansystolic murmur. A_2, aortic component of second heart sound; S_1, first heart sound; S_2, second heart sound.

Investigation

Investigation of VSDs includes:

- Chest radiography – this may show an enlarged left ventricle with prominent pulmonary vascular markings. Pulmonary oedema may be seen in infants.
- Echocardiography – used to assess the VSD's size and location, and can help to evaluate the effects on cardiac function.
- MRI – can be used if further assessment is needed, or if the VSD is not well seen on echocardiography.
- Cardiac catheterization – can be used if further assessment is required, as with ASD.

Management

Approximately 30% of cases close spontaneously, most of these by 3 years of age. Some do not close until 10 years of age. Defects near the valve ring or near the outlet of the ventricle do not usually close. Patients should be treated at an early stage to avoid development of pulmonary hypertension and Eisenmenger syndrome.

Operative closure is the treatment of choice (if there is a significant left-to-right shunt) and is recommended for all lesions that have not undergone spontaneous closure. Some small lesions are managed conservatively; such patients have loud pansystolic murmurs (and may be seen in OSCE exams)!

Patients with VSDs may be at higher risk of developing infective endocarditis but routine antibiotic prophylaxis is no longer recommended.

Patent ductus arteriosus

In the fetus, most of the output of the right ventricle bypasses the lungs via the ductus arteriosus. This vessel runs from the pulmonary trunk (artery) to the aorta, connecting just distal to the left subclavian artery (Fig. 18.7). The ductus arteriosus normally closes about 1 month after birth in full-term infants and takes longer to close in premature infants.

The factors that determine the nature of the clinical features are the same as in VSD and ASD (i.e., the size of the defect, the size of the shunt, the presence of pulmonary hypertension and the development of Eisenmenger syndrome).

A PDA is more likely in babies born at high altitude, probably due to the low atmospheric oxygen concentration. This lesion is also common in babies who have congenital rubella syndrome.

History

A small PDA is asymptomatic but a large defect causes a large left-to-right shunt and may lead to LVF with pulmonary oedema causing failure to thrive and tachypnoea.

Adults with undiagnosed PDA may develop pulmonary hypertension and present with dyspnoea.

In adults, reversal of the shunt may occur, with venous blood entering the systemic circulation. As blood enters

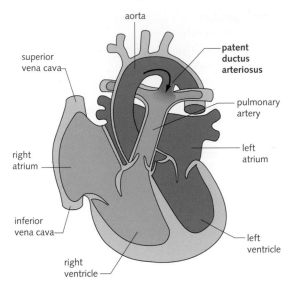

Figure 18.7 Patent ductus arteriosus. This allows mixing of systemic and pulmonary blood. Movement of blood within the ductus can occur in both directions depending upon the relative pressures in the aorta and the pulmonary trunk. (Courtesy Lissauer T, Clayden G. *Illustrated textbook of paediatrics*, 2nd edn. London: Mosby, 2001.)

below the subclavian arteries, this can result in cyanosis and clubbing of the lower extremities, whereas the arms remain pink. This is called differential cyanosis.

Examination

The classic findings in a patient who has PDA (Fig. 18.8) are:

- Collapsing high-volume pulses – this is due to the effect of the run-off of blood back down the ductus.
- A loud continuous machinery murmur heard in the second left intercostal space – a palpable thrill may be associated.

Management

The management of PDA involves two stages:

1. Pharmacological closure in neonates – indomethacin may induce closure if given early (by inhibiting prostacyclin production).
2. Operative closure – this can be performed as an open procedure where the PDA is ligated or divided. Alternatively, a percutaneous approach can be performed with the introduction of an occluding device via a cardiac catheter. Antibiotic prophylaxis is not routinely recommended.

RIGHT-TO-LEFT SHUNTS

These conditions will generally cause cyanosis from early in life.

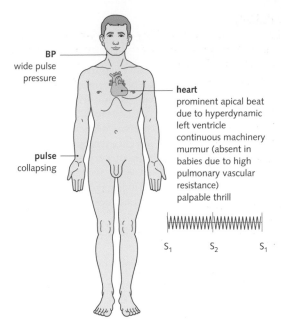

Fig. 18.8 Possible physical findings in a patient with patent ductus arteriosus (PDA). Patients with a large PDA have a loud pulmonary component of the second heart sound (P_2) due to pulmonary hypertension and the murmur is soft or absent. In those who have Eisenmenger syndrome, there is differential cyanosis and the toes are clubbed.

Tetralogy of Fallot

Tetralogy of Fallot (Fig. 18.9) is a congenital heart condition where the following four defects are seen:

1. Large VSD.
2. Pulmonary stenosis.
3. Right ventricular hypertrophy.
4. Aorta overriding the interventricular septum.

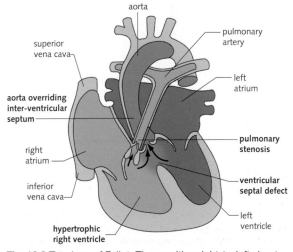

Fig. 18.9 Tetralogy of Fallot. The resulting right-to-left shunt causes cyanosis. (Courtesy Lissauer T, Clayden G. *Illustrated textbook of paediatrics*, 2nd edn. London: Mosby, 2001.)

Clinical features

Most children present within the first year of life with the following features:

- Central cyanosis (progressive hypoxaemia is the main feature and may not be present in the neonate if right ventricular pressure has not yet exceeded left ventricular pressure).
- 'Tet spells' and reduced exercise tolerance – intermittent cyanosis (and even syncope in some cases) can occur, characteristically after crying or feeding, due to increase in right-to-left shunt. Symptoms may be relieved by squatting or bringing the legs to the chest, which increases systemic resistance and reduces right-to-left shunt.
- Failure to thrive – difficulty feeding, behind on growth charts, etc.

Examination findings are described in Fig. 18.10.
After repair:

- Most patients are asymptomatic.
- Some may experience palpitations as patients are prone to arrhythmias.
- Some may develop exertional dyspnoea (reoccurrence of right ventricular outflow tract obstruction or pulmonary regurgitation).
- There may be signs of residual right ventricular outflow tract obstruction, pulmonary regurgitation or VSD if the repair is not complete.

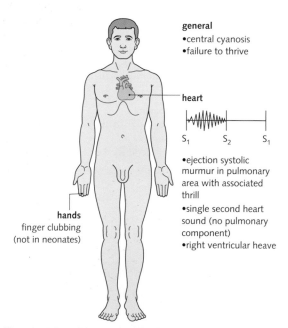

general
- central cyanosis
- failure to thrive

heart

S_1 S_2 S_1

- ejection systolic murmur in pulmonary area with associated thrill
- single second heart sound (no pulmonary component)
- right ventricular heave

hands
finger clubbing (not in neonates)

Fig. 18.10 Possible physical findings in a patient with tetralogy of Fallot. Central cyanosis may not be present in neonates if right ventricular pressure has not exceeded left ventricular pressure; finger clubbing takes time to develop and therefore is not seen in neonates.

Investigation

Investigations include:

- Blood tests – patients may be polycythaemic in response to prolonged hypoxia.
- Electrocardiogram – this may show signs of right ventricular hypertrophy.
- Chest X-ray (CXR) – may show a 'boot shaped heart' due to right ventricular hypertrophy and a small pulmonary artery.
- Echocardiogram – visualization of abnormal anatomical features of tetralogy.

Management

Corrective surgery is required, with total correction the treatment of first choice. Surgery can be carried out at an early age (starting at 4–6 months). In very young infants with severe pulmonary atresia, a palliative operation (Blalock-Taussig shunt) may be undertaken to increase pulmonary flow. This is usually done by creating an anastomosis from the subclavian artery to the pulmonary artery, with the intention that a definitive procedure can be carried out later.

Transposition of the great arteries

During development of the heart, the truncus arteriosus is divided by the aortic septum. This develops towards the proximal end of the truncus arteriosus, spiralling as it develops to meet what will become the ventricles. Transposition of the great arteries occurs when the truncus arteriosus develops normally but the normal spiral does not occur.

In complete transposition of the great arteries, the morphological left ventricle pumps blood into the pulmonary trunk and the morphological right ventricle pumps blood into the aorta, creating two closed systems (Fig. 18.11). There is usually also an ASD, VSD or PDA, allowing blood from the two systems to mix, otherwise this would be incompatible with life.

Clinical features

Symptoms are less severe in infants who have a large communication between the two sides.

Early cardiac failure and cyanosis are the most common presenting features.

Examination findings are variable and dictated by the nature of the communication between the two sides – whether it is the result of PFO, ASD, VSD or PDA and the size of this communication.

Investigation

Diagnosis is made through:

- Echocardiography – can demonstrate abnormal anatomy, including the anatomy of the coronary arteries. Can also readily diagnose any additional associated lesions.

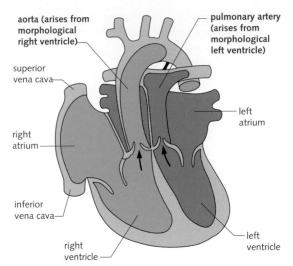

Fig. 18.11 Transposition of the great arteries. This is incompatible with life without a ventricular (VSD) or atrial septal defect (ASD) or a patent ductus arteriosus. (Courtesy Lissauer T, Clayden G. *Illustrated textbook of paediatrics,* 2nd edn. London: Mosby, 2001.)

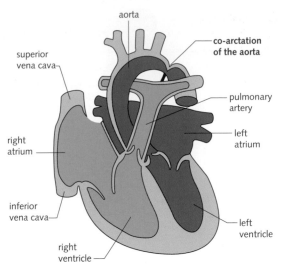

Fig. 18.12 Coarctation of the aorta, causing stenosis. (Courtesy Lissauer T, Clayden G. *Illustrated textbook of paediatrics,* 2nd edn. London: Mosby, 2001.)

- Cardiac catheterization – can provide additional information if echocardiography imaging is insufficient, e.g., as part of surgical planning.
- Cardiac MRI – can provide additional information and direct three-dimensional (3D) reconstruction of abnormal anatomy if required.
- CXR – not diagnostic but can demonstrate abnormal cardiac contour (classically described as an 'egg on a string').

Management

Management involves:

- Use of prostaglandin E1 to prevent postnatal closure of ductus arteriosus if this is the communication between the two sides.
- Operative management – surgical correction of the transposition is the definitive treatment. In some patients, arterial switch is not possible and an atrial switch operation is carried out instead. An operative procedure to create a large ASD may provide benefit in the short term while awaiting definitive corrective surgery.

OBSTRUCTIVE CONGENITAL DEFECTS

Coarctation of the aorta

In this condition, there is a congenital narrowing of the aorta, usually beyond the left subclavian artery around the area of the ductus arteriosus (Fig. 18.12). There are two main types:

1. Infantile type – this presents soon after birth with heart failure.
2. Adult type – the obstruction develops more gradually and presents in early adulthood. This type is associated with a high incidence of bicuspid aortic valve.

An adaptive response to the coarctation develops in those patients who do not present in infancy. This involves the development of collateral blood vessels, which divert blood from the proximal aorta to other peripheral arteries, bypassing the obstruction. These collaterals are seen around the scapula as tortuous vessels that can sometimes be palpated and as prominent posterior intercostal arteries that cause rib notching, visible on chest radiography. These collaterals take some years to develop and are rarely seen before 6 years of age.

History

Infants may present with failure to thrive and tachypnoea secondary to LVF. Alternatively, coarctation may present as rapid severe cardiac failure with the infant in extremis.

Adults whose condition is not diagnosed in childhood may present with:

- Hypertension diagnosed at routine medical testing – always consider in the young patient with hypertension.
- Symptoms of leg claudication.
- LVF.
- Subarachnoid haemorrhage – due to the association with berry aneurysm.
- Angina pectoris due to premature heart disease.

Examination

The physical findings in patients who have coarctation of the aorta are shown in Fig. 18.13. Check for:

- Blood pressure – it is important to take blood pressure in both arms whenever performing the cardiovascular

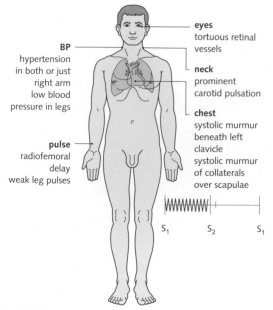

BP
hypertension
in both or just
right arm
low blood
pressure in legs

pulse
radiofemoral
delay
weak leg pulses

eyes
tortuous retinal
vessels

neck
prominent
carotid pulsation

chest
systolic murmur
beneath left
clavicle
systolic murmur
of collaterals
over scapulae

S_1 S_2 S_1

Fig. 18.13 Possible physical findings in a patient with coarctation of the aorta. If the coarctation is severe, there may be a continuous murmur beneath the left clavicle and signs of left ventricular failure (bilateral basal crepitations and audible third heart sound).

examination. Aortic dissection and coarctation both cause a pressure differential between the arms if the obstruction is proximal to the left subclavian artery. The blood pressure in the legs is also lower than in the arms.

- Radiofemoral delay and weak leg pulses – it is important to always look for radiofemoral delay because it is diagnostic of this condition.
- A heaving displaced apex beat due to left ventricular hypertrophy.
- Murmurs – the coarctation may cause a systolic murmur (or a continuous murmur if the narrowing is very tight). This is located below the left clavicle. The collaterals cause an ejection systolic murmur that can be heard over the scapulae. There may be a murmur associated with a bicuspid aortic valve, which is ejection systolic in nature and is located over the aortic area.

Investigation

Investigation of coarctation includes:

- Electrocardiography – may reveal signs of left ventricular hypertrophy and often right bundle branch block.

- Chest radiography – rib notching might be seen in children over 6 years of age. (Because the first and second intercostal arteries arise from the vertebral arteries, there is no rib notching on these ribs.) The aortic knuckle may be absent or a double knuckle may be seen (made up of the dilated subclavian artery above and the post-stenotic dilatation of the aorta below).
- Echocardiography – the coarctation and any associated lesion may be visualized but imaging the thoracic aorta can be difficult even with a transoesophageal echocardiogram. Coarctation is associated with a number of other congenital abnormalities (e.g., bicuspid aortic valve, transposition of the great arteries, septum primum ASD, VSD and mitral valve disease).
- Cardiac catheterization – localizes the coarctation accurately and also provides more information on associated lesions.
- MRI – can provide 3D reconstruction of the coarctation and is a useful tool prior to treatment to correct the coarctation.

Management

First-line treatment is traditionally surgery to relieve the obstruction. There are a number of different procedures, including resection of the coarctation and end-to-end anastomosis repair, bypass grafting, etc.

Balloon angioplasty and stenting may be carried out as an alternative first-line treatment, avoiding the need for sternotomy and cardiopulmonary bypass; these techniques can also be used to treat coarctation that recurs after surgery.

Without correction, the prognosis is extremely poor and most patients die before the age of 50.

OTHER LESIONS IN CONGENITAL HEART DISEASE

The conditions discussed above are those most likely to be seen. There are, however a number of less common congenital cardiac abnormalities and these are detailed in Table 18.1.

Table 18.1 Other less common causes of congenital cardiac abnormalities.

Congenital cardiac defect	Anatomical abnormality	Clinical features	Management
Congenital aortic stenosis (acyanotic)	• Stenosis may be valvular (most common), subvalvular, or supravalvular. • Note: Williams syndrome – an autosomal dominant condition with hypercalcaemia and supravalvular aortic stenosis.	• More common in males. • The child may be hypotensive, dyspnoeic and sweaty. • Increased incidence of angina and sudden death. • Ejection systolic murmur heard in the second right intercostal space. • May be signs of left ventricular strain (heaving apex) or failure (S3, tachycardia and bilateral basal crackles).	• Operative correction of stenosis is the treatment of choice. • In very small infants, valvuloplasty may be preferred in the first instance.
Pulmonary artery stenosis (cyanotic only if severe)	• Stenosis at one or many points along the pulmonary arteries. • Note: associated with tetralogy of Fallot in some cases; also a complication of maternal rubella infection.	• If mild, the patient may be asymptomatic with signs of right ventricular hypertrophy (i.e., left parasternal heave) and a pulmonary ejection systolic murmur. • If severe, blood flows from the right side to the left through the foramen ovale and the child is cyanosed and dyspnoeic.	• Diagnosis is confirmed by echocardiography. • Pulmonary angioplasty may provide a definitive cure. • If there is a recurrence or the lesion is not suitable for angioplasty, the obstruction may be removed surgically.
Hypoplastic left heart (cyanotic)	• Underdevelopment of all or part of the left side of the heart – there is generally significant hypoplasia of the left ventricle, with atresia, hypoplasia or stenosis of the left-sided heart valves. There may also be hypoplasia of the ascending aorta.	• The child is often cyanosed at birth. • Heart failure occurs in the first week of life. • Echocardiography is diagnostic.	• Surgical treatment is the only option – this can be done with staged reconstruction or transplantation. The mortality rate is extremely high. • Use of prostaglandin E1 to keep the ductus arteriosus open while awaiting surgery.
Ebstein anomaly (cyanotic if associated with PFO or ASD – occurs in 50%)	• Apical displacement of the tricuspid valve into the right ventricle, tricuspid regurgitation, and 'atrialization' of the right ventricle. • Wide range of associated cardiac abnormalities. • Accessory pathway in 25%; high rate of arrhythmias.	• If severe, infants present with right heart failure and failure to thrive. • If moderate, may present in adolescence or adulthood with reduced exercise tolerance, palpitations, or heart failure. If right-to-left shunt present, may also present with cyanosis or paradoxical emboli. • Pansystolic murmur at tricuspid area, widely split S1 and S2 (due to RBBB). • If mild, may be asymptomatic.	• If intervention is required, tricuspid repair is preferable to tricuspid replacement.

● Chapter Summary

- Congenital heart disease is associated with a number of genetic conditions (particularly chromosomal abnormalities) and environmental factors (particularly intrauterine exposure to alcohol/drugs/other toxins and maternal rubella).
- Understanding the changes that occur in the cardiac cycle and which shunting mechanism occurs with each defect will aid understanding of how each condition presents.
- There are a number of complications associated with congenital heart disease (e.g., heart failure, arrhythmia, pulmonary hypertension, Eisenmenger syndrome and paradoxical emboli).
- Some conditions present with a left-to-right-shunt (e.g., atrial septal defect, ventricular septal defect and patent foramen ovale). These conditions are the most common types of congenital heart disease and the patient will initially be acyanotic.
- Left-to-right shunts can cause pulmonary hypertension and eventually shunt reversal (i.e., it becomes a right-to-left shunt). This results in deoxygenated blood entering the arterial circulation, causing cyanosis. This is known as Eisenmenger syndrome.
- The aim should be to identify and correct left-to-right shunts before pulmonary hypertension has developed. By the time Eisenmenger syndrome has developed, the maladaptive changes are irreversible – definitive treatment requires either a lung transplant with correction of shunt or a heart-lung transplant.
- Some conditions result in a right-to-left shunt from birth (or soon after birth), such as tetralogy of Fallot or transposition of the great arteries. Infants with these conditions will be cyanosed.
- Tetralogy of Fallot is the combination of a large ventricular septal defect, aorta overriding the interventricular septum, pulmonary stenosis and right ventricular hypertrophy.
- There are a number of methods of investigating congenital heart abnormalities but echocardiogram is one of the most important. It can provide the vast majority of information required when planning treatment.
- Some patients with congenital heart disease will require palliative surgery while planning or awaiting definitive surgery.

SELF-ASSESSMENT

Single best answer (SBA) questions

Chapter 1 Cardiac anatomy, physiology and development

1. During your cardiothoracic surgery attachment, the consultant asks about the mediastinum and its contents. Which of these link the mediastinal compartment to the contents correctly?
   A Anterior mediastinum – sympathetic chain.
   B Anterior mediastinum – trachea.
   C Middle mediastinum – oesophagus.
   D Posterior mediastinum – internal thoracic artery.
   E Superior mediastinum – thymus.

2. Which of the following statements regarding the coronary vessels is true?
   A From the coronary veins, blood drains into the coronary sinus and then into the right atrium.
   B In the majority of people the SA node and the AV node are supplied with blood from the left coronary artery.
   C The coronary arteries arise just distal to the pulmonary valve.
   D The left coronary artery usually gives rise to the posterior descending artery.
   E The right coronary artery usually gives rise to the circumflex artery.

3. Which of the following statements regarding cardiac myocytes is true?
   A They are longer than skeletal muscle fibres.
   B They are multinucleated.
   C They have a branched structure.
   D They never have the ability to generate a spontaneous action potential.
   E Troponin is contained within the thick filaments.

4. Which of these most accurately describes the circulation changes occurring after birth?
   A Pulmonary vascular resistance increases.
   B There is increased blood flow through the umbilical vessels.
   C The foramen ovale immediately closes and fuses between the two atria.
   D The ductus arteriosus closes and becomes the ligamentum arteriosum.
   E Foetal haemoglobin continues to be produced for 3 months.

Chapter 2 The cardiac cycle, control of cardiac output, and haemodynamic regulation

1. Regarding hormonal control of the cardiovascular system, which of the following statements is correct?
   A Angiotensin-converting enzyme is predominately found in the vascular bed of the gastrointestinal tract.
   B Antidiuretic hormone is released when a rise in osmolarity is detected.
   C Adrenaline is secreted from the adrenal cortex.
   D Adrenaline/epinephrine causes vasodilatation in skeletal muscle by acting on β_1 receptors.
   E Renin is converted to angiotensin I by angiotensinogen.

2. Which of the following is true of the baroreceptor reflex?
   A Baroreceptors in the carotid body are innervated by the glossopharyngeal nerve.
   B Constriction of cutaneous arterioles brought about by the baroreceptor reflex can be overcome by thermoregulatory changes in vascular tone.
   C Decreased loading of baroreceptors increases venous tone by reducing parasympathetic activity.
   D Increased stretch in the arterial wall causes a decrease in baroreceptor firing.
   E It is central to the long-term regulation of blood pressure.

3. A tall, thin 38-year-old gentleman attends the GP with progressive breathlessness on exertion and when lying down at night. He is noted to have a blood pressure of 185/68 mmHg, a heart rate of 55 beats per minute. What is the most likely cause of his wide pulse pressure?
   A Aortic regurgitation.
   B Aortic stenosis.
   C Cardiac tamponade.
   D Hypovolaemia.
   E Sepsis.

4. A 75-year-old lady attends her GP for some routine blood tests after feeling generally lethargic for a number of weeks. Her haematocrit is noted to be 0.61. Her blood tests were normal 6 months ago. What is the most likely diagnosis?
   A Acute myeloid leukaemia.
   B Asthma.

C   Cardiac failure.
D   High altitude living.
E   Polycythaemia rubra vera.

5. Which of the following cardiovascular reflexes results in an increased parasympathetic outflow and can be used to terminate supraventricular tachycardia?
A   Alerting response.
B   Baroreceptor reflex.
C   Chemoreceptor reflex.
D   Diving reflex.
E   Hepatojugular reflex.

Chapter 3 ECG interpretation

1. A 72-year-old man is brought into hospital after a fall and lying for 8 hours outside in the cold overnight. His observations on arrival include a temperature of 33.9°C, a heart rate of 48 beats per minute and a blood pressure of 104/56 mmHg. Which of these abnormalities might be found on the ECG?
A   Downsloping ST segment.
B   J waves.
C   Raised ST segment.
D   'Tented' T waves.
E   U waves.

2. A 56-year-old man with a history of hypertension and a smoking history of 40–50 pack years presents with a 6-hour history of central chest pain. His ECG shows 1mm ST elevation in leads II, III and aVF. What is the likely diagnosis?
A   Anterior ST elevation myocardial infarction.
B   Inferior ST elevation myocardial infarction.
C   Lateral ST elevation myocardial infarction.
D   Posterior ST elevation myocardial infarction.
E   Septal ST elevation myocardial infarction.

3. 32-year-old woman undergoes a period of cardiac monitoring as the result of a number of episodes of transient loss of consciousness. During the monitoring, the following arrhythmia is seen. What abnormality is most likely to be seen on the resting ECG?
A   Broad QRS complexes.
B   Delta waves.
C   Long PR interval.
D   Long QT interval.
E   'Tented' T

4. A 72-year-old lady is admitted to the acute medical unit following a fall at home. As part of the clerk-in process, an ECG is carried out. This shows a cardiac axis of −45 degrees. Which one of the following might cause this abnormality?
A   Chronic lung disease.
B   Left ventricular hypertrophy.
C   Pulmonary embolus.
D   Right bundle branch block.
E   Ostium secundum atrial septal defect.

5. A 75-year-old man is admitted to the respiratory ward with a lower respiratory tract infection. He has prominent Q waves on his admission ECG. Which of the following is true of Q waves?
A   In leads I and aVL, they suggest old inferior myocardial infarction.
B   They are always pathological.
C   They are usually transient.
D   They may suggest transmural myocardial infarction.
E   They are due to depolarization current towards the lead.

Chapter 4 Other common investigations

1. What is the gold standard investigation for assessing coronary artery disease?
A   Coronary angiography.
B   CT coronary angiogram.
C   Dobutamine stress echocardiogram.
D   Electrocardiogram.
E   Exercise tolerance test.

2. A 57-year-old male smoker with a history of hypertension and dyslipidaemia presents to the chest pain clinic with 3 months of exertional chest pain. This occurs predictably when he runs 3 miles (previously able to run 5 miles twice a week). His father had an MI aged 50 and his brothers have had MIs aged 48 and 59. His GP started aspirin, amlodipine, bisoprolol, and atorvastatin last week, with little improvement. What investigation is most appropriate
A   Coronary angiogram.
B   CT coronary angiogram.
C   Exercise ECG test.
D   Dobutamine stress echocardiogram.
E   Myocardial perfusion MRI scan.

3. A 24-year-old IV drug user is admitted with a 1-month history of fevers, night sweats and rigors. On examination, he has splinter haemorrhages, a raised jugular venous pressure (JVP), a pansystolic murmur and mild pedal oedema.

Which investigation below is most likely to give a definitive diagnosis?

A   Blood cultures.
B   ECG.
C   Chest X-ray.
D   Routine bloods.
E   Urine sample.

4. A 67-year-old lady was referred to the cardiology clinic when her GP incidentally found a murmur. She is in good health without any cardiac symptoms and still regularly goes country dancing. There are no known ischaemic risk factors. On examination, she has an ejection systolic murmur, but there are no signs of cardiac failure. ECG is unremarkable. Which investigation would be most appropriate?

A   Cardiac MRI scan.
B   CT coronary angiogram.
C   Echocardiography.
D   Exercise ECG.
E   MUGA scan.

Chapter 6 Chest pain

1. A 28-year-old male is admitted with sharp chest pain that is eased by lying down. An ECG showed ST elevation in all leads. What is the most likely diagnosis?

A   Pericarditis.
B   Pleurisy.
C   Pneumothorax.
D   Pulmonary embolus.
E   ST elevation myocardial infarction.

2. A 45-year-old male presents acutely unwell to the emergency department. He is pale and sweaty. He complains of chest pain going through to between the shoulder blades. He has a difference in blood pressure of 50/30 mmHg between left and right arms. What is the most likely diagnosis?

A   Acute aortic regurgitation.
B   Acute myocardial infarction.
C   Aortic dissection.
D   Pulmonary embolus.
E   Tension pneumothorax.

3. A 63-year-old male presents to the emergency department with chest pain 4 weeks after presenting with an ST elevation myocardial infarction (STEMI). He complains of a sharp pain that is worse on deep breaths and eased on sitting forward. Temperature is 38.1°C. ECG shows ST elevation in all leads. What is the most likely diagnosis?

A   Aortic dissection.
B   Dressler syndrome.
C   Further ST elevation myocardial infarction.
D   Pulmonary embolus.
E   Unstable angina.

4. A 45-year-old woman is admitted with chest pain and ST elevation in all leads of her ECG 1 week after a viral illness. What is the most appropriate treatment?

A   Aspirin 300 mg and clopidogrel 300 mg.
B   Ibuprofen.
C   Paracetamol.
D   Primary percutaneous coronary intervention.
E   Thrombolysis.

5. Which of the following statements regarding cardiac enzymes/biomarkers is correct?

A   A negative troponin at the time of presentation and 12 hours later excludes myocardial infarction.
B   A raised troponin (I or T) concentration is always due to myocardial infarction.
C   Creatine kinase, lactate dehydrogenase and troponin I are all raised in unstable angina.
D   If a patient presents 48 hours after onset of chest pain, it is too late to measure troponin.
E   Troponin is found in cardiomyocyte cell membranes.

6. A 36-year-old man presents with heavy central chest pain that started 1 hour after taking cocaine. He is a smoker, but has no other known atherosclerotic risk factors. He is pale and sweaty, but examination is otherwise normal. Anterolateral ST elevation is seen on the ECG, and troponin is positive. What is the most likely diagnosis?

A   Aortic dissection.
B   Myocardial infarction.
C   Myocarditis.
D   Pulmonary embolus.
E   Takotsubo cardiomyopathy.

Chapter 7 Breathlessness and peripheral oedema

1. Cardiovascular system examination is a common OSCE station in finals. Which of the following is true when examining the jugular venous pressure (JVP)?

A   A JVP with a vertical height greater than 2 cm above the manubriosternal angle is abnormal.
B   Gentle pressure over the abdomen elicits the hepatojugular reflex and causes a transient increase in the JVP.
C   The height of the JVP above the manubriosternal angle gives an estimate of right atrial pressure in mmHg.
D   The internal jugular vein should be visualized and is usually located just lateral to the sternocleidomastoid.
E   The patient should be lying flat with their head turned slightly away from the examiner.

2. A 72-year-old lady attends the cardiology clinic with isolated ankle swelling over the past year. She is not troubled by breathlessness. Her only medical history of note is hypertension, indigestion and migraine. She has been started on a number of medicines recently. She has an unremarkable echocardiogram that day. Which of her medicines is most likely to blame?
A Amlodipine.
B Bendroflumethiazide.
C Furosemide.
D Lansoprazole.
E Propranolol.

3. A 71-year-old lady presents with dyspnoea and a cough. Her only past medical history is hypertension and 2 previous myocardial infarctions. Her observations include a heart rate of 110 bpm, blood pressure of 96/64 mmHg, oxygen saturations of 91% on room air and a temperature of 38.6°C. She has increased airspace opacification at the left base on the chest X-ray. ECG shows new atrial fibrillation. What is the most appropriate immediate management?
A Antibiotic therapy as per local guidelines.
B Oral digoxin loading.
C Oxygen therapy, aiming for saturations 94%–98%.
D Intravenous fluid administration.
E Referral to cardiology for urgent assessment.

4. A 64-year-old gentleman presents to the hospital with a syncopal episode and ongoing dyspnoea. He has a sharp left sided chest pain that is pleuritic in nature. Pulmonary embolism (PE) is suspected. Which of these chest radiograph features is associated with PE?
A Bat's wing shadowing.
B Increased cardiothoracic ratio.
C Oligaemic lung fields.
D Kerley B lines.
E Upper lobe blood diversion.

5. A 74-year-old lady comes in to the emergency department complaining of breathlessness. She is distressed and tachypnoeic at 28 breaths per minute, but her other observations are normal. On examination her chest sounds clear and she has mild bilateral pitting oedema to the mid-shins. She has an arterial blood gas (ABG) which shows the following results (on room air):

$$H+ = 33\,nmol/L,\ PO2 = 13\,kPa,$$
$$PCO2 = 3.6,\ HCO3- = 25\,mmol/L.$$

What is the most likely diagnosis
A Acute left ventricular failure (LVF).
B Exacerbation of chronic obstructive pulmonary disease (COPD).

C Exacerbation of interstitial lung disease.
D Psychogenic hyperventilation.
E Pulmonary embolism.

Chapter 8 Palpitation

1. A 28-year-old man comes into the emergency department with palpitations and breathlessness. He has a past medical history of irritable bowel syndrome and brittle asthma. He has a heart rate of 180 bpm and ECG confirms a supraventricular tachycardia (SVT). Which of the following is an appropriate first line treatment?
A Rapid bolus of intravenous adenosine.
B Intravenous verapamil infused over 2 minutes.
C Ocular pressure.
D Defibrillation.
E Isoprenaline infusion.

2. A 64-year-old lady presents with a number of episodes of rapid palpitations over the preceding 4 weeks. Which clinical feature allows differentiation between atrial fibrillation and SVT?
A Association with chest pain.
B Irregularly irregular pulse.
C Normal resting ECG.
D Palpitations are less severe and less frequent.
E Precipitation by excessive coffee drinking.

3. A 75-year-old woman complains of palpitations. There are no visible P waves on her ECG. Which of the following conditions is associated with this ECG finding?
A Atrial fibrillation.
B Atrial flutter.
C Sick sinus syndrome.
D Third-degree atrioventricular block.
E Ventricular tachycardia.

4. On a routine ECG, a 67-year-old Brazilian man is found to have a prolonged PR interval. Which of the following is a common cause of this abnormality?
A ACE inhibitors.
B β-Blockers.
C Left bundle branch block.
D Pericarditis.
E Wolff-Parkinson-White syndrome.

5. A 46-year-old man presents to the emergency department with a collapse and a 30-minute history of sudden-onset palpitations. He is clammy, sweaty and looks unwell. ECG shows a narrow complex tachycardia. Which one of the following is an indication for urgent DC cardioversion?
A A blood pressure of 95 mmHg systolic.
B Central heavy chest pain.

C   A rate of >200 bpm.
D   Breathlessness at rest.
E   Peripheral oedema.

Chapter 9 Syncope

1. A 28-year-old female presents to the emergency department following a faint. Which of the following is the most classic feature of cardiac syncope?
    A   Gradual onset.
    B   Precipitated by sudden turning of the head.
    C   Rapid recovery.
    D   Residual neurological deficit.
    E   Warning symptoms.

2. A 71-year-old man is brought in by ambulance. He complains of a collapse and sudden-onset, severe 'ripping' pain in his chest and upper back. He looks pale and his systolic blood pressure is 100 mmHg in his right arm and 70 mmHg in his left arm. Auscultation of his chest is unremarkable. ECG shows ST depression and T wave changes in leads II, III and aVF. What is the most likely underlying diagnosis?
    A   Aortic dissection.
    B   Myocardial infarction.
    C   Pericarditis.
    D   Pulmonary embolism.
    E   Tension pneumothorax.

3. A 26-year-old man who is otherwise fit and well presents to the GP a couple of days after collapsing while playing basketball. It occurred suddenly and without warning symptoms. He recovered quickly and feels back to normal. This has happened to him twice in the past and his father and uncle have also had similar problems. What condition might be suspected?
    A   Acute coronary syndrome.
    B   Hypertrophic cardiomyopathy.
    C   Orthostatic hypotension.
    D   Takotsubo cardiomyopathy.
    E   Vasovagal syncope.

4. A 81-year-old lady who is on holiday presents to the hospital in the evening complaining of ongoing fast palpitations and a number of episodes of feeling faint that day (without loss of consciousness). She had been out at a party the previous night and has little recollection of events but does remember drinking alcohol. What is the most likely cause of her symptoms?
    A   Atrial fibrillation.
    B   Complete heart block.
    C   Ongoing intoxication.
    D   Sinus tachycardia.
    E   Ventricular tachycardia.

5. A 67-year-old lady presents to the hospital reporting a number of events of presyncope over the last few days. She had a non-ST elevation myocardial infarction around 3 months ago and was started on a number of medications following this, including aspirin, bisoprolol, ramipril and atorvastatin. Her blood pressure is 104/67 mmHg. ECG shows sinus bradycardia at a rate of 45 bpm but is otherwise unremarkable. Which of the following options is most appropriate initially?
    A   Insertion of temporary pacing wire.
    B   List patient for permanent pacemaker.
    C   Start digoxin for its positive inotropic effect.
    D   Treat bradycardia with intravenous atropine.
    E   Withhold bisoprolol and ramipril.

Chapter 10 Heart murmurs

1. A 45-year-old female is found to have a pansystolic murmur. Which of the following causes this?
    A   Aortic regurgitation.
    B   Aortic stenosis.
    C   Atrial septal defect.
    D   Mitral regurgitation.
    E   Tricuspid stenosis.

2. A 45-year-old lady presents with a fever. She has not had any recent illnesses. On examination, she has digital clubbing, and auscultation reveals a mid-diastolic murmur and a diastolic 'plop'. What is the most likely diagnosis?
    A   Atrial myxoma.
    B   Infective endocarditis.
    C   Mitral valve prolapse.
    D   Pericarditis.
    E   Rheumatic fever.

3. A keen medical student examining a patient on the ward palpates a tapping apex beat. What is the cause?
    A   Mitral regurgitation.
    B   Mitral stenosis.
    C   Left ventricular aneurysm.
    D   Left ventricular hypertrophy.
    E   Pericardial effusion.

4. A 35-year-old male presents with fever, clubbing, haematuria and a murmur. What is the most likely diagnosis?
    A   Haemolytic uraemic syndrome (HUS).
    B   Infectious mononucleosis.
    C   Infective endocarditis.
    D   Rheumatic fever.
    E   Tetralogy of Fallot.

5. Which of the following are correct with respect to the character of the arterial pulse?
    A   Collapsing pulse can be a feature of mitral regurgitation.
    B   Pulsus alternans is a feature of atrial fibrillation.

C   Pulsus paradoxus may be found in restrictive cardiomyopathy.
D   Radio-femoral delay occurs in atrial septal defect.
E   Slow rising pulse is a feature of aortic regurgitation.

6. At a neonatal check, the paediatrician hears a loud systolic murmur at the lower left sternal edge. The baby seems otherwise well. Which of the following is most likely to be the cause?
A   Acute mitral regurgitation.
B   Congenital aortic stenosis.
C   Hypertrophic cardiomyopathy.
D   Large ventricular septal defect.
E   Small ventricular septal defect.

7. A 25-year-old woman who is being investigated for exertional shortness of breath is found to have a pulmonary venous pressure of 48 mmHg on echocardiography. Which of the following is a feature of pulmonary hypertension?
A   Corrigan's pulse.
B   Heaving apex beat.
C   JVP not visible.
D   Mid-diastolic murmur.
E   Palpable second heart sound.

8. Which of the following is a correct association?
A   Continuous murmur – atrial septal defect.
B   Early diastolic murmur – aortic stenosis.
C   Mid-diastolic murmur – tricuspid regurgitation.
D   Pansystolic murmur – mitral stenosis.
E   Physiological splitting of the second heart sound – inspiration.

Chapter 11 Atherosclerosis

1. A previously fit 55-year-old male smoker presents with sudden onset central chest heaviness and breathlessness. Troponin is raised and ECG demonstrates sinus rhythm 55 bpm with new inferior T wave inversion. What is the diagnosis?
A   Pulmonary embolus (PE).
B   NSTEMI.
C   Stable angina.
D   STEMI.
E   Unstable angina.

2. The following patients have presented on a busy day in the emergency department. Which of these is most likely due to embolus rather than atherosclerotic plaque rupture?
A   A 45-year-old male smoker with a history of hypertension, type 1 diabetes and severe deforming rheumatoid arthritis, who presents with sudden severe central chest pain.

B   A 76-year-old man with previous ischaemic stroke and angina, with normal heart sounds and ECG, who attends with a suddenly painful left leg that is cold and pale.
C   An 82-year-old female smoker with sudden onset severe abdominal pain, nausea and diarrhoea. Pain is out of keeping with abdominal examination findings, cardiovascular examination is normal and CT demonstrates bowel ischaemia.
D   A 34-year-old lady with a new diagnosis of atrial fibrillation and ischaemic stroke.
E   A 63-year-old man with hyperlipidaemia and a strong family history of MI presents with change from predictable exertional angina to prolonged chest pain at rest.

3. A 62-year-old man with a history of hypertension, type 2 diabetes and intermittent claudication presents to A&E with a 1-hour history of crushing central chest pain. An ECG shows ST segment elevation in the anterior leads. Which of the following is likely to be responsible?
A   60% stenosis of the left main coronary artery by a stable atherosclerotic plaque.
B   Complete occlusion of the circumflex artery following erosion of an atherosclerotic plaque.
C   Complete occlusion of the left anterior descending artery following rupture of an atherosclerotic plaque.
D   Complete occlusion of the right coronary artery following rupture of an atherosclerotic plaque.
E   Severe anaemia.

Chapter 12 Risk factors

1. Which of these is an indicated therapy for primary prevention of ischaemic heart disease (IHD)?
A   Aspirin for a 30-year-old male with type 1 diabetes mellitus.
B   A statin for a 54-year-old male smoking 9 cigarettes/day, brother had MI aged 50, BP 140/78 mmHg, total cholesterol 7.0 and HDL cholesterol 1.1.
C   Amlodipine for a 48-year-old Caucasian male who smokes 5 cigarettes/day and has an ABPM of 162/91 mmHg.
D   A statin for a 54-year-old female who has never smoked, no family history of IHD, BP 140/78 mmHg, total cholesterol 7.0 and HDL cholesterol 1.1.
E   A β-blocker for a 30-year-old male with BP 170/90 mmHg.

2. Which of these would be most suitable for primary prevention in a patient with hypercholesterolaemia and a 23% 10-year-risk of a cardiovascular event?
A   Atorvastatin 20mg nocte.
B   Cholestyramine 4g daily.

C Niacin 1g.
D Pravastatin 20mg nocte.
E Simvastatin 20mg nocte.

3. A 56-year-old Caucasian lady visits her GP after she has a blood pressure reading of 186/98mmHg at her work medical. The GP repeats her blood pressure and it is 182/110 mmHg. She feels well and full examination including fundoscopy is normal. What should the GP do next?
   A Arrange ambulatory or home BP monitoring.
   B Bloods and urinalysis.
   C Send to hospital for an urgent assessment.
   D Start an ACE inhibitor.
   E Start amlodipine.

4. A 28-year-old Caucasian man has a BP of 198/110 mmHg on his mother's BP machine at home. He visits his GP and his BP is 224/126 mmHg. He says he is probably just more nervous today as he has been worrying about his blood pressure and has been having palpitations and headaches as a result. The GP notes that he has a background of anxiety and looks tremulous. It is difficult to visualize his fundi in a bright room with no blinds. What should the GP do?
   A Ask a detailed family history.
   B Bloods and urinalysis.
   C Send to hospital for an urgent assessment.
   D Start an ACE inhibitor.
   E Tell him it is likely due to anxiety, not to worry and to come back for a repeat BP.

5. Your colleague comes to you to ask you about a pre-operative ECG for a patient attending for elective knee replacement. She is 76-years-old with a background of hypertension for 30 years. She has never had any chest pain and currently feels entirely well. You cannot find any previous ECGs to compare. What do you advise?

A She has had a lateral MI in the past.
B She is having a heart attack.
C This demonstrates an electrolyte abnormality.
D This is a normal variant.
E This is likely due to hypertension.

6. A 54-year-old man with autism is diagnosed with essential hypertension by his GP. He has always been terrified of needles and does not wish to have regular blood tests. Which anti-hypertensive would be most suitable?
   A Amlodipine.
   B Bendroflumethiazide.
   C Candesartan.
   D Indapamide.
   E Ramipril.

Chapter 13 Stable angina and acute

coronary syndromes

1. Which of the following drugs should be used in the management of STEMI but not NSTEMI?
   A β-Blocker.
   B Thienopyridine derivative.
   C Recombinant tissue plasminogen activator (tPA).
   D Aspirin.
   E Glyceryl trinitrate.

2. A 68-year-old lady with central dull chest pain has a raised troponin and anterolateral T-wave inversion on her ECG. She has no past medical history or allergies and otherwise normal bloods. Which treatment combination would be given to reduce thrombus extension?
   A Aspirin and clopidogrel.
   B Aspirin, ticagrelor and fondaparinux.
   C Aspirin, ticagrelor and metoprolol.
   D Aspirin, clopidogrel and oxygen.
   E Clopidogrel, ticagrelor and tirofiban.

3. A 56-year-old man with a history of hypertension is complaining of central chest pain on exertion that resolves with rest. He is currently taking an ACE inhibitor for his hypertension and a salbutamol inhaler for asthma. His doctor makes a diagnosis of angina pectoris and wants to start him on a medicine to decrease frequency of angina attacks. His heart rate is 88 bpm and his BP is 140/85 mmHg. What would be the most appropriate drug for this patient?
   A Atenolol.
   B Digoxin.
   C Diltiazem.
   D GTN spray.
   E Nifedipine.

4. A 73-year-old lady presented 24 hours after developing chest pain, is diagnosed with an anterior STEMI and received percutaneous coronary intervention with standard medical care. She was a smoker but had no other risk factors. You see her in clinic 3 months later. She has not had any further chest pain but tells you she has not been walking as far after the heart attack. On palpation of her precordium she has a slight rocking or dyskinetic cardiac impulse but examination is otherwise unremarkable. Routine ECG shows anterior Q waves and ST elevation, with no other abnormalities. What is the most likely complication?
   A Further ST elevation myocardial infarction.
   B Left ventricular aneurysm formation.
   C Left ventricular hypertrophy.
   D Pericarditis.
   E Ventricular septal defect.

5. An 81-year-old gentleman underwent percutaneous coronary intervention for an inferior NSTEMI 3 days ago. Whilst having breakfast, he suddenly collapses. He is found to have no pulse. CPR and airway management has been started by your colleagues and a resuscitation team is on its way. Which of the following is next most urgent?
   A Arterial blood gas (ABG).
   B Blood glucose.
   C Cardiac monitoring via defibrillator pads.
   D Portable chest X-ray (CXR) urgently.
   E Urgent bedside echocardiography.

6. A 74-year-old gentleman is admitted with a late presentation of inferior STEMI 3 days ago. He had been initially stable on the cardiology ward but has suddenly become breathless at rest. His oxygen saturations have fallen from 98% to 92% on air, and you start him on oxygen therapy. BP has fallen slightly to 110/75 mmHg. Examination reveals a quiet pansystolic murmur radiating to the left axilla, third heart sound and bilateral crepitations. There is nothing of note on the recent cardiac monitor trace, and 12-lead ECG demonstrates sinus rhythm at 99 bpm and anterior Q waves and T wave inversion. What is the most likely complication?
   A Acute mitral regurgitation.
   B Arrhythmia.
   C Myocardial free wall rupture.
   D Complete heart block.
   E Ventricular septal rupture.

Chapter 14 Heart failure

1. A 65-year-old man develops worsening ankle swelling and is found to have right ventricular failure. Which other clinical sign is most likely to be elicited on examination?
   A Bilateral basal crepitations.
   B Hepatomegaly.
   C Hypertension.
   D Mid-diastolic murmur.
   E Wheeze.

2. A 74-year-old male is admitted with shortness of breath. On examination, crepitations are heard up to the mid-zones. A diagnosis of acute left ventricular failure is made. Which of the following treatments would be started first?
   A β-Blockers.
   B Continuous positive airway pressure (CPAP).
   C Diuretics.
   D Morphine.
   E Oxygen.

3. A 72-year-old lady who is breathless on even mild exertion attends the cardiology clinic. Her ECG shows sinus rhythm with a left bundle branch block (LBBB) pattern and QRS duration of 155 ms. Echocardiogram shows severe left ventricular systolic dysfunction (LVSD). She is already on appropriate medications. Which of the following treatments is most likely to be considered?
   A Biventricular pacemaker.
   B Dual chamber pacemaker.
   C Left ventricular assist device.
   D Single lead atrial pacemaker.
   E Single lead ventricular pacemaker.

4. A 54-year-old man with heart failure develops diarrhoea and vomiting. Which of the following medications is it most important to withhold?
   A Amlodipine.
   B Aspirin.
   C Atorvastatin.
   D Bisoprolol.
   E Candesartan.

5. An 81-year-old-lady with worsening breathlessness is referred for an echocardiogram and diagnosed with moderate left ventricular systolic dysfunction. Which one of the following is classic of left ventricular failure?
   A Ascites.
   B Bilateral pitting peripheral oedema.
   C Dyspnoea due to poor pulmonary perfusion.
   D Nocturia.
   E Paroxysmal nocturnal dyspnoea.

Chapter 15 Arrhythmias

1. A 72-year-old man on the cardiology ward complains of palpitations and lightheadedness. An ECG is performed and a diagnosis of ventricular tachycardia is made. Which of the following is correct regarding

ventricular tachycardia?

A   It is a narrow complex tachycardia.
B   It should always be treated with immediate defibrillation.
C   It should be treated with atropine.
D   It is a life-threatening condition.
E   It may be caused by hyponatraemia.

2. An 81-year-old lady is prescribed digoxin for atrial fibrillation. Which of the following is correct regarding digoxin?

A   It acts to slow conduction of the sinoatrial node.
B   It is contraindicated in Wolff–Parkinson–White syndrome.
C   Its main route of excretion is by the liver.
D   It has a very short half-life.
E   Its effects are enhanced by hyperkalaemia.

3. A patient suffers a cardiac arrest whilst on the cardiology ward. Resuscitation is unfortunately unsuccessful. Which of the following are true regarding advanced life support?

A   Pulseless ventricular tachycardia(VT) requires an immediate synchronized DC shock.
B   Adrenaline is administered at a dose of 1 μg every 3–5 min of CPR.
C   Atropine is given in cases of PEA/asystole.
D   Pulseless VT/Ventricular fibrillation cardiac arrest has a better prognosis than asystole.
E   A defibrillator energy setting of 75 J should be used in the first instance for adults with ventricular fibrillation.

4. A 67-year-old male is admitted in extremis to the emergency department. His ECG shows a broad complex tachycardia. The staff are unsure whether this represents VT or SVT with aberrancy. Which of the following features/treatments are correct?

A   Concordance is present in VT.
B   Capture beats are present in SVT with aberrancy.
C   Fusion beats are seen in SVT with aberrancy.
D   Intravenous verapamil can safely be used to differentiate between the VT and SVT with aberrancy.
E   If in doubt, treat as SVT.

5. A 57-year-old man on the medical ward is struggling with his breathing. He has an elevated jugular venous pressure and crepitations bilaterally to the mid zones on auscultation. Blood pressure is 92/55 mmHg and his ECG shows atrial fibrillation at a rate of 160 beats/min. He was admitted for treatment of cellulitis and noted to be in sinus rhythm the previous day. Which of the following is the most appropriate initial management?

A   Oral bisoprolol and warfarin.
B   Oral digoxin.

C   Intravenous furosemide.
D   Intravenous amiodarone.
E   Urgent synchronized direct current cardioversion.

Chapter 16   Valvular disease

1. A 62-year-old woman is reviewed in clinic. She is known to have previous rheumatic fever. Which of the following is a feature of the disease?

A   It only affects mitral and aortic valves.
B   It is by far the most common cause of mitral regurgitation.
C   It is caused by valve infection with group B streptococci.
D   Requires antibiotic prophylaxis to prevent endocarditis.
E   Results in cusp and commissural fusion.

2. A 67-year-old man goes to his GP with exertional shortness of breath and chest tightness and is found to have an ejection systolic murmur. Which of the following is a feature of severe aortic stenosis?

A   Fixed splitting of S2.
B   Loud S2.
C   S4.
D   Thrusting displaced apex beat.
E   Wide pulse pressure.

3. A 45-year-old woman is found to have mitral stenosis on echocardiography. Which of the following is a feature of the condition?

A   A displaced apex beat.
B   A pansystolic murmur heard best at the apex.
C   An early diastolic murmur best heard with the diaphragm of the stethoscope.
D   An end-diastolic murmur best heard with the bell of the stethoscope.
E   Malar flush.

4. Which of the following statements is true regarding mitral valve prolapse?

A   Affects 0.1% of the population.
B   Frequently leads to severe heart failure.
C   It is always associated with mitral regurgitation.
D   It is associated with a mid-diastolic click.
E   More common in women.

5. A 63-year-old man is reviewed in the cardiology clinic. On examination he has a median sternotomy scar. Which of the following operations would fit with his scar?

A   Aortic valve replacement.
B   Closed mitral valvotomy.
C   Implantable cardiac defibrillator (ICD) insertion.
D   Mitral valvuloplasty.
E   Temporary pacemaker insertion.

6. Which is correct regarding causative organisms in infective endocarditis?
   A A negative blood culture rules out infective endocarditis.
   B Enterococci are very rare.
   C Fungal infections are common causes of infective endocarditis.
   D Staphylococcus aureus is associated with severe and destructive infection.
   E The most common causative organisms in developed countries are the Streptococcus viridans group.

7. A 74-year-old lady is admitted with a 2 week history of fever, malaise and progressive breathlessness. During assessment, findings include an ejection systolic murmur, an early diastolic murmur and bibasal crepitations. She had a prosthetic aortic valve replacement 4 years ago. Which clinical sign is most likely to be found on examination?
   A First-degree AV block.
   B Janeway lesions.
   C Microscopic haematuria.
   D Roth spots.
   E Splenomegaly.

8. A 28-year-old IV drug user is thought to have endocarditis. Which of the following is a minor criterion for the diagnosis of infective endocarditis?
   A Erythema multiforme.
   B Growth of Staphylococcus aureus in sputum culture.
   C IV drug use.
   D Prolonged QRS duration.
   E Vegetations visualized on echocardiography.

Chapter 17 Diseases of the myocardium and pericardium

1. A 63-year-old male presents to the emergency department with chest pain 3 weeks after presenting with an ST elevation myocardial infarction (STEMI). He complains of a sharp left-sided chest pain that is worse when lying flat. ECG shows ST elevation in all territories. What is the most likely diagnosis?
   A Aortic dissection.
   B Dressler Syndrome.
   C Further ST elevation myocardial infarction.
   D Pneumothorax.
   E Unstable angina.

2. A 32-year-old man with hypertrophic cardiomyopathy attends the cardiology clinic. He is thinking of starting a family and is asking about the risk of passing on the condition to his children. What is the most common mode of inheritance of hypertrophic cardiomyopathy?
   A Autosomal dominant.
   B Autosomal recessive.

   C Non-Mendelian.
   D X-linked dominant.
   E X-linked recessive.

3. A 32-year-old female attends the emergency department with sharp chest pain. Pericarditis is suspected. Which of these clinical signs is associated with pericarditis?
   A Clubbing.
   B Conjunctival haemorrhages.
   C Janeway lesions,
   D Pericardial rub,
   E Parasternal heave.

4. A man has been involved in a road traffic accident and is brought in by ambulance to the emergency department with suspected cardiac tamponade. What does Beck's triad of signs in tamponade consist of?
   A Hypoxia, decreased level of consciousness and impalpable apex beat.
   B Low arterial blood pressure, jugular venous distension and muffled heart sounds.
   C Poor capillary refill, tachycardia and decreased level of consciousness.
   D Narrow pulse pressure, exaggerated reduction in systemic blood pressure during inspiration and presence of gallop rhythm.
   E Raised jugular venous pressure which drops with inspiration, pericardial friction rub and impalpable apex beat.

5. A 58-year-old lady is admitted with chest pain, a week after the death of her mother. As part of the investigation of her condition she has an echocardiogram which shows ballooning of the left ventricular apex and a diagnosis of Takotsubo cardiomyopathy is made. Which of the following is true regarding this condition?
   A It carries a 30% mortality rate in the acute phase.
   B It is more common in young men.
   C It should be treated with fluid resuscitation.
   D It may be misdiagnosed as ST elevation myocardial infarction (STEMI).
   E It was first described in Japanese lobster fishermen.

6. A 24-year-old man is referred for an echocardiogram after attending the emergency department with chest pain. His ECG at the time showed changes consistent with left ventricular hypertrophy. Which of the following statements is true of hypertrophic cardiomyopathy (HCM)?
   A Disopyramide is contraindicated.
   B It does not present after the third decade.
   C It may be treated with percutaneous myomectomy.
   D Prognosis is better if diagnosed at an earlier age.
   E Obstruction occurs in a minority of patients.

Chapter 18 Congenital heart disease

1. A murmur is found at the 6-week post-natal check, and the GP wonders about congenital heart disease. Which of the following cardiac malformations is most common?
   A   Atrial septal defect (ASD).
   B   Ebstein anomaly.
   C   Patent ductus arteriosus (PDA).
   D   Tetralogy of Fallot.
   E   Ventricular septal defect (VSD).

2. A mother brings her 6-week-old baby boy to see her GP as she is concerned his lips, hands and feet look blue. Which of the following congenital heart defects causes cyanosis early in life?
   A   Atrial septal defect (ASD).
   B   Coarctation of the aorta.
   C   Patent ductus arteriosus (PDA).
   D   Tetralogy of Fallot.
   E   Ventricular septal defect (VSD).

3. A 62-year-old lady reports a 3-year history of worsening breathlessness to her GP. She is found to be significantly cyanosed and is known to have a ventricular septal defect. Which one of the following may be associated with Eisenmenger syndrome?
   A   Anaemia.
   B   Left-to-right shunt.
   C   Paradoxical emboli.
   D   Decreased pulmonary vascular resistance.
   E   Splinter haemorrhages.

4. A 28-year-old woman presents with sudden-onset left-sided weakness. As part of her investigations, echocardiography raised a suspicion of a patent foramen ovale (PFO). About a quarter of the population have a PFO. Which of the following may be associated?
   A   Left bundle branch block.
   B   Migraine.
   C   Mitral prolapse.
   D   Mitral stenosis.
   E   Right axis deviation.

5. A worried mother takes her 6-month-old baby to the GP as she is worried he looks blue. The GP hears a murmur and wonders whether this might be tetralogy of Fallot. Which of the following is true of this condition?
   A   Feeding improves symptoms.
   B   It includes patent ductus arteriosus.
   C   Left ventricular hypertrophy is a feature.
   D   Pulmonary hypertension is a prominent feature.
   E   Squatting helps ease symptoms.

6. A 38-year-old gentleman is found to have Ebstein anomaly on echocardiography during a private medical assessment. Which of the following describes Ebstein anomaly?
   A   Apical displacement of the tricuspid valve.
   B   Overriding aorta.
   C   Pulmonary stenosis.
   D   Right ventricular hypertrophy (RVH).
   E   Ventricular septal defect (VSD).

Extended-matching questions (EMQs)

Each option may be used once, more than once or not at all.

Chapter 1 Cardiac anatomy, physiology and development

Anatomy and physiology

A. BNP
B. Coronary veins
C. Endocardium
D. Epicardium
E. Mediastinum
F. Myocardium
G. Pericardium
H. Troponin

For each description below, choose the most appropriate structure or protein from the list given above.

1. A hormone that is secreted when the ventricles are stretched, and can be used to monitor heart failure.
2. A protein within cardiomyocytes, therefore measured in serum as a sensitive marker of cardiomyocyte injury.
3. Coronary arteries are contained within this layer of the heart.
4. Produces serous fluid to allow the heart to move smoothly.
5. This structure contains the heart and provides a passageway for other structures.

Chapter 2 The cardiac cycle, control of cardiac output, and haemodynamic regulation

Cardiac electrophysiology

A. L-type Ca^{2+} channels.
B. Voltage-gated K^+ channels.
C. Na^+/Ca^{2+} exchanger.
D. Na^+/K^+ ATPase.
E. Voltage-gated Na^+ channels.
F. Sarcoplasmic reticulum Ca^{2+}ATPase.
G. Ligand-gated membrane Ca^{2+} channel.
H. Gap junction.

For each description below, choose the most appropriate answer from the list given above.

1. Responsible for phase 0 of the fast cell action potential.
2. Responsible for the rapid conduction of depolarization between adjacent cells in the ventricular myocardium.
3. Acts to bring about relaxation of cardiomyocytes and removes the majority of the calcium from the cytosol.
4. May be abnormal in long QT syndrome.
5. Inhibited by digoxin.

Chapter 3 ECG interpretation

Components of the ECG trace

A. P wave.
B. PR interval.
C. Q wave.
D. QRS complex.
E. ST segment.
F. T wave.
G. QT interval.
H. U wave.
I. J wave.

For each description below, choose the most appropriate answer from the list given above.

1. Prolonged in bundle branch block.
2. Represents phase 2 (the plateau phase) of the cardiac action potential.
3. Represents ventricular repolarization.
4. May be shortened if there is an accessory pathway.
5. If prolonged increases risk of polymorphic ventricular tachycardia.

ECG leads

Each of the limb leads looks at the heart's electrical activity in a particular direction in the frontal plane. For each limb lead below, choose the answer that most corresponds to that lead with reference to the diagram.

1. I
2. II
3. III
4. aVF
5. aVL
6. aVR

Chapter 4 Other common investigations

CXR signs related to cardiology

A. Abnormal aortic contour.
B. Air bronchograms.
C. Continuous diaphragm sign.
D. Double density sign.
E. Kerley B lines.
F. Median sternotomy wires.
G. Water bottle sign.
H. Widened mediastinum.

For each description below, choose the most appropriate radiographic sign from the list given above.

1. Heart failure.
2. Left atrial enlargement.
3. Pericardial effusion.
4. Pneumomediastinum.
5. Previous cardiac surgery.

Chapter 5 History and examination of the cardiovascular system

Clinical Signs

A. Collapsing pulse.
B. Crepitations at lung bases.
C. Ejection-systolic murmur.
D. Elevated jugular venous pressure.
E. Janeway lesions.
F. Mid-diastolic murmur.
G. Osler nodes.
H. Pansystolic murmur.
I. Radiofemoral delay.
J. Roth spots.
K. Tendon xanthomata.

For each description below, choose the most appropriate clinical sign from the list given above.

1. Classically associated with infective endocarditis; the result of septic emboli in the skin.

2. Sign most classically associated with coarctation of the aorta.
3. Common examination finding in those with isolated left ventricular failure.
4. Classically associated with aortic stenosis.
5. Classically associated with aortic regurgitation.

Chapter 6 Chest pain

Causes of chest pain

A. Angina.
B. Aortic dissection.
C. Arrhythmia.
D. Boerhaave syndrome.
E. Indigestion.
F. Myocardial infarction.
G. Myocarditis.
H. Pericarditis.
I. Pneumonia.
J. Pneumothorax.
K. Pulmonary embolus.

For each description below, choose the most appropriate cause of chest pain from the list given above.

1. A 16-year-old with no past medical history is admitted to A&E with 1 day of chest pain and 3 days of progressive fatigue, exertional dyspnoea, and orthopnoea. During your systemic enquiry, he reports having had a flu-like illness 2 weeks ago which he felt was unrelated as it had already resolved. On examination, he has a mild tachycardia of 108 bpm, a tachypnoea of 22 breaths/min, a raised JVP, a 3rd third heart sound, and bilateral crepitations. ECG demonstrates sinus tachycardia with inferior T wave flattening, and troponin is mildly raised.

2. A 26-year-old gentleman has a 1 day history of severe vomiting, and presents with severe sudden onset central chest pain and breathlessness. On admission, he is tachycardic at 117 bpm, with otherwise normal observations. Examination reveals a dull left base, a left lateral rasping sound, and subcutaneous emphysema.

3. A 55-year-old gentleman who has never smoked presents to A&E at midnight with burning central chest pain. He reports it started 5 hours ago after a big dinner out with colleagues, and became worse when he went to bed. He has taken some Rennies on the way to the hospital, with some improvement.

4. An 80-year-old lady is admitted with breathlessness and sharp right-sided chest pain on inspiration. She was diagnosed with breast cancer 2 weeks ago. On examination, her left leg is markedly swollen and erythematous. Her oxygen saturations on air are

93%, and ECG demonstrates sinus tachycardia at 104 bpm.

5. A normally fit and well 34-year-old lady has just returned from a sun and alcohol-filled holiday, and has had 4 days of dysuria, loin pain, fever and rigors. She presents to the A&E with 2 hours of palpitations, chest pain, and lightheadedness. Her heart rate is 190 bpm and seems irregular, her blood pressure is 102/70 mmHg, and her temperature is 39.8°C.

Chapter 7 Breathlessness and peripheral oedema

Causes of oedema

A. Cardiac failure.
B. Hepatic failure/cirrhosis.
C. Hypoalbuminaemia.
D. Infection.
E. Medication-related.
F. Renal failure.
G. Venous compression or thromboembolism.

For each patient below, choose the most likely diagnosis from the list given above.

1. A 54-year-old man attends his GP with a 5-day history of left leg swelling and discomfort. He has recently returned from holiday in South America. He is otherwise well. His left calf is tender on palpation and he has pitting ankle oedema on the left side only.
2. A 49-year-old lady with a long history of intravenous drug misuse presents to the GP with nausea and swelling of the abdomen and legs. She reports lethargy and feeling itchy. She is icteric and has a number of large bruises on her arms.
3. A 66-year-old man attends the GP out-of-hours with bilateral ankle swelling and headache for the past couple of weeks. He reports he saw his own GP 1 month ago for 'an MOT' and was started on treatment for high blood pressure.
4. An 81-year-old lady presents with an approximately 4-month history of right leg swelling and abdominal bloating. Despite this, she reports approximately 2 stone weight loss over the past year. She has a past medical history of asthma, hypertension and previous breast cancer a number of years ago. Blood tests show a microcytic anaemia with a haemoglobin level of 98 g/dL, but no other abnormalities. An echocardiogram from 6 weeks ago showed good ventricular function and no valvular abnormalities.
5. A 72-year-old gentleman presents with a 6-month history of breathlessness on exertion and swelling of his lower legs. He is particularly troubled by breathlessness when lying down overnight and

has found himself waking up gasping for breath on occasion – because of this he is sleeping in his recliner chair and he finds this helps. He has bilateral crepitations on auscultation of his chest. His blood tests are unremarkable.

Chapter 8 Palpitation

Causes of palpitation

A. Anaemia.
B. Anxiety.
C. Hypoglycaemia.
D. Hypovolaemia.
E. Sepsis.
F. Pregnancy.
G. Supraventricular tachycardia.
H. Thyrotoxicosis.
I. Ventricular ectopic beats.
J. Ventricular fibrillation.
K. Ventricular tachycardia.

For each patient below, choose the most likely cause of the patient's palpitations from the list given above.

1. A 24-year-old lady is studying for her final exams at university. She has recently broken up with a long-term partner. She has had a number of episodes of rapid palpitations over the preceding week. She also has associated tingling in her fingers, bilaterally. Systemic enquiry is unremarkable.
2. A 62-year-old gentleman with a history of alcohol excess reports lethargy and frequent palpitations for the past 2 months. He also reports dark stools over the past 6 months. He has epigastric tenderness, but examination is otherwise unremarkable.
3. A 16-year-old boy attends the GP with his mother. She is concerned as he has mentioned a number of episodes where his heart appears to miss a beat. This has been going on for a number of years. There are no obvious precipitants, but he feels it occurs more at night. His ECG is completely normal.
4. A 67-year-old gentleman is being monitored on the cardiology ward following a recent myocardial infarction. A 10-second period of a broad complex tachycardia at a rate of 130 bpm is noted on the cardiac monitor. He reports being aware of palpitations at the time. His ECG following this was unremarkable except for unchanged T wave inversion in leads V4–V6.
5. An 82-year-old lady who lives alone presents to the hospital with a 5-day history of diarrhoea and vomiting. Her diarrhoea and vomiting has settled over the last day but she has been having palpitations for

the past 2 days and has been finding it difficult to mobilize at home. Her blood pressure when supine is 145/87 mmHg and 108/61 mmHg when erect. ECG is unremarkable.

Chapter 9 Syncope

Causes of syncope

A. Acute coronary syndrome.
B. Aortic stenosis.
C. Atrial fibrillation.
D. Complete heart block.
E. Hypertrophic cardiomyopathy.
F. Long QT syndrome.
G. Orthostatic hypotension.
H. Pulmonary embolism.
I. Subarachnoid haemorrhage.
J. Vasovagal syncope.
K. Wolff-Parkinson-White syndrome.

For each patient below, choose the most appropriate cause of syncope from the list given above.

1. A 32-year-old lady has episodes of rapid, regular palpitations associated with dizziness and a collapse on one occasion. These episodes tend to last several minutes at a time and occur every couple of months on average. ECG shows a PR interval of 89 ms, QRS interval of 94 ms and a QTc of 405 ms.
2. An 89-year-old man who has recently become very short of breath on exertion. He is also frequently lightheaded on exertion and has had two syncopal episodes recently. He has been troubled with angina for a number of years. His blood pressure is 115/95 mmHg and his heart rate is 78 bpm.
3. A 54-year-old lady with a background of depression and previous intravenous drug use is admitted for treatment of pneumonia with co-amoxiclav and clarithromycin. Her regular medications include citalopram and methadone. She has a number of episodes of rapid palpitations associated with lightheadedness and one 'faint'.
4. An 86-year-old man is admitted to the hospital after being stuck in bed due to dizziness and a number of syncopal episodes on standing. He has had diarrhoea and vomiting for the past week and has been struggling to cope at home. ECG shows sinus rhythm at 95 bpm and blood pressure is 103/62 mmHg.
5. A 54-year-old man admitted with an anterior myocardial infarction 2 days ago reports dizziness and lightheadedness for the past day. He has collapsed on 2 occasions. ECG shows a heart rate of 40 bpm and no relationship between P waves and QRS complexes.

Chapter 10 Heart murmurs

History and examination

A. Aortic area.
B. Apex.
C. Axilla.
D. Continuous murmur.
E. Early diastolic murmur.
F. Ejection systolic murmur.
G. Late diastolic murmur.
H. Left lower sternal border.
I. Pansystolic murmur.
J. Pulmonary area.
K. Right sternal border.
L. Weak carotid artery pulse.
M. Weak femoral artery pulse.
N. Weak radial artery pulse.

For each description below, choose the most appropriate answer from the list given above.

1. A 26-year-old lady who is 7 months pregnant visits her GP due to tiredness. The GP identifies anaemia and a murmur. What is the most likely timing of this murmur?
2. A 67-year-old lady becomes extremely short of breath 3 days after a large myocardial infarction. Doctors suspect that she has ruptured the papillary muscles in the left ventricle. A loud murmur is heard throughout the chest. What is the most likely timing of this murmur?
3. A young child presents to his GP with pain in both legs when he runs. He is found to have a blood pressure of 176/104 mmHg. Which of the clinical signs is most likely to be present on examination?
4. The murmur of aortic regurgitation is best heard with the patient leaning forward at end expiration. Where on the chest should a stethoscope be placed to best hear this murmur?
5. The murmur of mitral stenosis is best heard with the patient in the left lateral position at end expiration. Where on the chest should a stethoscope be placed to best hear this murmur?

Causes of pulmonary hypertension

A. Aortic regurgitation.
B. Chronic obstructive pulmonary disease (COPD).
C. Mitral regurgitation.
D. Mitral stenosis.
E. Primary pulmonary arterial hypertension.
F. Pulmonary embolism.
G. Pulmonary stenosis.
H. Rheumatoid arthritis.
I. Systemic sclerosis.

For each patient with pulmonary hypertension below, choose the most appropriate cause from the list given above.

1. A 24-year-old lady with no significant past medical history presents with gradually worsening breathlessness on exertion. The only findings of note on examination are a prominent parasternal heave, loud pulmonary second sound and a third heart sound.
2. A 38-year-old lady on the combined oral contraceptive pill who describes a sudden onset left-sided chest pain which is worse on inspiration. She was recently in plaster having fractured her ankle.
3. A 44-year-old lady with a history of dysphagia, joint pain and cold extremities. On examination it was noted that she had taut skin over her fingers, and over her face giving rise to a pursed mouth appearance.
4. A 55-year-old gentleman has a history of rheumatic fever, and has had frequent episodes of acute pulmonary oedema. On examination his pulse is irregularly irregular, he has a loud first heart sound and rumbling mid-diastolic murmur on auscultation.
5. A 64-year-old gentleman who is a heavy smoker, has a chronic cough productive of grey sputum and has become gradually breathless and wheezy on minimal exertion.

Chapter 11 Atherosclerosis

Antiplatelets and anticoagulants

A. Aspirin.
B. Clopidogrel.
C. Fondaparinux.
D. Ticagrelor.
E. Tirofiban.
F. Unfractionated heparin.

For each description below, choose the most appropriate medication from the list given above.

1. Reversible platelet ADP receptor $P2Y_{12}$ antagonist.
2. GPIIb/IIIa inhibitors.
3. Irreversible platelet ADP receptor $P2Y_{12}$ antagonist.
4. Directly inhibits factor Xa.
5. Antithrombin III enhancer.

Chapter 12 Risk factors

Management of hypertension

A. Start ACE inhibitor
B. Start α-blocker
C. Start angiotensin II receptor antagonist
D. Start calcium channel blocker
E. Refer to specialist

F. Send to A&E
G. Start spironolactone
H. Start thiazide-like diuretic

For each description below, choose the most appropriate management from the list given above.

1. A 61-year-old lady has a BP of 160/94 mmHg at routine annual review. She is already taking maximum doses of amlodipine and ramipril. What is the next step?
2. A 49-year-old black Sudanese gentleman with an ambulatory BP monitoring average of 150/90 mmHg comes to discuss starting an antihypertensive. He is asymptomatic and examination and bloods and urinalysis are normal. What is the next step?
3. A 67-year-old gentleman has been taking maximum doses of amlodipine, ramipril and bendroflumethiazide for over 10 years. Recently, during his elective cholecystectomy, he was told his blood pressure was high. His creatinine was 77 μmol/L with an eGFR > 60 mL/min per 1.73 m^2, and his K$^+$ was 4.8 μmol/L. On repeat today, his BP is 178/102 mmHg. He is referred for specialist advice. What else should be done?
4. A 54-year-old Caucasian lady has not tolerated an ACE inhibitor for hypertension due to a dry cough. However, her BP and bloods on monitoring have remained satisfactory. What should be the next step?
5. A 30-year-old gentleman was started on an ACE inhibitor for hypertension a month ago. His BP today is 145/90 mmHg, but since repeating his bloods, his creatinine has risen from 80 μmol/L to 130 μmol/L and his K$^+$ has risen to 5.7 mmol/L. His ACE inhibitor is stopped immediately. What should be done next?

Causes of secondary hypertension

A. Aortic coarctation
B. Cushing syndrome
C. Hyperthyroidism
D. Hypothyroidism
E. Phaeochromocytoma
F. Polycystic kidney disease
G. Primary hyperaldosteronism
H. Renal artery stenosis

For each description below, choose the most likely cause for secondary hypertension from the list given above.

1. An 82-year-old gentleman with a history of MI and intermittent claudication presents with increasingly difficult to control hypertension despite four antihypertensives at good doses. He has a loud abdominal bruit.

2. A 36-year-old lady complains of increasing cramps in her legs whilst at the gym, and recent headaches and nosebleeds. She has hypertension in her past medical history. On examination her legs seem cold peripherally, and she has a continuous murmur in her chest.
3. A 31-year-old gentleman presents with hypertension. He is not entirely sure about his family history, but his 56-year-old father required 'a kidney removed for a kidney problem', dialysis and had a stroke last year. His sister has just recently had problems with her kidneys too.
4. A 46-year-old lady presents with weakness, tremor, irritability and weight loss despite a good appetite. She has borderline tachycardia and hypertension.
5. A 52-year-old gentleman complains of new weakness and muscle cramps at the gym. He also finds intermittent headaches and nocturia more of a problem. He has hypertension but little else to find on examination, and bloods demonstrate eGFR >60, urea 3.5 mmol/L, K$^+$ 3.3 mmol/l and Na$^+$ 147 mmol/L.

Chapter 13 Stable angina and acute coronary syndromes

Medication side effects 1

A. Angioedema.
B. Cold extremities.
C. Constipation.
D. Dry cough.
E. Gynaecomastia.
F. Headache.
G. Leg oedema.
H. Muscle pain.
I. Pulmonary fibrosis.
J. Thrombocytopenia.

For each drug below, choose the most well-recognized side effect from the list given above.

1. Carvedilol.
2. Glyceryl trinitrate.
3. Simvastatin.
4. Spironolactone.
5. Tirofiban.

ECG changes

A. Concave ST elevation in all leads except AVR.
B. Prolonged QT interval.
C. Q waves in V1–V4. Right axis deviation.
D. Short P waves and tall T waves.
E. ST elevation in leads II, III and aVF with ST depression in V2–V4.

F. ST elevation in V1–V4.
G. ST depression V1–V4.
H. S wave in V1 + R wave in V5 > 35 mm.
I. VT/VF.

For each clinical diagnosis below, match the most likely ECG changes in the list given above.

1. Acute inferior myocardial infarction.
2. Hyperkalaemia.
3. Longstanding hypertension.
4. Old anterior myocardial infarction.
5. Pericarditis.

Medication side effects 2

A. Amiodarone.
B. Amlodipine.
C. Aspirin.
D. Atenolol.
E. Bendroflumethiazide.
F. Clopidogrel.
G. Isosorbide mononitrate.
H. Lisinopril.
I. Choose not to discontinue any drug.

From the list of drugs above, select which one you would consider discontinuing as a result of the adverse effect described.

1. A patient troubled by ankle swelling after starting treatment for hypertension.
2. Acute deterioration in renal function after starting this treatment for the first time.
3. Recent coronary angioplasty, itchy rash, but constitutionally well.
4. Development of pulmonary fibrosis.
5. Erectile dysfunction having started new treatment from GP for hypertension.

Chapter 14 Heart failure

Pharmacological treatment of heart failure

A. Bisoprolol.
B. Candesartan.
C. Digoxin.
D. Eplerenone.
E. Hydralazine.
F. Isosorbide mononitrate.
G. Ivabradine.
H. Ramipril.
I. Sacubitril/valsartan.
J. Spironolactone.

For each description below, choose the most appropriate medication from the list given above.

1. A mineralocorticoid receptor antagonist that is not associated with gynaecomastia.
2. A medication that may be of use if patients cannot tolerate enalapril due to dry cough.
3. An I_f channel inhibitor.
4. A medication that is negatively chronotropic but positively inotropic.
5. A medication to which tolerance develops rapidly if used without breaks.

Causes of heart failure

A. Pulmonary hypertension.
B. Aortic regurgitation.
C. Aortic stenosis.
D. Chemotherapy.
E. Mitral stenosis.
F. Systemic hypertension.
G. Viral myocarditis.
H. Alcohol.
I. Atrial septal defect.
J. Mitral regurgitation.

For each patient presenting with heart failure described below, choose the most appropriate diagnosis from the list given above.

1. 19-year-old male with a recent flu-like illness. He has a third heart sound and cardiomegaly was noted on the chest radiograph.
2. 44-year-old diabetic with renal impairment. Fundoscopy revealed arteriovenous nipping, silver wiring and small haemorrhages.
3. 56-year-old male with ankylosing spondylitis. A collapsing pulse was noted on peripheral examination.
4. 78-year-old male with an ejection systolic murmur loudest in the aortic area, radiating to the neck.
5. 65-year-old female with pansystolic murmur.

Starting medications in heart failure/after myocardial infarction

A. ACE inhibitor.
B. α-Blocker.
C. Angiotensin II receptor antagonist.
D. Calcium channel antagonist.
E. Cardioselective β-blocker.
F. Eplerenone.
G. Hydralazine and nitrate.
H. Loop diuretic.
I. Spironolactone.

For each clinical scenario below, choose the most appropriate medication from the list given above.

1. 60-year-old male, 1 day following uncomplicated angioplasty following myocardial infarction. Already prescribed aspirin, clopidogrel, statin and bisoprolol.
2. 68-year-old female, day 1 post-myocardial infarction, who is taking ramipril, simvastatin, aspirin and clopidogrel. Her heart rate is 90 beats/min, blood pressure 140/70 mmHg and there are no signs of heart failure.
3. 70-year-old male with chronic heart failure, seen in the clinic. He is in NYHA class III despite already taking bisoprolol, ramipril and furosemide at optimal doses.
4. 72-year-old male, whose heart failure symptoms have not improved despite treatment with bisoprolol, ramipril, spironolactone and furosemide.
5. 64-year-old male whose heart failure symptoms are well controlled on treatment with ramipril, bisoprolol, spironolactone and furosemide. He has noticed some breast enlargement and discomfort since the spironolactone and furosemide were started.

Chapter 15 Arrhythmias

ECG appearances

A. Left bundle branch block.
B. Atrial flutter.
C. Accelerated idioventricular rhythm.
D. Mobitz Type I heart block.
E. Mobitz Type II heart block.
F. Right bundle branch block.
G. Hypothermia.
H. Accessory pathway.
I. Atrial fibrillation.
J. Complete heart block.

For each ECG finding described below, choose the single most likely diagnosis from the above list of options.

1. RSR' pattern in lead V1.
2. P waves which have no fixed relationship with the QRS complexes. The QRS complexes are broad and the heart rate is 35 beats/min.
3. J waves.
4. Delta wave.
5. Progressive prolongation of PR interval followed by a dropped beat.

Treatment of arrhythmia

A. Intravenous adenosine.
B. Urgent synchronized DC cardioversion.
C. Intravenous atropine.

D. Insertion of permanent pacemaker.
E. Oral digoxin.
F. Intravenous amiodarone.
G. Intravenous verapamil.
H. Intravenous magnesium.
I. Immediate defibrillation.
J. Intravenous adrenaline.

For each scenario described below, choose the single most appropriate treatment from the above list of options.

1. A 28-year-old man with a history of poorly-controlled asthma presents to the emergency department with palpitations. ECG shows a narrow complex tachycardia at a rate of 160 bpm. Vagal manoeuvres and carotid sinus massage have been tried without success.
2. A 24-year-old man who has recently started on treatment for schizophrenia is on cardiac monitoring for a prolonged QT interval. He has a transient loss of consciousness and the monitor at the time demonstrated a broad complex tachycardia of varying amplitude.
3. A 75-year-old lady with COPD is referred to hospital by her GP after developing a productive cough and breathlessness. She is noted to have a narrow complex, irregularly irregular tachycardia on ECG, at a rate of 130 bpm.
4. A 69-year-old lady who is on the cardiology ward following a myocardial infarction has a cardiac arrest. Basic life support is commenced. After the defibrillator pads are applied asystole is seen on the monitor.
5. An 82-year-old man with a 2-week history of breathlessness on exertion and lethargy has been referred to the hospital after his GP noticed he was profoundly bradycardic. His only regular medications are paracetamol and omeprazole. ECG shows no relationship between P waves and QRS complexes and a rate of 36 bpm.

Chapter 16 Valvular disease

Examination findings

A. Aortic stenosis.
B. Atrial septal defect.
C. Coarctation of the aorta.
D. Hypertrophic cardiomyopathy.
E. Mild mitral stenosis.
F. Mitral valve prolapse.
G. Pulmonary hypertension.
H. Tricuspid regurgitation.
I. Ventricular septal defect.

For each clinical finding below, choose the most likely diagnosis from the list given above.

1. Double apical impulse.
2. Left parasternal heave.
3. Mid-systolic click and late systolic murmur.
4. Opening snap and mid-diastolic murmur with pre-systolic accentuation.
5. Pulsatile liver.

Underlying pathology in endocarditis

A. *Aspergillus.*
B. *Candida albicans.*
C. Coagulase-negative Staphylococci.
D. *Coxiella burnetii.*
E. HACEK organisms.
F. Libman-Sacks endocarditis.
G. *Pseudomonas aeruginosa.*
H. *Streptococcus gallolyticus (Streptococcus bovis).*
I. *Staphylococcus aureus.*
J. Viridans group Streptococci.

For each patient below, choose the most likely cause from the list given above.

1. A 32-year-old male with a 2-day illness presents with collapse. He looks unwell. He is pyrexial at 38.9 °C, tachycardic at 118 beats/min and has a murmur. He has a history of intravenous drug use (IVDU).
2. A 37-year-old male who, following initial results, is believed by the microbiologist to have contracted infective endocarditis due to work with farm animals.
3. A 48-year-old male who has been unwell for 6 weeks, has a murmur, finger clubbing and poor dental hygiene. He has a history of rheumatic heart disease but no recent infections or previous surgery.
4. A 57-year-old female who is noted to have vegetations on her mitral valve on echocardiogram. She has a history of systemic lupus erythematosus. She is otherwise well and remains so at clinic follow-up; there is no other recent past medical history, and blood cultures are negative.
5. Endocarditis in an 82-year-old male. Blood cultures show a gram-positive cocci in chains; this bacteraemia is believed to be linked with his recent diagnosis of colon cancer.

Chapter 17 Diseases of the myocardium and pericardium

Causes of chest pain

A. Acute pericarditis.
B. Cardiac tamponade.

C. Constrictive pericarditis.
D. Dilated cardiomyopathy.
E. Hypertrophic cardiomyopathy.
F. Infective endocarditis.
G. Myocarditis.
H. Non-ST elevation myocardial infarction.
I. Takotsubo cardiomyopathy.

For each scenario below, choose the most likely corresponding diagnosis from the list given above.

1. A 67-year-old man attends the emergency department following a collapse. He was discharged 1 week ago following a myocardial infarction. He is hypotensive and his jugular venous pulse is raised. He has cold peripheries and quiet heart sounds.
2. A 45-year-old man presents with a 3-day history of central, sharp chest pain that is relieved by sitting forward. He is pyrexial at 38.7°C. Auscultation reveals a scratching sound audible over the precordium.
3. A 63-year-old woman attends with a 12-hour history of chest pain. She has no significant past medical history. She reports, however, struggling to cope since being fired from her job 2 days ago. ECG shows ST elevation across anterior leads. Angiography shows normal coronary arteries but left ventricular apical ballooning is noted.
4. An ambulance is called to a 29-year-old man who has collapsed while playing football. He is pronounced dead at the scene. Two of his relatives had passed away in a similar manner.

5. A 34-year-old woman presents with a 5-day history of fever and malaise. She reports a history of mechanical aortic valve replacement. She is noted to have a number of erythematous lesions on her hands and feet and a systolic murmur on auscultation.

Chapter 18 Congenital heart disease

Causes of congenital heart disease

A. Absent tricuspid valve.
B. Aortic root dilatation.
C. Bicuspid aortic valve.
D. Coarctation of the aorta.
E. Dextrocardia.
F. Patent ductus arteriosus.
G. Pulmonary stenosis.
H. Tetralogy of Fallot.
I. Septal defects.
J. Options B, C or D.
K. Options F, G or I.
L. Options F, H or I.

For each scenario below, choose the best correlated option from the list of congenital heart lesions given above.

1. Kartagener syndrome.
2. Maternal alcohol use.
3. Maternal rubella.
4. Trisomy 21.
5. Turner syndrome.

SBA answers

Chapter 1 Cardiac anatomy, physiology and development

1. E. The thymus is contained within the superior and anterior mediastinal compartments and can extend up into the neck; however, it involutes (becomes smaller) after puberty and may be hardly identifiable in old age. The sympathetic chain is part of the autonomic nervous system and sits to either side of the spinal cord. As the trachea travels posteriorly, it bifurcates at the border of the superior and inferior mediastinal compartments and therefore does not extend into the posterior mediastinum. The oesophagus sits behind the trachea and travels through both the superior and posterior mediastinal compartments and through the diaphragm to join the stomach. The internal thoracic arteries arise from the subclavian arteries, travel down the interior surface of the anterior chest wall and through the anterior mediastinum.

2. A. The coronary veins drain via the coronary sinus into the right atrium. In most people, the SA and AV nodes are supplied by the right coronary artery. The coronary arteries arise from the aorta just distal to the aortic valve. The right coronary artery usually gives rise to the posterior descending artery, but a small proportion of patients have a left dominant circulation where the circumflex also supplies the posterior descending artery. The left coronary artery gives rise to the circumflex artery.

3. C. Cardiac myocytes have a branched structure, are shorter than skeletal muscle fibres and have a single central nucleus. Pacemaker cells exist in the SA node, AV node, Purkinje fibres, and ventricular cardiomyocytes, and unlike other cardiomyocytes, these do not require external stimulation to initiate their action potential but are capable of self-generating rhythmic depolarization – this is known as automaticity. Troponin is a complex of proteins which are present at intervals along the thin actin filaments.

4. D. The ductus arteriosus is maintained by prostaglandin E during pregnancy, and closes after birth to become the ligamentum arteriosum. Pulmonary vascular resistance decreases immediately after birth. The umbilical vessels vasoconstrict during and after birth, and the cord is then clamped, therefore blood flow stops. The foramen ovale quickly closes (functionally) between the atria due

to the shift in atrial pressures when the pulmonary circulation opens up with the first breaths after birth – however fusion only occurs about 3 months later, and interestingly, anatomic closure is incomplete (known as patent foramen ovale) in about a quarter of the normal population. Foetal haemoglobin continues to be produced for around 6 months.

Chapter 2 The cardiac cycle, control of cardiac output, and haemodynamic regulation

1. B. Increased plasma osmolarity will stimulate antidiuretic hormone release. Angiotensin-converting enzyme (ACE) is predominantly found in the endothelium of the pulmonary vascular bed. Adrenaline is secreted from the adrenal medulla. Adrenaline causes vasodilatation in skeletal muscle by acting on β_2 receptors. Renin converts angiotensinogen to angiotensin I.

2. B. The baroreceptor reflex is important in the cutaneous circulation if the temperature is neutral, but can be overcome if there is peripheral vasodilation due to high temperature. The carotid sinus, not the carotid body, contains baroreceptors; these are innervated by a branch of the glossopharyngeal nerve. Decreased baroreceptor loading increases venous tone by increasing sympathetic activity. Increased stretch in arterial walls increases baroreceptor firing. The baroreceptor reflex is important for minute-to-minute control of the blood pressure but little use for long-term regulation (as it adjusts to the new set point in chronic hypertension/hypotension).

3. A. Aortic regurgitation is the most likely cause of this gentleman's symptoms. All of the other options are causes of a narrow pulse pressure.

4. E. Polycythaemia rubra vera is a well-documented cause of an elevated haematocrit. Acute myeloid leukaemia will generally cause a reduction in haematocrit. Chronic hypoxia can cause an elevated haematocrit but the asthmatic patient should not be chronically hypoxic. Cardiac failure does not generally cause an elevated haematocrit (although may cause lethargy). Haematocrit may be elevated in high altitude living, but this is unlikely to be the cause in this case!

5. D. The diving reflex causes intense vagal (parasympathetic) inhibition decreasing the slope

of the pacemaker action potential and slowing heart rate, possibly terminating supraventricular tachycardias (SVTs). The alerting (fight or flight) response will increase heart rate. The baroreceptor reflex acts to maintain blood pressure at a set point and is not involved in the treatment of SVTs. Under normal circumstances, chemoreceptor activation (via hypoxaemia or hypercapnia) will increase heart rate (and respiratory rate). The hepatojugular reflex is used to augment the jugular venous pressure, not to treat SVT.

Chapter 3 ECG interpretation

1. B. J waves may be seen in hypothermia. A downsloping ST segment or 'reverse tick' may be seen in digoxin therapy. A raised ST segment is most commonly associated with myocardial infarction (but may be seen in other conditions such as pericarditis). 'Tented' T waves are a common finding in hyperkalaemia, as are U waves in hypokalaemia.

2. B. Inferior ST elevation myocardial infarction (STEMI) is classically seen as ST elevation in leads II, III, aVF. Anterior STEMI may be seen on the ECG as ST elevation in leads V3–V4. A lateral STEMI would be seen as ST elevation in leads I, aVL and leads V5–V6. Posterior STEMI may be seen as ST elevation in leads placed on the posterior chest wall (V7–V9) or as reciprocal depression in leads V1–V2. Septal MI would be seen as ST elevation in leads V1–V2. Infarcts may commonly cover more than one of these territories, such as with anteroseptal or anterolateral infarcts, for instance.

3. D. This ECG rhythm strip shows torsades de pointes, a polymorphic ventricular tachycardia. Episodes of torsades are generally self-terminating, but occasionally may lead to ventricular fibrillation and death. The ECG in between these episodes typically shows a long QT interval. Broad QRS complexes are generally seen in bundle branch block and ventricular rhythms – they are seen here during the arrhythmia, but are unlikely to be present between arrhythmias in a woman of this age. Delta waves (a slurred upstroke of QRS complex) are seen in Wolff-Parkinson-White syndrome, a common cause of supraventricular tachycardia. A long PR interval describes first degree heart block and is not associated with torsades de pointes. 'Tented' T waves are a common feature of hyperkalaemia – this can predispose to arrhythmia but generally not torsades de pointes.

4. B. This lady has left axis deviation. One of the possible causes of this is left ventricular hypertrophy. All the other conditions above are potential causes of *right* axis deviation.

5. D. Small Q waves represent normal left to right depolarisation of the interventricular septum and small Q waves are often seen in the left-sided leads (I, aVL, V5, V6). Pathological Q waves are wider than two small squares (0.08 s) and/or >25% of the corresponding R wave. Pathological Q waves suggests previous transmural infarction. Pathological Q waves in leads I and aVL suggest an old high lateral infarct, whereas previous inferior myocardial infarction is suggested by pathological Q waves in II, III and aVF. They are usually permanent and are due to ventricular depolarization away from the lead (resulting in a negative deflection).

Chapter 4 Other common investigations

1. A. Coronary angiography is the most sensitive and specific test, as it allows direct visualization of the coronary arteries using contrast and continuous X-ray scanning, and therefore demonstrates the location and extent of any stenosis or obstruction. However, there are serious but rare complications. CT coronary angiograms provide indirect imaging. Stress tests may indirectly demonstrate reduced perfusion in a coronary artery territory. An ECG may demonstrate evidence of reduced perfusion during chest pain, or evidence of a previous MI.

2. B. An exercise ECG is unlikely to demonstrate symptoms as the Bruce protocol does not achieve the level of workload his symptoms are occurring at. This man presents with typical angina, and as per the NICE guidelines, should be initially investigated with a CT coronary angiogram.

3. A. All of the above investigations will be helpful in this classic description of infective endocarditis with signs of right heart failure. ECG may demonstrate atrioventricular block if there is aortic root abscess formation, or occasionally MI secondary to septic emboli. Chest X-ray (CXR) may demonstrate cardiac failure or spread of septic emboli to the lungs from right heart infective endocarditis. Urinalysis may demonstrate microscopic haematuria. Both CXR and urine culture will look for other sources of infection. Routine bloods include inflammatory markers and renal function, which may be deranged if there is associated glomerulonephritis (a minor Duke's criteria). Echocardiogram is not mentioned here but will be required to demonstrate vegetations as the source of infection (in this case most likely affecting the tricuspid valve given the presentation and history of IV drug abuse). Although equally important in Duke's criteria, blood cultures are possibly more important here when there is already a strong suspicion of infective endocarditis prior to echocardiogram. Blood cultures

are crucial to identify the causative organism and its antimicrobial sensitivities, both for diagnosis and to ensure effective treatment, and ideally three sets of cultures should be taken prior to starting antibiotics urgently. See Chapter 16 for further details.

4. C. This lady is likely to have asymptomatic aortic stenosis. An echo will demonstrate site and severity of valvular disease and resultant size and function of the myocardium. This is also a safe and widely available investigation. If there was suspicion of hypertrophic cardiomyopathy, echocardiography would still be the first-line investigation and would confirm the diagnosis, but in certain cases MRI can provide more information. There is no suggestion of coronary artery disease here therefore CT coronary angiography and exercise testing are not required. A MUGA scan is a test using radionuclides to evaluate ventricular function.

3. B. Dressler syndrome is an immune-mediated pericarditis that usually occurs weeks to months after acute myocardial infarction. Aortic dissection can be associated with STEMI if the ostia are involved, and rarely pericarditic ECG changes, but you would then expect the patient to be more unwell, and dissection

is not at increased risk following MI. Further STEMI would cause regional rather than widespread ST elevation. Pulmonary embolus may cause pleuritic chest pain and pyrexia, but would usually present with cough and dyspnoea and would not cause widespread ST elevation. Unstable angina would not cause ST elevation.

4. B. This lady is presenting with pericarditis, which causes saddle-shaped ST elevation in all ECG leads. The treatment of choice is a nonsteroidal antiinflammatory drug, such as ibuprofen. ST elevation myocardial elevation causes ST elevation only within coronary artery territories, therefore treatments for acute coronary syndrome are inappropriate. Paracetamol may be helpful but is less likely to be beneficial than ibuprofen.

5. A. A negative troponin at the time of presentation and 12 hours later excludes myocardial infarction. Troponin may also be raised for many other reasons (e.g. arrhythmia, heart failure etc.). There is not muscle damage (by definition) in unstable angina, therefore cardiac biomarkers would not be elevated. Troponin levels may be elevated for at least 1 week post myocardial infarction. Troponin is found in the thin filaments of the myofibrils, not on cell membranes.

6. B. Although cocaine use is a risk factor for drug-induced myocarditis and aortic dissection, myocardial infarction is by far the most likely cause given the presentation and prevalence – this can be secondary to plaque rupture or severe coronary vasoconstriction secondary to cocaine. In myocarditis, nonspecific ECG changes and raised troponin may also be seen. Aortic dissection is rare in itself, and can rarely be associated with STEMI (inferior more likely than anterior), and would require to be ruled out if there is a high clinical suspicion. Not surprisingly, Takotsubo cardiomyopathy is possible with cocaine use given it is thought to be due to a catecholamine surge, and cocaine is a potent sympathomimetic. It can also cause a raised troponin, but would also be associated with apical left ventricular dyskinesis in a territory unrelated to a single coronary artery. Cocaine is not known to be a risk factor for pulmonary embolism.

Chapter 7 Breathlessness and peripheral oedema

1. B. If identification of the JVP is difficult, the hepatojugular reflex may be helpful. The JVP is considered raised if >4 cm above the manubriosternal angle. Height of the JVP above the manubriosternal angle gives an estimate of right atrial pressure in cm H2O (not mmHg). The internal jugular vein lies deep

arms in comparison to the legs — femoral delay; however, if the coarctation occurs before the left subclavian artery, it can cause a BP differential between the arms and radioradial delay.

to the sternocleidomastoid; the external jugular vein may be visualized lateral to sternocleidomastoid. The patient should be lying at approximately 45 degrees with their head turned slightly away.

2. A. Calcium channel blockers of the dihydropyridine class (amlodipine, nifedipine, etc.) commonly cause ankle swelling as a side effect. Bendroflumethiazide and furosemide are diuretics and may be used in the treatment of ankle swelling/oedema. Ankle swelling is not a common side effect of propranolol or lansoprazole.

3. C. This lady is dyspnoeic and has low oxygen saturations; her presentation is in keeping with a pneumonia. Always perform an A–E assessment on unwell patients. She will likely need antibiotics and intravenous fluids but oxygenation is the first priority. Digoxin treatment for atrial fibrillation if it persists is not unreasonable, but again is not the priority. Despite her cardiac history there is nothing to indicate she warrants urgent assessment by a cardiologist.

4. C. Oligaemic lung fields (decreased pulmonary vascular markings) may sometimes be seen on chest X-rays in patients presenting with PE. X-rays are, however, often normal in PE. All of the other radiograph features mentioned are characteristic of pulmonary oedema/left ventricular failure.

5. D. Psychogenic hyperventilation is the most likely option as she is hyperventilating despite normal oxygenation. She has an alkalaemia secondary to loss of CO_2. She does have pitting oedema which may fit with a degree of cardiac failure but note this is a common finding and a clear chest on auscultation and normal oxygen saturations would not support a diagnosis of acute LVF. Exacerbation of COPD or interstitial lung disease would be seen as hypoxia +/− hypercapnoea on the ABG. Pulmonary embolism may be seen as a low CO_2 and resultant alkalosis but is unlikely given her entirely normal oxygenation.

Chapter 8 Palpitation

1. B. Intravenous verapamil is an appropriate choice of treatment in this circumstance. Adenosine slows conduction through the AV node and is a valid treatment of SVT, but should be avoided in asthmatics as may precipitate bronchospasm. Ocular pressure is a vagotonic procedure, but should not be used as it carries a risk of retinal detachment. Defibrillation is inappropriate here; if the patient shows adverse features of arrhythmia then sedation and synchronized DC cardioversion may be appropriate. Isoprenaline is used in the treatment of bradycardia, not tachycardia.

2. B. SVT is generally rapid but regular, whereas AF is irregularly irregular. Both AF and SVT may cause chest pain. In both cases, resting ECG may be normal (apart from SVT due to Wolff-Parkinson-White syndrome, which has characteristic resting ECG changes). AF with a fast ventricular response may be similar to SVT with respect to frequency and severity of the palpitations. Both AF and SVT may be precipitated by coffee.

3. A. Atrial fibrillation is the only condition where P waves are not seen on the ECG. Although sometimes difficult to see, P waves are not absent in atrial flutter or ventricular tachycardia. Intermittent P waves are seen in sick sinus syndrome. P waves are independent of the QRS complexes in complete heart block and ventricular tachycardia.

4. B. β-Blockers (and calcium channel blockers) are well-recognized causes of first degree heart block (long PR interval) whereas ACE inhibitors are not. Although left bundle branch block and first-degree heart block may be the result of the same underlying process (e.g., age-related fibrosis), left bundle branch block itself does not cause first degree heart block. Pericarditis may result in PR segment depression but is not a common cause of prolonged PR interval, unless in association with myocarditis. Wolff-Parkinson-White syndrome classically causes a short PR interval rather than a prolonged one.

5. B. The four adverse features that would warrant urgent DC cardioversion are shock (systolic BP <90 mmHg), syncope, myocardial ischaemia and heart failure. Typical ischaemic sounding chest pain would warrant synchronized DC cardioversion. Other means of reverting his arrhythmia can be trialled while this is arranged. This blood pressure is not low enough to warrant DC cardioversion. A rate of >200 bpm is not an indication for DC cardioversion unless the rapid rate results in other adverse features. Breathlessness at rest and peripheral oedema are not necessarily adverse features; pulmonary oedema is, however, as this is a sign of heart failure. The peripheral oedema is also unlikely to be secondary to the arrhythmia, given the short duration.

Chapter 9 Syncope

1. C. Classic cardiac syncope (due to a paroxysmal arrhythmia for example) is of sudden onset and with rapid recovery. Patients generally have no warning symptoms and no neurological deficit. Persistent neurological deficit may indicate an intracranial event. Syncope precipitated by sudden turning of the head may indicate carotid sinus hypersensitivity.

2. A. A sudden onset 'tearing' or 'ripping' chest pain that radiates to the back with a difference in blood pressure between arms is classical of aortic dissection. A variety of ECG changes may be seen in dissection, including T wave inversion, ST depression or even ST elevation (the inferior territory is most commonly affected) due to involvement of the right coronary artery in the dissection; the ECG changes here are much more likely to be indicative of this than an acute myocardial infarction. The typical history in pericarditis is a sharp stabbing pain that is relieved by sitting forward; the ECG findings and blood pressure discrepancy are not consistent with pericarditis. Pulmonary embolism (PE) would not be associated with a blood pressure discrepancy between arms; in PE you might expect a sharp, pleuritic pain and hypoxia. Examination of the chest would not be unremarkable in tension pneumothorax and again, pain is more likely to be sharp and pleuritic.

3. B. The family history and exertional syncope that sounds cardiac (sudden onset without warning, rapid recovery) in a young person has to raise suspicion of hypertrophic cardiomyopathy (HCM). This man may have had dynamic obstruction from HCM or paroxysmal arrhythmia and requires urgent investigation. There is little to suggest that this is an acute coronary syndrome. Orthostatic (postural) hypotension generally occurs shortly after standing. Takotsubo cardiomyopathy is a sudden, transient weakness and ballooning of the ventricular myocardium (often in response to stress) and can be a mimic of myocardial infarction – it does not fit with this history. This patient's episodes are not in keeping with vasovagal syncope as they are occurring suddenly and without warning.

4. A. Alcohol (especially when drinking to excess) is a very well recognized trigger of atrial fibrillation and this seems the most likely cause of her symptoms given her ongoing rapid palpitations. Complete heart block may cause presyncope, but not rapid palpitations. She is unlikely to still be intoxicated and this does not explain her symptoms (plus she probably wouldn't appreciate the suggestion)! Alcohol is associated with sinus tachycardia but this is not likely to persist for this length of time and is also unlikely to be the cause of presyncope. Alcohol generally predisposes to supraventricular arrhythmias rather than ventricular arrhythmias.

5. E. Withholding her medications is the most sensible first option out of those listed – both these medications will lower blood pressure and the bisoprolol will slow her heart rate. Given she is bradycardic, hypotensive and is having episodes of presyncope, these should be withheld (and perhaps later restarted at a lower dose). There are no adverse features of bradycardia (myocardial ischaemia, shock, heart failure, and syncope) to suggest she requires atropine and no indication for pacing at this stage. Digoxin *is* positively inotropic but is also negatively chronotropic and likely to slow her heart rate further and should not be given to such patients.

Chapter 10 Heart murmurs

1. D. Mitral regurgitation is a classical cause of a pansystolic murmur. Aortic regurgitation is associated with an early diastolic murmur. Aortic stenosis is associated with an ejection systolic murmur. Atrial septal defects cause fixed splitting of the second heart sounds and possibly an ejection systolic pulmonary flow murmur. Tricuspid stenosis is associated with a mid-diastolic murmur.

2. A. Atrial myxoma is very rare; however, it is the most common cardiac tumour, and is almost always benign. It is characteristically associated with a 'tumour plop' due to tumour impacting on the endocardial wall and can cause a mitral stenosis murmur if the tumour obstructs the mitral valve. It can present with fever (and other constitutional symptoms) and heart failure due to tumour obstruction. The 'plop' is not associated with any of the other conditions above. All except mitral valve prolapse can cause fever; mitral valve prolapse also produces a systolic murmur. Cardiac causes of clubbing are Atrial myxoma, Bacterial endocarditis and Cyanotic congenital heart disease (ABC). Infective endocarditis more often causes regurgitant murmurs (due to valve destruction or distortion) rather than stenotic murmurs (due to obstruction). Pericarditis is classically associated with a pericardial rub and chest pain. Rheumatic fever characteristically occurs 2–3 weeks after a streptococcal sore throat, and can be associated with multiple organ involvement, including joints, skin and brain.

3. B. When the first heart sound is loud and palpable in mitral stenosis, this is described as a tapping apex beat. Mitral regurgitation is associated with a thrusting, displaced apex beat. Left ventricular aneurysm may cause diffuse asynchronous or double apex beat as the aneurysm can cause a second outward bulge in systole. Left ventricular hypertrophy is associated with a heaving non-displaced apex beat, which can be seen due to hypertension, aortic stenosis and HCM. In pericardial effusion, the apex beat may be reduced or impalpable. Other causes of an impalpable apex beat include anything that increases the distance between your fingers and the apex (e.g., obesity, emphysema, pneumothorax, massive pleural effusion) or because the apex is not where you expect it. Therefore, it is important to

check not only for lateral and inferior displacement, but if still impalpable, also check the other side – the patient may have dextrocardia!

4. C. In a patient with clubbing, haematuria, fever and a murmur, suspect a subacute presentation of bacterial endocarditis (clubbing takes time to develop). HUS is a thrombotic microangiopathy which tends to occur in children, often secondary to infection. Thrombosis occurs in the damaged microcirculation of the kidney to cause haemolytic anaemia, thrombocytopenia and acute kidney injury. Fever and microscopic haematuria is expected, a murmur due to increased cardiac output in sepsis may be found, but clubbing is not associated. Infectious mononucleosis (AKA glandular fever) is due to Epstein-Barr virus infection, and typically presents in young adults with a sore throat, lymphadenopathy, fever and fatigue, with later hepatomegaly and splenomegaly. Complications are most commonly haematological or neurological, but carditis and renal complications are rare. Rheumatic fever is a delayed immune reaction to *Streptococcus* A throat infection and can affect any valve and therefore can cause a range of murmurs along with fever, arthritis and skin manifestations. However, it is not associated with clubbing or haematuria. Tetralogy of Fallot is a congenital heart condition which presents within the first few years of life and survival to adulthood is rare without surgery. Clubbing can develop, but it is not associated with fever or haematuria.

5. C. Systolic blood pressure normally falls with inspiration, but an exaggerated fall of >10 mmHg is termed pulsus paradoxus. This can occur in cardiac tamponade, restrictive cardiomyopathy, constrictive pericarditis and severe obstructive lung disease. In most of these conditions Kussmaul's sign may also be observed, where the JVP paradoxically rises with inspiration due to impaired right ventricular filling. These terms can be misleading and confusing, as pulsus paradoxus is an exaggeration of the normal trend, whereas Kussmaul's sign is a reversal of the normal fall in JVP during inspiration. Collapsing pulse can be a feature of aortic regurgitation, large arteriovenous malformations/fistulas, or marked peripheral vasodilatation. Pulsus alternans is associated with severe heart failure. Radio-femoral delay can be found in aortic coarctation or dissection. Slow rising pulse is a feature of aortic stenosis.

6. E. A small VSD produces a louder murmur than a larger one. Small VSDs are unlikely to cause significant haemodynamic derangement and are more likely to close spontaneously without requiring intervention. Acute mitral regurgitation is likely to present with heart failure or cardiogenic shock, and the baby is unlikely to be so well; the murmur is loudest at the apex and radiates to the left axilla. Aortic stenosis typically causes a murmur in the second right intercostal space (upper left sternal edge). Hypertrophic cardiomyopathy does not usually present until later in life.

7. E. A loud palpable second heart sound is a feature of pulmonary hypertension. A parasternal right ventricular heave can be found in pulmonary hypertension, but the apex beat is not affected. Other features include an elevated JVP and an early diastolic murmur. Corrigan's pulse is a feature of aortic regurgitation.

8. E. Physiological splitting of the second heart sound increases on inspiration and disappears on expiration. A continuous 'machinery' murmur may be due to patent ductus arteriosus. Aortic stenosis and atrial septal defect both cause an ejection systolic murmur. Early diastolic murmur may be due to aortic or pulmonary regurgitation Tricuspid regurgitation can cause a pansystolic murmur. Mid-diastolic murmurs may be due to mitral or tricuspid stenosis.

Chapter 11 Atherosclerosis

1. B. This fulfils the criteria of non-ST elevation myocardial infarction (NSTEMI). Inferior MI is frequently associated with bradycardia. A massive pulmonary embolus may give similar symptoms and can cause troponin rise in right ventricular strain, but tends to cause more anterior T wave or ST changes and tachycardia, and is less likely without other known additional PE risk factors. If there is any doubt, urgent bedside echocardiography may be helpful to differentiate between evidence of right heart strain (PE) or localized hypokinetic segment (MI). Angina alone would not cause a rise in troponin.

2. D. Atrial fibrillation suggests an embolic source to the stroke, and as a 34-year-old female, patient D is unlikely to have significant enough atherosclerosis to cause a stroke. This is therefore the best answer. Patient A has a number of established risk factors for MI including smoking, hypertension and diabetes; rheumatoid arthritis is an additional risk factor for MI. Patient B has known atherosclerotic disease and is at high risk of peripheral arterial disease.
With patient C, although acute mesenteric ischaemia is more frequently due to embolus than thrombosis-in-situ, there is no obvious source of embolus and she clearly has a higher risk of atherosclerotic disease than the lady in answer D.
Patient E's presentation is in keeping with unstable angina or MI.

3. C. The anterior myocardium is supplied by the left anterior descending artery, and complete occlusion will cause an anterior MI. 60% stenosis of a coronary artery would not be sufficient to cause myocardial infarction. The circumflex supplies the lateral wall, and the right coronary supplies the posterior/inferior surfaces. Severe anaemia can cause decompensation from pre-existing stenosis but is very unlikely to cause ST elevation. It tends to cause worsening angina, or very rarely, type 2 MI (defined as myocardial injury not caused by an acute coronary artery event, instead due to ischaemia from other causes of imbalance of myocardial supply and demand).

Chapter 12 Risk factors

1. B. For patient B, calculate the 10-year risk using online calculators (e.g., https://www.qrisk.org/; http://www.assign-score.com/estimate-the-risk/). Using either calculator, 10-year risk is over 10% and primary prevention with a statin is warranted. Using the same calculators for patient D, 10-year risk is below 10% and therefore statin therapy is not indicated.
   Patient A should not be started on aspirin as current guidelines do not recommend routine use for primary prevention. Evidence of overall benefit from prevented heart attacks (and cancer!) does not clearly outweigh the increased risk of haemorrhage. Adults with type 1 and type 2 diabetes are not recommended to have aspirin as primary prevention in NICE guidelines NG17 and NG28 (2015). However, some experts argue aspirin should be considered in some high-risk groups (e.g., hypertensive patients >50 years with CKD).
   Patient C would not require amlodipine treatment. He should receive antihypertensive treatment for stage 2 hypertension, but first choice at this age (if not black) would be an ACE inhibitor.
   Patient E would not be started on a ß-Blockers. ß-Blockers are used as anti-anginal treatment but are not used for primary prevention of IHD. ß-Blockers are also no longer one of the preferred options for hypertension management (however certain ß-Blockers such as labetalol use may be considered in some hypertensive emergencies).

2. A. NICE recommends a high-intensity statin treatment for both primary and secondary prevention, which equates to a >40% reduction in LDL. This dose of atorvastatin falls into this category and is appropriate for primary prevention.
   Cholestyramine is a bile acid binding resin, which binds bile acids in the intestine, and as these are synthesized from cholesterol, they reduce plasma LDL. However, these drugs can aggravate hypertriglyceridaemia, and there is no clear evidence that these show benefit; therefore, they are no longer recommended for primary or secondary prevention. Niacin was thought to inhibit adipose tissue breakdown, thereby decreasing free fatty acid and therefore plasma cholesterol levels. However, large studies have not shown any benefit, and there is increased risk of statin side-effects when used in combination. Preparations have been withdrawn. This dose of pravastatin is considered to be low intensity cholesterol lowering and would not be recommended.
   This dose of simvastatin is medium intensity cholesterol lowering.

3. B. Bloods and urinalysis are the next step. With this level of hypertension, there is no need to confirm hypertension with further monitoring, and there are no signs of end-organ dysfunction requiring A&E. At this level of blood pressure, you would be keen to start an oral antihypertensive quickly and arrange prompt review. If the urinalysis demonstrated glucose and a large quantity of protein, instead of starting amlodipine as per hypertension guidelines, there may be benefit in starting an ACE inhibitor instead if diabetic nephropathy was suspected.

4. C. This patient requires a full assessment including fundoscopy as his blood pressure is very high. It should not be put down to anxiety without further assessment for hypertensive emergency; therefore the most appropriate place for ongoing monitoring and careful treatment of blood pressure is a hospital. Given he is young, he will need to be investigated for secondary causes of hypertension, and indeed anxiety, palpitations and headache may be symptoms of phaeochromocytoma.

5. E. This ECG meets the voltage criteria for LVH. The lateral ST depression and asymmetric T wave inversion is typical of the strain pattern seen in LVH (ST change in the opposite direction of the QRS complex), as expected in longstanding hypertension. It is not a normal ECG, but there is no suggestion of a current or previous MI. This is not typical of any electrolyte abnormality.

6. A. Calcium channel blockers do not require blood test monitoring. ACE inhibitors, Angiotensin II receptor blockers, thiazide and thiazide-like diuretics all require monitoring of renal function and electrolytes.

Chapter 13 Stable angina and acute coronary syndromes

1. C. tPA is only used in STEMI, in the absence of contraindications and when primary percutaneous

coronary intervention is not available within 90 minutes. The other treatments are used in both NSTEMI and STEMI.

2. B. To prevent thrombus extension, patients should be started on dual antiplatelet therapy and an anticoagulant (assuming no contraindications) and therefore option B is correct. Options A, C and D are missing anticoagulants.

    A ß-blocker is important in NSTEMI to minimize myocardial demand but will not help with thrombus extension. Oxygen may be appropriate if the patient is hypoxic to minimize ischaemia but will not impact on thrombus size. Option E includes two separate P2Y12 antagonists; this should be avoided due to bleeding risk, and there are no high-risk features suggested to warrant an additional GPIIb/IIIa inhibitor.

3. C. Digoxin is the only drug here not used to treat angina. ß-blockers (e.g. atenolol) are contraindicated due to asthma. Nifedipine is likely to cause reflex tachycardia without a concurrent β-blocker, which would increase myocardial demand when his heart rate is already higher than desirable. Diltiazem would be preferable in reducing heart rate and myocardial demand. A GTN spray would be useful during attacks or to prevent attacks before exercise, but would not have as much effect on decreasing frequency of angina attacks as diltiazem.

4. B. Left ventricular aneurysm is the most likely reason for persistent ST elevation in the anterior territory alone, explains the paradoxical cardiac impulse in systole, and will increase her risk of heart failure, ventricular arrhythmias and mural thrombus. Although she will be at further risk of cardiac events and could develop in-stent thrombosis, further STEMI is very unlikely without chest pain or sudden deterioration. Left ventricular hypertrophy is unlikely here given the history; however, it can give a 'strain pattern' of ST depression in the lateral leads and ST elevation in the anterior leads almost similar to left bundle branch block. There would be excessively high left ventricular voltages, however. Pericarditis is unlikely without symptoms or signs and given the timeframe after the initial STEMI, plus her ECG would show widespread concave ST elevation rather than in a single coronary artery territory. There is no murmur or signs of right heart failure to suggest ventricular septal defect.

5. C. Whilst all of these will be required, remember ABCDE and your basic life support/advanced life support training. Application of defibrillator pads is required to determine the rhythm to direct resuscitation down the shockable or non-shockable pathways, and remember arrhythmia is one of the most common post-MI complications. ABG will be helpful to determine whether there are possible reversible causes (e.g., hypoxia, electrolyte abnormalities). Blood glucose can be checked very quickly and is easily treatable if abnormal, therefore should be checked within the ABCDE structure. CXR may demonstrate pulmonary oedema and helps rule out other reversible causes (e.g., tension pneumothorax); however, you would look for clinical signs of these initially. Urgent echo may demonstrate other post-MI complications that can cause collapse (e.g., myocardial free wall rupture and cardiac tamponade, rupture of the interventricular wall, acute mitral regurgitation), as well as demonstrate evidence for other causes of collapse, e.g., pulmonary embolus.

6. A. Whilst both acute mitral regurgitation (due to rupture of chordae tendineae or papillary muscles) and ventricular septal defect can cause a pansystolic murmur and haemodynamic compromise, acute mitral regurgitation is much more frequent and often causes pulmonary oedema. Ventricular septal defect however is more associated with right heart failure and a pansystolic murmur radiating to the right sternal border. In practice, this is often difficult to differentiate; in any case, diagnosis will require Doppler echocardiography for confirmation. The ECG changes are normal evolving changes after anterior STEMI and although arrhythmia is a common complication, there is no evidence for it on the cardiac monitor. Heart block is not demonstrated on the ECG and is usually temporary if it occurs after inferior MI. Free wall rupture can present with signs of cardiac tamponade (hypotension, raised JVP, muffled heart sounds) or sudden cardiac death.

Chapter 14   Heart failure

1. B. Hepatomegaly occurs in right ventricular failure due to hepatic congestion. Bilateral basal crepitations and wheeze are signs of left ventricular failure and pulmonary congestion (or possibly respiratory disease). The patient is more likely to be hypotensive than hypertensive; right ventricular failure (with reduced right ventricular stroke volume) leads to poor filling of the left ventricle and reduced cardiac output and therefore reduced blood pressure as a result. Mid-diastolic murmur suggests mitral stenosis (which may lead to right ventricular failure) but is not a sign of right ventricular failure as such; mitral stenosis is also uncommon and almost always the result of rheumatic heart disease.

2. E. Remember to assess patients presenting with left ventricular failure in an A–E manner. The patient is breathless and therefore oxygen is the priority. They

will more than likely require intravenous diuretics but this takes longer to prepare (and to act) than giving oxygen. ß-Blockers should not be started until the patient is stable (no longer requiring intravenous diuretics). CPAP may be required in some patients (but certainly not all); consider if the patient is severely dyspnoeic and acidaemic. Opiates are no longer routinely recommended in acute left ventricular failure due to limited evidence of benefit and some evidence of increased harm.

3. A. Patients like this lady with heart failure secondary to severe LVSD and LBBB on ECG may be candidates for biventricular pacing (also known *as cardiac resynchronization therapy; CRT*), sometimes using a device that has a defibrillator function in addition (CRT-D). Biventricular pacing has a lead into both ventricles and one to the right atrium. The other types of pacemaker are used in the treatment of atrioventricular blocks, sinus node dysfunction and certain other causes of bradycardia; they are unlikely to be helpful here. A left ventricular assist device (LVAD) is an implantable pump that assists left ventricular function – it is not likely to be considered at this stage as LVADs are used as a 'bridge' e.g., to transplantation or recovery (if the issue is a transient one).

4. E. Candesartan is an angiotensin II receptor blocker and (as with ACE inhibitors), should be withheld during intercurrent illness, especially diarrhoea and vomiting, due to risk of renal impairment and hyperkalaemia. None of the other medications would be expected to cause significant harm if continued in this setting.

5. E. Paroxysmal nocturnal dyspnoea (PND) is classically seen in left ventricular failure. It is thought to be the result of pulmonary oedema due to gradual resorption of interstitial fluid overnight and nocturnal depression of respiratory function. All of the other options are more typical of right ventricular failure than left ventricular failure; the dyspnoea in left ventricular failure is the result of pulmonary oedema rather than poor pulmonary perfusion.

Chapter 15 Arrhythmias

1. D. Ventricular tachycardia (VT) is a life-threatening arrhythmia. If the patient is conscious with no haemodynamic compromise, treatment may be with antiarrhythmic drugs. In cases of conscious patients with evidence of compromise, urgent synchronized DC cardioversion is used. In the unconscious patient without a pulse (pulseless VT), immediate unsynchronized cardioversion (defibrillation) is indicated. VT is a broad-complex tachycardia.

Atropine may be given as part of the treatment of certain patients with bradycardia, but not tachycardia. VT can be caused by hypokalaemia.

2. B. Digoxin use in Wolff–Parkinson–White can result in rapid conduction through the accessory pathway and resultant haemodynamic compromise. Digoxin acts to slow conduction through the atrioventricular node. Digoxin's main route of excretion is renal. The half-life of digoxin is long, approximately 36–48 hours. The effects of digoxin are enhanced by *hypo*kalaemia and, as such, hypokalaemic patients are at increased risk of digoxin toxicity.

3. D. The 'shockable' rhythms have a better prognosis than 'non-shockable rhythms'. For pulseless VT *a non-synchronized* DC shock (i.e., defibrillation) is administered. Adrenaline is given at a dose of 1 mg every 3–5 minutes of CPR. Atropine is no longer used in a cardiac arrest situation. In the case of ventricular fibrillation, the defibrillator initial energy setting should be at least 150 J; synchronized DC cardioversion (e.g., in supraventricular tachyarrhythmias) uses lower energy settings.

4. A. Concordance means precordial leads with entirely positive (R) or entirely negative (QS) complexes, with no RS complexes seen. Capture and fusion beats are pathognomonic of VT. Verapamil can be hazardous in VT and should never be used to differentiate between SVT with aberrancy and VT. If in doubt, always treat as VT.

5. E. This man has evidence of heart failure in association with tachycardia. This is an adverse feature suggesting an unstable rhythm and warrants urgent synchronized direct current cardioversion. The other treatments may all have a part to play in management of atrial fibrillation or heart failure but are not the priority in an unstable patient.

Chapter 16 Valvular disease

1. E. Rheumatic fever is an autoimmune process is triggered by pharyngeal infection with group A β-haemolytic streptococci; the Aschoff nodules with initial inflammatory infiltrate are gradually replaced by fibrous tissue and scarring which leads to distortion of the cusps and commissures. Rheumatic fever can affect all heart valves, although the mitral and aortic are most frequently affected. It is not the most common cause of mitral regurgitation, but is the cause of the vast majority of mitral stenosis. Antibiotic prophylaxis for infective endocarditis is no longer recommended; however, patients will require long-term antibiotics to prevent recurrent rheumatic fever.

2. C. A fourth heart sound is heard when blood from atrial contraction strikes the non-compliant hypertrophied left ventricle, which can develop in severe aortic stenosis. Left ventricular hypertrophy also gives rise to a heaving non-displaced apex beat. Severe aortic stenosis is associated with paradoxical splitting of S2 (not present if aortic closing sound absent); fixed splitting is found in atrial septal defect. S2 becomes quieter in severe aortic stenosis as the thickened valves become less pliable and less able to coapt forcefully. Severe stenosis also limits stroke volume, and is associated with a narrow pulse pressure. Other severity markers include a thrill, a slow-rising or low-volume pulse, a later-peaking murmur and signs of left ventricular failure.

3. E. Malar flush (a red/purple discolouration across the cheeks) is classically associated with mitral stenosis. Mitral stenosis causes a mid-diastolic murmur best heard with the bell of the stethoscope. It may result in a 'tapping' apex beat but in pure mitral stenosis, the apex beat will not be displaced.

4. E. Mitral valve prolapse affects around 2%–3% of the population and has a female preponderance. Patients are usually asymptomatic, and it is often found incidentally on examination due to a mid-systolic click. This can be followed by a systolic murmur if there is associated mitral regurgitation. Mitral valve prolapse tends to follow a benign course and does not tend to progress towards severe mitral regurgitation or heart failure in the majority of cases.

5. A. Aortic valve replacement is performed through a median sternotomy incision. Closed mitral valvotomy is performed through a left thoracotomy incision. Mitral valvuloplasty, ICD insertion and temporary pacemaker insertion are performed percutaneously.

6. D. *Staphylococcus aureus* is associated with destructive infections and higher complication and mortality rates. It has overtaken Viridans streptococci as the most common causative organism in developed countries. Enterococci are the third most common cause of bacterial endocarditis. Fungal infections remain rare and are usually seen in immunocompromised patients, IV drug abusers, and after valve surgery. A significant proportion of cases will be culture-negative (~5% of infective endocarditis affecting native valves); this may be due to fastidious organisms that do not grow in normal blood cultures, or antibiotic therapy prior to blood cultures. Other components of the modified Duke criteria may be present to make the diagnosis.

7. C. Whilst a systolic flow murmur is present in all prosthetic aortic valves, the early diastolic murmur of aortic regurgitation is not normal. This presentation of prolonged fever and new heart failure should ring alarm bells as infective endocarditis of prosthetic valves has a poor prognosis – this must be identified and treated early. The most common findings in infective endocarditis are a murmur, pyrexia and microscopic haematuria (~90%). Splenomegaly is common (30%–40%), finger clubbing is less so (~10%); both are only present in subacute endocarditis. The well-known signs such as Osler nodes, Janeway lesions, and Roth spots are much less common (5% or less). Heart failure complicates ~50% of cases; conduction disorders are a less common complication (10%–20%). Stroke is a complication in ~20% of cases, but more subtle neurological abnormalities may be found in 30%–40% of patients.

8. C. Predisposition to infective endocarditis is a minor criterion. Others are fever, vascular phenomena, immunological phenomena and microbiological evidence not meeting a major criterion. Blood culture (not sputum culture) growth of *Staphylococcus aureus* and vegetations seen on echo are major criteria. Endocarditis may be associated with prolonged PR interval and occasionally AV dissociation; however, prolonged PR interval and erythema multiforme are criteria for rheumatic fever (revised Jones criteria), not infective endocarditis (modified Duke criteria).

Chapter 17 Diseases of the myocardium and pericardium

1. B. Dressler syndrome is a pericarditis that usually occurs 3-8 weeks after acute myocardial infarction. Pericarditis frequently causes widespread ST elevation in a distribution that does not fit with coronary artery territories. The description of his pain is classic for pericarditic pain. In contrast, the pain of an aortic dissection is classically 'ripping' or 'tearing' in nature, sudden in onset, often radiates to the back and is not normally positional; the ECG in aortic dissection may be normal or may show signs of STEMI if the dissection involves the coronary ostium. His pain is not classic for ischaemic pain and therefore not likely to represent further STEMI or unstable angina; there would also not be ST elevation in all territories in these conditions. Pneumothorax may cause sharp left-sided chest pain but will generally be worsened by inspiration rather than lying flat and it would not be associated with widespread ST elevation.

2. A. Hypertrophic cardiomyopathy (HCM) is inherited in the vast majority of cases in an autosomal dominant pattern (there are exceptions) and is attributed to mutations in a number of genes coding for sarcomere proteins. One could expect 50% of his children to inherit the mutation. Family members of affected patients are often offered screening. Some very rare, non-sarcomeric causes of HCM may follow other modes of inheritance.

3. D. Pericardial friction rubs are scratching sounds heard on auscultation and are associated with pericarditis. Janeway lesions, clubbing and conjunctival haemorrhages are features of endocarditis. Parasternal heave is a sign suggestive of right ventricular hypertrophy and pulmonary hypertension.

4. B. Beck's triad consists of muffled heart sounds (due to effusion), along with raised jugular venous pressure and low arterial blood pressure. Other signs such as delayed capillary refill, hypoxia, reduced consciousness, absent apex beat and pulsus paradoxus may occur in tamponade but these are not part of the classical triad. A friction rub may be heard if there is co-existing pericarditis.

5. D. Takotsubo cardiomyopathy is often initially misdiagnosed as ECG features may mimic those of STEMI. Takotsubo cardiomyopathy is also known as 'broken heart syndrome'. It affects far more women than men and treatment is generally supportive in nature. Fluid resuscitation may be indicated in some cases but patients frequently have evidence of fluid overload due to systolic dysfunction. Long-term prognosis is generally very good with a low mortality rate and up to 95% of patients achieving full recovery. The name 'Takotsubo' comes from the Japanese word for a kind of octopus trap because of the shape the left ventricle takes on rather than it being first described in Japanese fishermen.

6. E. Obstruction is a feature in only around 25% of patients. Disopyramide is sometimes used in patients with obstruction to reduce resting pressure gradients and improve symptoms. HCM has many variants and can present at any age. Myomectomy may be indicated in some patients with HCM but this is not a percutaneous procedure. Those diagnosed as children have a poorer prognosis and a higher risk of sudden cardiac death, whereas those who remain asymptomatic and are diagnosed at a later age, as adults, generally have a better prognosis.

Chapter 18 Congenital heart disease

1. E. VSD is the most common of the traditional congenital cardiac abnormalities (or second most common if bicuspid aortic valve is included).

2. D. Tetralogy of Fallot presents with progressive cyanosis early in life. ASD, VSD and PDA do not present initially with cyanosis as the shunt is from left to right; however, cyanosis can occur later if Eisenmenger syndrome develops. Coarctation is not associated with cyanosis.

3. C. Eisenmenger syndrome develops when a long standing left-to-right shunt reverses into a cyanotic right-to-left shunt due to increased pulmonary vascular resistance and therefore there is the potential for paradoxical emboli. It is associated with polycythaemia and fingernail clubbing but not anaemia or splinter haemorrhages.

4. B. PFO is thought to be associated with migraine, along with paradoxical emboli causing stroke/transient ischaemic attack and decompression sickness. The others are not believed to have a positive association.

5. E. Squatting may relieve symptoms as it increases systemic vascular resistance, thereby decreasing right-to-left shunting. Exertion, such as feeding or crying, may worsen right ventricular outflow obstruction and precipitate a 'tet' spell, where cyanosis worsens, and syncope may even occur. Pulmonary artery pressure is usually low because pulmonary stenosis protects the pulmonary circulation. Patent ductus arteriosus and left ventricular hypertrophy are not included in the four defects seen in tetralogy of Fallot.

6. A. Downward/apical displacement of the septal tricuspid leaflet is common to all cases of Ebstein anomaly. In around half of patients with Ebstein anomaly, PFO or ASD is associated, and accessory conduction pathway is seen less commonly. VSD and right ventricular outflow tract obstruction are infrequently associated; however, these, along with overriding aorta and RVH, are the four features of tetralogy of Fallot.

Chapter 1 Cardiac anatomy, physiology and development

Anatomy and physiology

1. A   Although it seems a misnomer, brain natriuretic peptide was thus named as it was first identified in the brains of pigs.

2. H   Myocardial cell injury must occur for cardiac troponin to be detected in the bloodstream.

3. D   This is the outermost layer of the heart, and if the coronary artery is perforated during angioplasty (a rare complication), this leads to tamponade. The middle and innermost layers of the heart are the myocardium and endocardium respectively.

4. G   The balance between fluid production and reabsorption by the serous pericardium can be disturbed due to certain conditions (e.g., pericarditis, malignancy), and fluid can accumulate (pericardial effusion).

5. E   The mediastinum contains a number of structures including the heart, great vessels, thymus, and trachea, and separates the two pleural cavities.

Chapter 2 The cardiac cycle, control of cardiac output, and haemodynamic regulation

Cardiac electrophysiology

1. E   Phase 0 of the action potential is the result of rapid Na^+ influx through voltage-gated Na^+ channels after the threshold potential is reached.

2. H   The gap junction is an intercellular connection between adjacent cells. These junctions allow rapid conduction of action potentials through the myocardium.

3. F   Around 90% of cytosolic calcium is removed by $Ca2^+$ATPase on the sarcoplasmic reticulum. The remainder is removed by $Na^+/Ca2^+$ exchangers on the plasma membrane.

4. B   Long QT syndrome is most frequently caused by defects in voltage-gated K^+ channels – defective K^+ channels delay repolarization and lengthen the QT interval.

5. D   Digoxin inhibits the Na^+/K^+ATPase, which increases intracellular sodium levels, reducing activity of the $Na^+/Ca2^+$ exchanger and therefore increasing intracellular calcium. This prolongs phase 4 and phase 0 of the action potential, slowing heart rate and increasing contractility.

Chapter 3 ECG interpretations

Components of the ECG trace

1. D   The QRS complex represents ventricular depolarization. In bundle branch block, the QRS complex is prolonged due to delayed conduction down the affected bundle branch.

2. E   The ST segment correlates with phase 2 (the plateau phase) of the cardiac action potential. During the plateau phase, there is generally no (or very limited) net current flow, hence the reason why the ST segment is normally isoelectric with the ECG baseline.

3. F   The T wave is the result of ventricular repolarization.

4. B   The PR interval may be short in conditions with an additional conducting pathway (for example Wolff-Parkinson-White syndrome).

5. G   The QT interval when prolonged (e.g., either congenitally, or as the consequence of a number of different drugs) increases the risk of developing an arrhythmia known as torsades de pointes (a polymorphic ventricular tachycardia).

ECG leads

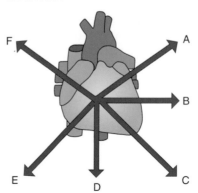

1. B   Lead I is represented by line B and is said to be at an angle of 0 degrees.

2. C   Lead II at +60 degrees.

3. E   Lead III is at +120 degrees.

4. D   Lead aVF is at +90 degrees.

5. A   Lead aVL is at −30 degrees.

6. F   Lead aVR is at −150 degrees.

Chapter 4 Other common investigations

CXR signs related to cardiology

1. E   In heart failure, there are multiple useful signs. Cardiomegaly is defined as a cardio-thoracic ratio >50% in posterior-anterior (PA) films. Alveolar oedema is usually seen as patchy bilateral opacification radiating from the hila ('bat's wing appearance'), and interstitial oedema can be seen as septal (e.g., Kerley B) lines and fluid in the horizontal fissure. Upper zone pulmonary vessel congestion can be seen. Pleural effusion may be seen as blunting (indistinctness) of the cardiophrenic angle or the meniscus sign. The (imperfect) ABCDE mnemonic can be helpful to remember CXR signs of left-ventricular failure: Alveolar oedema, Kerley B lines, Cardiomegaly, upper venous Diversion, pleural Effusion.

2. D   The upper left heart border is usually flat or slightly concave; when the left atrium is enlarged, the left atrial appendage can look convex and protruding, and sometimes the right side of the left atrium pushes behind the right cardiac shadow to indent the lung and form a separate right heart border silhouette known as the double density sign. This is different to left-ventricular enlargement which usually causes the lower left heart border to displace downwards or laterally.

3. G   In pericardial effusion, the cardiac silhouette is symmetrically enlarged. This is described as a globular enlargement, and with massive effusion can appear like a water bottle. Sometimes this can be difficult to distinguish from cardiomegaly.

4. C   Usually the centre of the diaphragm is obscured by the heart and not visible on CXRs; however, in pneumomediastinum (or occasionally pneumopericardium), air between the lower border of the heart and the diaphragm separates the tissues and allows the complete diaphragm to be visualized. This may be seen after e.g., chest trauma, Boerhaave syndrome.

5. F   Median sternotomy wires or mediastinal surgical clips can be seen after surgery. Heart valve replacements can sometimes be seen.

Chapter 5 History and examination of the cardiovascular system

Clinical Signs

1. E   Janeway lesions are a cutaneous manifestation of infective endocarditis as the result of septic emboli in the skin. Osler nodes are an immunological phenomenon. Osler nodes are painful, whereas Janeway lesions are not.

2. I   Coarctation of the aorta would classically cause a radiofemoral delay.

3. B   In isolated left ventricular failure, bibasal crepitations may be heard at the lung bases. Elevated JVP may be seen in the patient that also has right ventricular failure.

4. C   Aortic stenosis is classically associated with an ejection-systolic murmur.

5. A   Patients with aortic regurgitation may have a 'collapsing' pulse. Aortic regurgitation is classically associated with an early rather than mid-diastolic murmur.

Chapter 6 Causes of chest pain

1. G   This is typical of heart failure caused by viral myocarditis with the flu-like prodrome, although the presentation varies widely. ECG changes are variable, and commonly demonstrate nonspecific ST segment changes. Myocarditis can involve the pericardium (myopericarditis) and can result in widespread concave ST elevation on the ECG. At this young age, myocardial infarction is very unlikely.

2. D   Boerhaave syndrome describes a full-thickness oesophageal tear which occurs as a result of severe vomiting and is thought to occur due to uncoordinated forceful ejection of gastric contents against a closed glottis when the oesophagus is not relaxed. This allows caustic gastric contents to empty into the mediastinum and can leak into the pleural space causing pleural effusion and/or pneumothorax. The presentation is varied, and the classic Mackler's triad (vomiting, chest pain, and subcutaneous emphysema) is uncommon. The crunching/rasping sound in time with cardiac cycle due to pneumomediastinum is known as Hamman's sign. Aspiration pneumonia would be within the differentials, as would pneumothorax given the subcutaneous emphysema. Coexisting arrhythmia (e.g., atrial fibrillation (AF) in association with infection) is possible; however, at this degree of tachycardia it is not severe enough to cause

chest pain alone. Boerhaave syndrome is the best unifying diagnosis and important to diagnose early – untreated, it usually leads to severe sepsis and death.

3. E   Burning pain precipitated by food and lying down and improved with antacids is likely due to indigestion. Due to his age, you would want to ascertain whether he has any ischaemic risk factors, and check his ECG and troponin for reassurance.

4. K   This lady presents with dypsnoea, pleuritic chest pain, tachycardia, and a leg suggestive of DVT. She has a strong risk factor for venous thromboembolism given her recent diagnosis of cancer. The most likely diagnosis is therefore pulmonary embolus.

5. C   This lady is likely to have AF with a fast ventricular response, driven by bacteraemia from pyelonephritis. Cardiac monitoring and ECG is vital, as chest pain may indicate myocardial ischaemia (due to rapid ventricular rate), which is an adverse feature.

Chapter 7   Breathlessness and peripheral oedema

Causes of oedema

1. G   Deep venous thrombosis (DVT) seems the most likely diagnosis here given the unilateral leg swelling and discomfort on palpation of the calf and recent long-haul flight.

2. B   There are a number of factors here that would point towards liver disease. Intravenous drug use is a significant risk factor for infection with blood borne viruses (including hepatitis B and C) which may lead to cirrhosis. Itchiness, easy bruising and particularly her icterus/jaundice suggest hepatic failure.

3. E   It is likely that this man has been started on amlodipine for treatment of hypertension. Amlodipine is well recognized as a cause of ankle swelling (and headache).

4. G   This lady's history is strongly suspicious of a malignancy, given her significant weight loss, microcytic anaemia and other investigations not revealing the cause of her symptoms. The abdominal bloating raises the possibility of a pelvic malignancy. It is possible that this may be causing external compression of pelvic veins and resultant oedema. Active malignancy would also increase risk of developing a DVT, although the long history would be somewhat unusual.

5. A   This gentleman is reporting orthopnoea and paroxysmal nocturnal dyspnoea. He has dyspnoea on exertion and peripheral oedema. This history is strongly suggestive of cardiac failure; echocardiography would be useful to evaluate his ventricular function.

Chapter 8   Palpitation

Causes of palpitation

1. B   Palpitations that present in stressful situations and are associated with peri-oral or finger paraesthesia are most likely secondary to anxiety. Do not forget about other causes of palpitation; anaemia is common in young females, although perhaps less likely here given the short history and other predisposing factors.

2. A   Dark stools, epigastric discomfort, lethargy and alcohol excess would lead to a strong suspicion of gastrointestinal blood loss, e.g., from a duodenal ulcer. Anaemia is the most likely cause of this gentleman's palpitations.

3. I   This is most likely to represent ectopic beats (sometimes felt as missed or forceful beats).

4. K   Arrhythmias are common following myocardial infarction. In this case, the rhythm is most likely ventricular tachycardia. It is unlikely to be ventricular fibrillation as the gentleman was conscious throughout and the episode resolved spontaneously. Supraventricular tachycardia is unlikely as the arrhythmia showed broad complexes and there is no mention of aberrant conduction on the resting ECG.

5. D   Given the normal ECG, this lady's palpitations are most likely secondary to hypovolaemia from her recent illness. She has a significant postural drop.

Chapter 9   Syncope

Causes of syncope

1. K   This lady has a very short PR interval on the ECG and in the context of palpitations and collapse, Wolff-Parkinson-White syndrome is the most likely diagnosis.

2. B   This man has the classic triad of symptoms seen in aortic stenosis (angina, syncope and breathlessness). He also has a very narrow pulse pressure. Of the available options, aortic stenosis is the most likely diagnosis and his symptoms indicate it is likely severe.

3. F   Citalopram, methadone and clarithromycin all tend to prolong QT interval. The paroxysms of rapid palpitations and presyncope/syncope likely represent a polymorphic tachycardia (torsades de pointes).

4. G   This man is likely significantly hypovolaemic (due to increased losses and reduced intake). He will likely have a significant postural drop if tested; this is a classic story for syncope as the result of orthostatic hypotension.

5. D   Arrhythmias are common after a myocardial infarction. Complete heart block after anterior MI occurs due to septal infarction and necrosis of the conducting system; this will require permanent pacing.

Chapter 10 Heart murmurs

History and examination

1. F   She is likely to have a flow murmur due to her current high-output state with the combination of anaemia and third trimester of pregnancy. These are generally ejection systolic.

2. I   Papillary muscle rupture causes acute mitral regurgitation and is a complication of myocardial infarction. She is likely to have a pansystolic murmur which classically radiates to the axilla. This can be difficult to differentiate from ventricular septal defect, which can also be a complication of myocardial infarction and cause a pansystolic murmur, which classically radiates to the right lower sternal border. Loud murmurs can frequently be heard throughout the precordium. An urgent echocardiogram will be required to confirm the diagnosis.

3. M   This boy presents with lower limb claudication and upper limb hypertension – this is a classic presentation of aortic coarctation. The femoral pulse may be weak or delayed, but pulses from aortic branches prior to the coarctation (e.g., radial, carotid) will have normal timing. The continuous hum heard on the lateral thoracic wall due to collateral vessels does not usually occur until late childhood.

4. H   Murmurs follow the direction of blood flow, therefore blood flow backwards from aortic regurgitation is heard loudest at the left lower sternal border.

5. B   The quiet low mid-diastolic rumbling of mitral stenosis is famously difficult to hear. Increase chances of hearing this by listening at the apex with the patient lying on their left side with their breath held in expiration.

Causes of pulmonary hypertension

1. E   Pulmonary hypertension with no identifiable precipitating factor is described as primary. It is rare, can be familial, and most commonly occurs in young women.

2. F   This clinical scenario suggests pulmonary embolism, with typical symptoms and risk factors (recent immobilization and oral contraceptive pill).

3. I   Systemic sclerosis (scleroderma) is a multisystem autoimmune disorder of the connective tissue. The description of tight thickened skin is classic of the type of systemic sclerosis which involves the skin. Systemic sclerosis, other autoimmune rheumatic disorders and vasculitides are important causes of pulmonary hypertension.

4. D   Rheumatic fever may result in rheumatic heart disease – most commonly affecting the mitral valve and causing mitral stenosis. The clinical signs are consistent with mitral stenosis. Atrial fibrillation is commonly seen in mitral stenosis, and is often a result of left atrial dilatation.

5. B   This history is typical of the insidious development of COPD. Pulmonary hypertension as a result of severe lung disease is known as cor pulmonale.

Chapter 11 Atherosclerosis

Antiplatelets and anticoagulants

1. D   Ticagrelor binds to the $P2Y_{12}$ component of the ADP receptor reversibly and induces conformational change to prevent the normal binding of ADP at high ticagrelor concentrations. It has now replaced clopidogrel as first-line treatment (together with aspirin) in the initial treatment of acute coronary syndromes (ACS).

2. E   Tirofiban, abciximab and eptifibatide belong to this group. They tend only to be given to high-risk ACS patients and during angioplasty.

3. B   Clopidogrel irreversibly blocks the $P2Y_{12}$ component of the ADP receptor for the lifetime of the platelet.

4. C   Fondaparinux directly inhibits factor Xa, while heparin catalyses antithrombin III which indirectly inhibits factor Xa. Both will therefore inhibit the coagulation cascade (see Fig. 11.3).

5. F   Unfractionated heparin inhibits thrombin and factor Xa through an antithrombin III-dependent mechanism. Inactivation of thrombin prevents thrombin-induced platelet activation and activation of multiple coagulation factors.

Chapter 12 Risk factors

Management of hypertension

1. H   Her hypertension has not been controlled by the medications at step 2 of the NICE and British

Hypertension Society guidelines; therefore proceed to step 3 and add a thiazide-like diuretic.

2. D   There is no suggestion of secondary hypertension, and as he is of African descent, at any age the first choice is a calcium channel blocker as per the hypertension guidelines.

3. B   He has uncontrolled hypertension on stage 3 of the hypertension guidelines; therefore he should be referred to a specialist and commenced on an additional antihypertensive as advised at stage 4. The options available from the list above are an α-blocker or spironolactone. Spironolactone can be a good antihypertensive especially in the context of heart failure, nephrotic syndrome or ascites. However, given his serum potassium is already at the high end of normal, starting spironolactone is likely to cause hyperkalaemia. An α-blocker is the best choice here and is best started at night in case he develops symptomatic first-dose hypotension.

4. C   10% of patients on an ACE inhibitor develop a dry cough due to increased bradykinin levels. An angiotensin II receptor antagonist also acts on the renin-angiotensin-aldosterone-system but does not inhibit bradykinin breakdown, and is the best alternative here.

5. E   This is an immediate indication to stop his ACE inhibitor, and he will require repeat blood tests – his renal function and mild hyperkalaemia will hopefully improve with cessation. Dramatic renal function decline after starting an ACE inhibitor can suggest renovascular hypertension, and warrants specialist review.

Causes of secondary hypertension

1. H   Renal artery stenosis is usually due to atherosclerosis in the elderly, may cause an upper abdominal bruit, and is typically associated with hypertension refractory to treatment.

2. A   Whilst headache and epistaxis are non-specific, they can be symptoms of aortic coarctation. Here, coarctation is strongly suggested by the lower limb relative hypoperfusion and the continuous murmur. Radiofemoral delay may also be found. The murmur may be palpable as a thrill, and there may be a prominent pulsation in the supraclavicular notch. If you request a CXR, it may demonstrate 'rib notching' from collateral vessels.

3. F   There are few indications for nephrectomy, as the kidney is not easily accessible and removal comes with risks. It is usually left in situ if it is non-functioning and kidney transplants are usually plumbed into the iliac vessels instead. The kidney is only removed if it is causing harm, such as from renal cell carcinoma or from surrounding pressure effects from a grossly enlarged kidney (e.g., polycystic kidneys). Autosomal dominant polycystic kidney disease is the most common inherited renal condition and is a different entity to autosomal recessive polycystic kidney disease, which affects infants. Although polycystic kidney disease and aortic coarctation are both associated with intracranial aneurysms and subarachnoid haemorrhage (the cause of the stroke here), the other aspects of the history in this case point to an inherited renal cause.

4. C   Weight loss despite a good appetite is a classic presentation of hyperthyroidism. Weakness, fine tremor, and irritability are also features. Tachycardia results from an increased basal metabolic rate. Hypertension is found both in hypothyroidism and (much more commonly) in hyperthyroidism.

5. G   Also known as Conn syndrome, primary hyperaldosteronism is due to excessive adrenal cortex production of aldosterone, which promotes sodium (and water) retention and potassium excretion. Hypokalaemia and hypernatraemia are classic findings; however, many patients may have normal or borderline results. Metabolic alkalosis is also typical. Weakness and cramps may result from hypokalaemia, or from other electrolytes that are lost (e.g., calcium and magnesium).

Chapter 13 Stable angina and acute coronary syndromes

Medication side effects 1

1. B   This is in common with other β-blockers. Other side effects include tiredness, bronchospasm, bradycardia and erectile dysfunction.

2. F   Other side effects of nitrates include flushing and postural hypotension.

3. H   Myalgia is an important side effect of all statins and should be investigated with serial assessments of creatinine kinase (CK) levels. A fourfold increase in the CK levels suggests that the drug should be discontinued. Liver and function tests should also be monitored.

4. E   Other side effects include hyperkalaemia, impotence and menstrual irregularities.

5. J   Bleeding with or without thrombocytopenia is a major side effect associated with the use of this glycoprotein IIa/IIIb inhibitor.

ECG changes

1. **E**   The leads II, III and aVF 'look' at the inferior wall of the heart, and ST elevation with reciprocal ST depression may be seen in the acute phase of myocardial infarction.

2. **D**   Hyperkalaemia is associated with tall T waves and short P wave amplitudes; the changes are dependent on the K^+ concentration. At higher concentrations, the PR interval becomes longer and QRS complexes become wider and eventually asystolic cardiac arrest occurs. Note that the ECG changes in hypokalaemia are the reverse, with larger P wave and smaller T amplitudes, leading to VT/VF as the terminal cardiac event.

3. **H**   Long-standing hypertension leads to left ventricular hypertrophy.

4. **C**   The chest leads V1–V4 'look' at the anterior wall of the left ventricle. The presence of Q waves supports the presence of old trans-mural myocardial infarction.

5. **A**   Widespread concave or saddle-shaped ST segment elevation occurs in pericarditis. Other ECG changes that may be seen include PR depression in the early stages and T wave inversion.

Medication side effects 2

1. **B**   Amlodipine can cause ankle swelling, and if this is troublesome, an alternative antihypertensive should be used instead.

2. **H**   Acute deterioration in renal function may result if the patient has renal artery stenosis. This is because the efferent renal arteriole is preferentially dilated compared to the afferent arteriole, so the perfusion pressure across the kidney falls.

3. **I**   A rash may result as a reaction to the contrast agent used for the angiogram, or as a reaction to clopidogrel. If the former is responsible, symptoms will resolve. If clopidogrel is the cause of the rash, this may resolve with time. Clopidogrel should not be discontinued without discussion with a consultant cardiologist, as this may predispose to acute stent thrombosis, which is potentially fatal.

4. **A**   Amiodarone may cause pulmonary fibrosis, liver derangement, hyper- or hypothyroidism, peripheral neuropathy, corneal microdeposits and prolonged QT. Patients must be warned they should shield their skin from sunlight as amiodarone causes photosensitivity.

5. **D**   Erectile dysfunction is a well-recognized side effect of β-blockers and unless essential can be discontinued – a calcium channel antagonist, such as verapamil or diltiazem, is often prescribed instead.

Chapter 14 Heart failure

Pharmacological treatment of heart failure

1. **D**   Eplerenone and spironolactone are mineralocorticoid receptor antagonists (or aldosterone antagonists). Spironolactone is associated with gynaecomastia, whereas eplerenone is not.

2. **B**   ACE inhibitors, such as enalapril, commonly (in around 5% of patients) cause a dry cough; patients who develop this adverse effect should be switched to an angiotensin II receptor blocker, such as candesartan.

3. **G**   Ivabradine inhibits the I*f* channel (the *f* is for 'funny').

4. **C**   Digoxin is negatively chronotropic (slows the heart rate) but positively inotropic (improves contraction strength), whereas bisoprolol for instance is negatively inotropic and chronotropic.

5. **F**   Tolerance to nitrate medications develops rapidly if there are no nitrate free periods – if isosorbide mononitrate is prescribed twice daily, it is generally done in an asymmetric manner (e.g., morning and lunchtime) to allow for a nitrate free period.

Causes of heart failure

1. **G**   Viral myocarditis is the most likely answer in a young male with recent flu-like illness and dilated cardiomyopathy. Other causes of dilated cardiomyopathy include idiopathic, excess alcohol and post-partum – note alcohol is unlikely to be the cause here given the young age of the patient.

2. **F**   The features mentioned indicate hypertensive retinopathy. Systemic hypertension is an important cause of heart failure.

3. **B**   The signs are of aortic regurgitation. Ankylosing spondylitis is associated with aortitis, aortic regurgitation and abnormalities of the cardiac electrical conduction system.

4. **C**   These signs are consistent with aortic stenosis – in the patient presenting with heart failure, surgical (or sometimes percutaneous) treatment may be warranted.

5. **J**   The murmur described is that of mitral regurgitation – in the patient presenting with heart failure surgical treatment may be warranted.

Starting medications in heart failure/after myocardial infarction

1. **A**   This man should also be started on an ACE inhibitor, as long as there is no contraindication. This has been shown to reduce mortality

in large randomised clinical trials. His renal function should be monitored.

2. E   This patient should be started on a β-blocker and this should be titrated upwards with the aim of reducing his heart rate to closer to 60 beats/min at rest. There is good evidence that β-blocker treatment reduces mortality after MI.

3. I   Patients who are still symptomatic despite treatment with an ACE inhibitor and a β-blocker, should be started on a mineralocorticoid receptor antagonist as the next step in their management – current guidelines recommend spironolactone initially unless contraindicated.

4. G   This man's symptoms have not improved despite first-line (ACE inhibitor and β-blocker) and second-line treatments (spironolactone). The next step would be third-line treatments of which the only option listed is hydralazine and nitrate in combination. An alternative here might be digoxin, particularly if he was tachycardic at rest.

5. F   Gynaecomastia and breast pain/discomfort is a commonly recognised side effect of spironolactone. Patients who experience these symptoms should be switched to eplerenone, which is also a mineralocorticoid receptor antagonist but does not have these adverse effects.

Chapter 15 Arrhythmias

ECG appearances

1. F   This is a typical feature of RBBB.

2. J   Complete heart block is exemplified by P waves which 'march' through the rhythm strip with no relationship to the QRS complexes. A ventricular escape rhythm is usually 30–40 beats/min and gives rise to wide QRS complexes.

3. G   J waves are classically seen in individuals with significant hypothermia.

4. H   Delta waves arise from the 'pre-excitation' of the ventricular myocardium. This results from antegrade conduction via the accessory pathway. The accessory pathway differs from the AV node in that it does not have a regulatory 'slowing down' function. Therefore, the PR interval is shortened.

5. D   Mobitz Type I heart block (or Wenckebach phenomenon) is characterized by progressive prolongation of PR interval until a beat is dropped and the cycle repeats. This is caused by fatigue of cells in the atrioventricular node and can be seen sometimes in healthy individuals.

Treatment of arrhythmia

1. G   This description is most likely of supraventricular tachycardia. Adenosine can cause bronchospasm in asthmatic patients and therefore is best avoided. Verapamil can be used as an alternative to return the patient to sinus rhythm if other interventions have failed.

2. H   This gentleman has likely been started on an antipsychotic medication, which can cause QT prolongation. This description is of an episode of torsades de pointes which is best treated with intravenous magnesium (even if magnesium levels are normal) and removal of the causative agent.

3. E   This is most likely atrial fibrillation with a fast ventricular response, possibly secondary to underlying lower respiratory tract infection. Of the above treatments, the most appropriate is treatment with digoxin (and treatment of underlying infection).

4. J   Asystole is a non-shockable rhythm with poor prognosis. There is no role for defibrillation in this cause. Treatment is with intravenous adrenaline, continued CPR and attempting to rule out a reversible cause of arrest.

5. D   Complete heart block in the absence of an obvious precipitant or pharmacological cause will require permanent pacing. If patients with complete heart block are unstable, they may require temporary pacing until this can be arranged. There is no clear indication for atropine at this stage.

Chapter 16 Valvular disease

Examination findings

1. D   A double apical impulse suggests hypertrophic cardiomyopathy. The left ventricle is stiff and this results in raised left-ventricular end-diastolic pressure. Therefore, the left atrium has to contract forcefully and it is this impulse (a palpable fourth heart sound) in addition to left-ventricular contraction that may be appreciated.

2. G   A left parasternal heave indicates right ventricular hypertrophy as the right ventricle sits anteriorly. Causes include pulmonary hypertension (most common), mitral valve disease and pulmonary stenosis. In pulmonary hypertension, the right ventricle is under strain against an increased pulmonary artery pressure. Mild mitral stenosis will not cause right ventricular hypertrophy. Right ventricular hypertrophy is unlikely in mitral valve prolapse

as the vast majority of patients remain asymptomatic and follow a benign long-term course.

3. F   These signs are suggestive of mitral-valve prolapse. This is usually idiopathic, but may occur in association with connective-tissue disorders.

4. E   An opening snap can precede the mid-diastolic murmur of mitral stenosis, and if the patient is in sinus rhythm, there can be pre-systolic increase in the murmur volume due to atrial contraction. Mitral stenosis is frequently associated with atrial fibrillation as the disease progresses, as AF risk increases with left atrial enlargement which occurs secondary to mitral stenosis.

5. H   The regurgitant jet causes back pressure in the right atrium and this is transmitted to the venous system causing hepatic congestion and (if severe) pulsatile hepatomegaly.

Underlying pathology in endocarditis

1. I   *Staph. aureus* is highly invasive and the most likely cause given the acute history and history of IVDU (and has become the most common cause overall). Fungi and pseudomonas are also more common in IVDU.

2. D   Q fever (and brucellosis) are associated with contact with farm animals.

3. J   This patient has a predisposition to infective endocarditis due to valve damage from previous rheumatic fever. Viridans group Streptococci are more likely than *Staphylococcus* in this case given subacute presentation, poor dentition and no suggestion of sources of *Staphylococcus* (skin or healthcare-associated infections). Bacteraemia from an oral or upper respiratory source can be due to chewing, brushing teeth, recent dental work, tonsillectomy or bronchoscopy.

4. F   Libman-Sacks endocarditis is seen in patients with systemic lupus erythematosus and is not related to infection. As there are no features of infection in this case, microbes that cause infective endocarditis but negative blood cultures are unlikely. These include *Bartonella, Coxiella, Chlamydia, Legionella* and *Brucella* species as well as fungi and the HACEK group (*Haemophilus sp., Aggregatibacter sp., Cardiobacterium sp., Eikenella corrodens, Kingella sp.*). Blood cultures may also be negative if antibiotics have been started before blood cultures are taken.

5. H   *Strep. gallolyticus* (or *Strep. bovis*) and *Strep. anginosus* (or *Strep. milleri*) are both gram-positive cocci in pairs or chains and are

associated with colorectal cancer. These are both Viridans group Streptococci but Option H is the better answer here.

Chapter 17   Diseases of the myocardium and pericardium

Causes of chest pain

1. B   This man has the classical signs of tamponade known as Beck's triad (hypotension, raised jugular venous pulse, muffling of heart sounds). This may be a presentation of myocardial rupture given this man's history of recent myocardial infarction.

2. A   The scratching sound may be a pericardial rub. This is a typical description of acute pericarditis. Sometimes patients may have evidence of co-existing myocarditis but there is no particular evidence to suggest this here.

3. I   Takotsubo cardiomyopathy may present similarly to acute coronary syndrome but coronary arteries are typically unremarkable on angiogram and left ventricular apical ballooning is the hallmark feature. This condition is often (but not always) preceded by a stressful life event.

4. E   Hypertrophic cardiomyopathy is the leading cause of sudden cardiac death in young athletes. A number of these conditions may be associated with sudden cardiac death but the family history suggests the underlying cause may be an inherited condition.

5. F   Infective endocarditis should always be suspected in patients presenting with fever. This lady is at increased risk due to previous valve replacement. The erythematous lesions may be Osler nodes or Janeway lesions.

Chapter 18   Congenital heart disease

Causes of congenital heart disease

1. E   Kartagener syndrome is a rare autosomal recessive condition that is characterized by situs inversus (mirror-image transposition of the viscera including dextrocardia), and effects of primary ciliary dyskinesia including bronchiectasis and sinusitis. Although other consequences are found, the classical triad involves the conditions underlined.

2. I   Maternal alcohol use can cause a number of congenital heart defects but most commonly ventricular septal defects, followed by atrial septal defects.

3. K   Maternal rubella can cause a patent (also called persistent) ductus arteriosus, pulmonary (valvular or artery) stenosis and atrial septal defect, as well as cataracts, deafness and microcephaly.

4. L   Down syndrome is associated with several congenital heart lesions and one or more of these occur in approximately 40% of cases.

5. J   The two most common cardiovascular malformations are bicuspid aortic valve (which can lead to aortic stenosis) and aortic coarctation – both obstructive lesions. Partial anomalous venous drainage and aortic dilatation are recognized, but less common.

Objective structured clinical examination (OSCE) stations

OSCE 1 Examination in the breathless patient

Mr White is a 75-year-old gentleman; he has been complaining of shortness of breath on exertion. Please examine his cardiovascular system:

Checklist

- Introduce yourself, check patient's details, obtain consent, and expose patient from the waist up.
- Observe the patient from the end of the bed.
- Examine the hands for splinter haemorrhages, clubbing, Osler nodes, Janeway lesions, and peripheral cyanosis.
- Palpate the radial pulse and comment on the rate and rhythm. Check for radioradial delay. Assess for a collapsing pulse by placing the flats of the fingers over the radial artery and raising the patient's arm above their head.
- State that you would like to measure the patient's blood pressure.
- Inspect the eyes, cheeks and mouth.
- Visualize the jugular venous pressure pulse and comment on its height.
- Palpate the carotid pulse and comment on the character and volume of the pulse.
- Inspect the precordium looking for scars, pacemakers, visual impulses.
- Palpate for the apex beat, heaves, and thrills over the valve areas.
- Auscultate the four valve areas, the axilla and neck.
- Auscultate for diastolic murmurs; left lateral position and then sitting forward in held expiration.
- Auscultate the lung bases, feel for sacral oedema and pedal oedema.
- Thank the patient and cover him up.
- To finish your examination, state that you would like to palpate all peripheral pulses, check for radiofemoral delay, perform fundoscopy, and order an ECG.

Questions

1. What signs might you find in right heart failure?
   - Peripheral oedema, elevated jugular venous pulse, hepatomegaly, ascites, murmur of tricuspid regurgitation (hepatomegaly may be pulsatile with tricuspid regurgitation).
2. How might you differentiate the jugular venous pulse (JVP) from the carotid pulsation?

- The JVP is a double pulsation and should not be palpable (whereas the carotid is a single, palpable pulsation). Pressing over the liver should augment the JVP (known as hepatojugular reflux). The height of the JVP varies with respiration and the position of the patient, whereas the carotid pulse does not vary.
3. What signs might you find in left heart failure?
   - Crepitations (particularly bibasally) on auscultation of the chest, evidence of pleural effusion, murmur of mitral regurgitation.
4. What findings might you find on an X-ray in left heart failure?
   - **A**lveolar oedema, Kerley **B** lines, **C**ardiomegaly, upper lobe venous **D**iversion and pleural **E**ffusion (ABCDE can be used to remember these findings).
5. What is the New York Heart Association (NYHA) classification of heart failure?
   - A grading system used to denote the symptoms and functional status of patients with heart failure. Patients are assigned a number (I to IV) with I meaning no limitation of physical activity due to symptoms, II meaning symptoms with ordinary activity, III meaning symptoms with minimal activity and IV meaning symptoms at rest.

OSCE 2 Examination in the cyanosed patient

Ms Clark is a 65-year-old lady who has been profoundly cyanosed for the last 3 years. She was previously known to have a murmur but did not ever have this investigated. She is not breathless at rest. Please examine her cardiovascular system.

See OSCE 1: Checklist.

Questions

1. How might central and peripheral cyanosis be differentiated clinically?
   - Central cyanosis can be seen in the lips and the tongue. Patients with central cyanosis will generally also be peripherally cyanosed; however peripheries are generally normal temperature unless there is associated poor peripheral circulation. *Pure* peripheral cyanosis will cause cold, blue hands and feet, but no cyanosis centrally, i.e., normal colour lips and tongue.

2. What is the differential diagnosis of central cyanosis and which is most likely in this patient?
   - The differential diagnosis here includes:
     i. Conditions that cause a right-to-left cardiac shunt (Eisenmenger syndrome and cyanotic congenital heart disease).
     ii. Pulmonary disease of any aetiology sufficient to cause hypoxia.
     iii. Abnormal haemoglobins e.g., methaemoglobinaemia (either acquired due to medications, toxins, etc., or rarely congenital causes).
     iv. Polycythaemia rubra vera (increased chance of cyanosis due to high haemoglobin and therefore greater oxygen requirement to fully oxygenate).

The most likely diagnosis in this case would be Eisenmenger syndrome, given the history of previous uninvestigated murmur and the fact that she has been cyanosed for the past 3 years (but not previously).

3. What is the aetiology of Eisenmenger syndrome?
   - Eisenmenger syndrome is the end result of a longstanding left-to-right cardiac shunt, generally caused by congenital heart disease (ventricular septal defect, atrial septal defect, or sometimes a patent ductus arteriosus), gradually leading to pulmonary hypertension and eventual reversal of the shunt. The now right-to-left cardiac shunt results in deoxygenated blood entering the systemic circulation and the patient becomes cyanosed at this point.

4. How is Eisenmenger syndrome managed?
   - By the time that Eisenmenger syndrome develops and the patient becomes cyanosed, there is unfortunately no known way to reverse these changes. Definitive treatment of this condition requires either a heart-lung transplant or lung transplant with repair of the underlying heart defect. Patients are, however, often managed conservatively as both these options have high mortality rates.

5. How might the development of Eisenmenger syndrome be prevented?
   - The main way to prevent this condition is through clinical examination and echocardiography to identify congenital heart defects early (before they cause pulmonary hypertension) and treating the underlying condition. For instance, ventricular septal defects can be closed either surgically or in some cases percutaneously.

OSCE 3 Examination of the patient with a valve replacement and implantable device

Mr Brown is a 74-year-old gentleman who has previously undergone a number of procedures, including a valve replacement and insertion of an implantable device. Please examine his cardiovascular system.

See OSCE 1: Checklist.

Questions:

1. What are the most common indications for a permanent pacemaker?
   - The most common indications are third-degree (complete) heart block, Mobitz type II second-degree heart block, and patients with symptomatic bradycardias, such as in sick sinus syndrome. Other indications include congenital heart disease, and patients with certain tachycardias (use of overdrive pacing to suppress abnormal rhythm).

2. In what situations might a biventricular pacemaker be used?
   - Biventricular pacing is also referred to as cardiac resynchronization therapy (CRT) and is generally used in patients with advanced heart failure and left bundle branch block (LBBB). In LBBB, the left ventricle depolarizes after the right ventricle and this results in the dyssynchrony of left and right ventricular contraction. With biventricular pacing, there is a separate lead into each of the ventricles and, generally, also one lead into the right atrium. This allows the pacemaker to deliver electrical impulses to each ventricle such that they contract in a synchronized manner. This hopefully improves the patient's symptoms.

3. What are the most common reasons for a patient to have a median sternotomy scar?
   - Median sternotomy is most commonly used for coronary artery bypass grafting and valve replacements. More rarely, this procedure may be used for transplantation and congenital heart defect repair.

4. How might a metal aortic valve replacement (AVR) be differentiated from a metal mitral valve replacement (MVR) clinically?
   - Patients with metal aortic valve replacements will have a normal S1, an opening click of the prosthetic aortic valve, and a metal prosthetic click instead of normal S2.
   - Patients with metal mitral valve replacements will have a metallic S1 (closure of the prosthetic valve), a normal S2, and a metallic opening snap in diastole.
   - Patients with MVR may have had the procedure done via lateral thoracotomy, whereas aortic valve replacement is via median sternotomy.

5. What are the main advantages and disadvantages of a bioprosthetic valve over a metal valve replacement?
   - The main benefit of bioprosthetic valves is that they do not require anticoagulation. However,

their lifetime is limited in comparison to mechanical valves – bioprosthetic valves may last, on average, 10 years (but failure may occur as early as 4–5 years or as late as 20 years), whereas mechanical valves may last 25 years or longer (and often may outlast the patient). Bioprosthetic valves are preferable in patients with a contraindication to anticoagulation and to the elderly (the valve is expected to outlast the patient), whereas mechanical valves may be preferable in younger patients.

OSCE 4 Incidental murmur (explanation and advice)

Ms Davidson is a 28-year-old lady who attends her GP after being told at a recent attendance to hospital that she has a murmur. She is asymptomatic but concerned that this may indicate serious pathology. Please explain to her the significance of an incidental murmur, with reference to possible causes and how this might be investigated:

Checklist

- Introduce yourself, check patient's details, and assess patient's pre-existing knowledge, including their ideas, concerns, and expectations.
- Explain that cardiac murmurs are generally the result of turbulent blood flow through the heart and its valves.
- Explain that cardiac murmurs are common and, in the young, often do not represent serious pathology. Some patients may wish to know that murmurs may be the result of a narrowed (stenosed) valve, a leaky (regurgitant) valve, or sometimes a hole in the heart muscle (septal defect), whereas other murmurs may occur without any underlying valve defect (functional or so called 'innocent' murmurs).
- Explain that sometimes murmurs may be the result of increased blood flow through the heart, such as can occur with anaemia and thyroid problems. Explain that these can be investigated for with simple blood tests.
- Explain that the definitive investigation of murmurs is mainly through echocardiography. Explain that this involves ultrasound scanning of the heart to look at the heart's valves and chambers and hopefully identify the source of the murmur.
- Ask the patient whether there are any areas that remain unclear or whether she has any questions.

Questions

1. Which common conditions may cause an 'innocent' flow murmur?
   - These murmurs may be seen in any hyperdynamic state, e.g., sepsis, anaemia, hyperthyroidism, exercise, and pregnancy.

2. Are systolic murmurs or diastolic murmurs more likely to be pathological?
   - Systolic murmurs can either be functional or can be secondary to underlying pathology. Diastolic murmurs are always due to underlying pathology.
3. Ms Davidson later reveals she is concerned because her brother has recently been diagnosed with hypertrophic cardiomyopathy (HCM). What is the usual mode of inheritance of this condition?
   - HCM is autosomal dominant in the vast majority of cases. There have been rare reports of autosomal recessive and X-linked inheritance.
4. HCM used to be called hypertrophic obstructive cardiomyopathy (HOCM). Why was it called this and why is it now commonly referred to as HCM?
   - Some individuals with HCM develop obstruction of the left ventricular outflow tract due to asymmetric septal hypertrophy of the myocardium. This occurs in only a minority of cases, and therefore the term hypertrophic cardiomyopathy is now used more commonly to represent those without obstruction.
5. How might HCM present?
   - The presentation of HCM varies widely. It may be asymptomatic and identified incidentally following examination/electrocardiography/ echocardiography. Symptoms of HCM include exertional chest pain, palpitation, exertional pre-syncope/syncope, symptoms of pulmonary congestion (e.g., breathlessness, orthopnoea, etc.). HCM may also present with sudden cardiac death.

OSCE 5 Aortic stenosis (explanation and advice)

Mr MacLeod is a 77-year-old gentleman who presents to the cardiologist complaining of exertional chest pain. His GP feels this is likely angina. He is noted to have a murmur. Echocardiography identifies moderate to severe aortic stenosis. He wants some more information about this condition:

Checklist

- Introduce yourself, check patient's details, and assess patient's pre-existing knowledge, including their ideas, concerns, and expectations.
- Explain that the echocardiogram has shown there is a narrowing of one of the valves in the heart.
- Explain blood leaves the heart through this narrowed valve to enter the main artery (aorta) to be carried to the rest of the body.
- Explain that this generally occurs due to wear and tear (degenerative change) over time and tends to progress as time goes on.

- Explain that this condition is often asymptomatic initially, but as the narrowing of the aortic valve progresses, this reduces blood flow through it and can cause certain symptoms, particularly when the body's requirements are higher, e.g., due to exercise or illness.
- Explain that the most common symptoms seen are chest pain, breathlessness, and dizziness or fainting (pre-syncope/syncope).
- Explain there are a number of possible treatments for this condition but these are not without their risks and additional tests may be helpful to identify the most suitable treatment. If he wants more information, explain that treatment can range from medications alone to heart surgery to replace the valve.
- Ask the patient whether there are any areas that remain unclear or whether he has any questions.

Questions

1. What is the classic triad of symptoms that might present in a patient with aortic stenosis?
   - Chest pain, syncope, and breathlessness.
2. What is the significance of a bicuspid aortic valve in the development of aortic stenosis?
   - Congenitally bicuspid valves are more prone to aortic stenosis than tricuspid aortic valves – this results in aortic stenosis presenting earlier.
3. What is meant by the term 'aortic sclerosis'?
   - Aortic sclerosis refers to calcification and thickening of the aortic valve leaflets, but without any restriction to valve leaflet movement or obstruction to the left ventricular outflow tract. This can cause an ejection-systolic murmur that classically *does not* radiate to the carotids and is associated with normal pulse pressure and pulse character. Aortic sclerosis is a symptomatic. In some patients, aortic sclerosis is a precursor to later aortic *stenosis*.
4. What are the treatment options in aortic stenosis?
   - There are a number of different options, including:
     - Medical management
     - Balloon aortic valvuloplasty (BAV)
     - Transcatheter aortic valve implantation (TAVI)
     - Aortic valve replacement (AVR) with either a mechanical valve or a bioprosthetic valve.
5. What are the reasons for using a TAVI over a conventional AVR?
   - Aortic valve replacement is a high-risk procedure that frailer patients with multiple comorbidities may not tolerate – it involves median sternotomy, cardiopulmonary bypass, and a longer recovery period. TAVI is a percutaneous method of delivering a replacement valve, generally via the femoral artery. This avoids many risks of conventional valve replacement and may allow frailer patients (who would previously have been unfit for treatment) to undergo a procedure that may significantly improve their symptoms and quality of life. In younger, healthier patients, conventional AVR is generally used over TAVI as need for re-intervention is lower and long-term TAVI valve durability is unknown (as it is a relatively new procedure).

OSCE 6 Angina explanation and advice

Mr Smith has been suffering from chest pain on exertion for the last 6 months. His GP told him that he has angina and prescribed medication to spray under his tongue when he gets chest pain. Explain to Mr Smith what angina is and the principles of treating it:

Checklist

- Introduce yourself, check patient's details, and assess patient's pre-existing knowledge, including their ideas, concerns and expectations.
- Angina is a result of inadequate blood supply to the heart when it is working harder, e.g., during exercise.
- It is usually caused by a narrowing of the arteries carrying blood to the heart muscle.
- Management of risk factors, such as hypertension, hyperlipidaemia, and diabetes, is important.
- Patients should stop smoking and reduce intake of salt and fatty foods to minimize progression of the disease.
- Medications aim to increase blood flow to the heart and to reduce the demand on the heart.
- Coronary artery stenting or bypass surgery can be performed when disease is severe.
- Ask the patient whether there are any areas that remain unclear or whether he has any questions.

Questions

1. Which side effects of glyceryl trinitrate (GTN) is it worth making patients aware of?
   - Palpitations, postural hypotension, lightheadedness, and other presyncopal symptoms are of particular importance. Rarely, patients may experience syncopal episodes. Patients also often develop an unpleasant throbbing headache.
2. What are the main risk factors for developing coronary artery disease?
   - Male sex, age, smoking, hypertension, hypercholesterolaemia, diabetes, physical inactivity, family history, and poor diet.

3. If Mr Smith presented to the Emergency Department with crushing central chest pain and was noted to have ST segment elevation in leads II, III and aVF, which coronary artery is most likely affected?
   - This situation is an inferior ST elevation myocardial infarction (STEMI) and the vast majority of the time is due to occlusion of the right coronary artery. Inferior STEMI can infrequently be the result of dominant left circumflex artery occlusion and very rarely due to occlusion of a 'wraparound' left anterior descending artery (anterior ST elevation would also generally be seen in this instance).

4. What clinical signs might you notice in the hypercholesterolaemic patient?
   - Tendon xanthomata, corneal arcus, and xanthelasma. Patients with none of these signs may still have elevated cholesterol.

5. In patients who have undergone coronary artery bypass surgery, what signs might be found on clinical examination?
   - The most obvious clinical finding would be a midline sternotomy scar. Other scars may be seen elsewhere due to harvesting of vessels for use as grafts (e.g., scars on the leg from saphenous vein grafting or the forearm from radial artery grafting).

OSCE 7 Chest pain history

Mrs Anderson has been having episodes of pain in her chest for the past 2 years. Please take a history from her:

Checklist

- Introduce yourself, check patient's details, and obtain consent.
- Fully explore the episodes of pain, e.g., using the SOCRATES method: Site, Onset, Character, Radiation, Associated features, Timing, Exacerbating and relieving factors, Severity. Assess to what extent Mrs Anderson is affected by her symptoms.
- Clarify patient's past medical (and surgical) history. Double check for hypertension, hypercholesterolaemia, diabetes, etc. as they may not always be mentioned.
- Take a drug history, remember allergies!
- Take a social history, including occupation, housing situation (asking about stairs is important), and whether the patient has any history of smoking, alcohol, or other recreational drug use.
- Ask about family history, particularly with regard to ischaemic heart disease (and age of presentation).
- Ask her ideas about what may be causing these episodes of pain, and if she has any particular concerns and expectations.
- Summarize findings and clarify whether the patient thinks there is anything else you need to know.

Questions

1. What is the typical description of angina?
   - Substernal chest discomfort that is of characteristic quality and duration (heavy, 'band-like' pain that lasts for minutes at a time). Pain is provoked by exertion or emotional stress and relieved by rest and/or nitrates within minutes.

2. What would you consider to be a positive family history of cardiovascular disease?
   - A positive family history is generally considered as diagnosis of cardiovascular disease in a male first-degree relative (father or brother) at under the age of 55 or in a female first-degree relative (mother or sister) at under the age of 65.

3. If an ECG was performed on Mrs Anderson, what might it show?
   - The ECG is normally unremarkable in patients with angina between episodes. During an attack, there may be evidence of ST segment depression or T wave inversion. There may also be unexpected findings, such as evidence of previous myocardial infarction, left ventricular hypertrophy, etc.

4. What are the main classes of anti-anginal medications?
   - Main classes of drugs include β-blockers (e.g., bisoprolol), calcium channel antagonists (e.g., amlodipine), and nitrates (e.g., isosorbide mononitrate). There are also a number of other medications that may be used, including nicorandil, ranolazine, and ivabradine.

5. If she has had a previous myocardial infarction, which other medications should she be taking for secondary prevention?
   - In addition to the medications mentioned above, patients should also be on aspirin, a high-intensity statin (e.g., atorvastatin), and an ACE inhibitor (e.g., ramipril) to reduce rates of cardiovascular morbidity and mortality.

OSCE 8 Hypertrophic cardiomyopathy and counselling

Mr and Mrs Jackson attend the GP. Mr Jackson was diagnosed with hypertrophic cardiomyopathy (HCM) 3 years ago. They are thinking of starting a family and are concerned the condition may be passed on to their children. Please advise them appropriately:

Checklist:

- Introduce yourself, check patient identification, and obtain consent.
- Check patient understanding and what information they are seeking.

- Explain that HCM is a genetic condition and can possibly be passed on to their children.
- Explain that in the vast majority of cases, the risk of a child inheriting the condition is 50%.
- Explain that there may be some benefits to genetic testing in an attempt to identify specific mutation(s) – e.g., it may be useful for prognostic purposes, prenatal or early diagnosis, screening other relatives, etc. It is worth explaining that a particular mutation may not be identified.
- Explain that even if a child is diagnosed with HCM, then prognosis is difficult to quantify as there is significant variation (even within families with known mutations).
- Clarify if there are any other questions/additional concerns.

Questions

1. What is the mode of inheritance of HCM (if not already stated)?
   - HCM is autosomal dominant in the vast majority of cases (there are a few rarer mutations that may be inherited in an autosomal recessive manner).
2. In individuals with known mutations, in which gene(s) are these found?
   - HCM is the result of mutations in a number of genes encoding sarcomeric proteins (most commonly in the β-myosin heavy chain gene or the myosin-binding protein C gene).
3. How does HCM generally present?
   - Presentation of HCM varies widely. Patients are often asymptomatic (and diagnosis is incidental). Patients may present with a range of symptoms, including breathlessness, angina, lightheadedness, palpitations, syncope, or even sudden cardiac death.
4. What clinical signs may be found in HCM?
   - Examination findings may include a 'jerky' peripheral pulse (if obstruction is present), a double apical beat, a systolic murmur (crescendo and decrescendo in nature) with a thrill felt at the lower left sternal edge. The murmur in hypertrophic cardiomyopathy is generally louder with Valsalva manoeuvre or with standing from squatting. Patients may have no signs on clinical examination.
5. If it was Mrs Jackson who had HCM, then what is her risk of complications during pregnancy?
   - Pregnancy is generally well tolerated in individuals with HCM although she would be at slightly higher risk than a patient without the condition. Patients at higher risk are those who have been symptomatic prior to pregnancy or if there is evidence of severe left ventricular outflow tract obstruction.

OSCE 9 Acute care scenario – acute pulmonary oedema

A 69-year-old patient on the cardiology ward becomes acutely breathless overnight. A nurse practitioner reviews him and arranges a portable chest X-ray. He is concerned the patient has acute pulmonary oedema and requests assistance.

Example assessment template (Note: local guidelines may vary):

	Assessment	Investigations	Management	
A	• Patient position. • Is the patient talking? In full/short sentences? • Any added sounds?	• Nil.	• Sit the patient up – may need adjuncts/airway manoeuvres if reduced Glasgow Coma Scale. • Oxygen 15L via non-rebreathe mask.	
B	• Respiratory rate and oxygen saturations. • Work of breathing, any cyanosis? • Trachea – is it central? • Chest expansion – equal and symmetrical? • Percussion. • Chest sounds – reduced air entry, wheeze, focal signs? *History – Any cough, respiratory disease or allergies?*	• Chest X-ray – look for ABCDE (**A**lveolar oedema, Kerley **B** lines, **C**ardiomegaly, upper lobe venous **D**iversion, **E**ffusions) • Arterial blood gases if patient is hypoxic.	• Oxygen 15L via non-rebreathe mask if not done. Titrate to arterial blood gas results if retaining carbon dioxide. • Consider nebulizers if wheezy and diagnosis in doubt (i.e., could this be an exacerbation of chronic obstructive pulmonary disease or asthma?).	

C	• Heart rate and blood pressure (can be set to auto cycle).
	• Capillary refill and peripheral perfusion.
	• Pulse rhythm and volume.
	• Jugular venous pressure.
	• Heart sounds – normal or additional sounds. Any murmurs?
	• Mucous membranes/ peripheral oedema.
	• Urine output.
	History – Any chest pain, previous cardiovascular disease?
		• Continuous cardiac monitoring.
		• ECG – arrhythmia may precipitate heart failure.
		• Blood tests to consider:
		  o *Full blood count* (for signs of anaemia or infection).
		  o *Urea and electrolytes*
		  o *Troponin* (acute coronary syndrome may present with heart failure – note troponin will also be elevated in heart failure itself, therefore history is important),
		  o *BNP/NT-proBNP* (to differentiate heart failure from other causes of dyspnoea),
		  o *Liver function tests* (may be deranged in right ventricular failure).
		  o *C-reactive protein* (if signs of infection).
		  o *Glucose*.
		  o *Venous blood gas* (if arterial sample not taken already).
			• Intravenous (IV) access
			• IV furosemide – 50mg is a reasonable starting dose; may need to be repeated. Caution is required as may lower blood pressure.
			• Catheter – useful for monitoring. Also, patients may have profound diuresis following IV furosemide and may not be able to manage otherwise.
			• Treat arrhythmia if present (e.g., with DC cardioversion/ atropine – heart failure is an adverse feature of arrhythmia and indicates cardiovascular instability).
				CALL FOR HELP early (or as soon as you identify an issue you may not be able to deal with yourself).
				
				REASSESS after interventions made.

D	• 'AVPU' (Alert/Responsive to pain/Responsive to Voice/ Unresponsive) or GCS (Glasgow Coma Scale). • Pupils/neurological exam if indicated (e.g., neurogenic pulmonary oedema).	• Capillary blood glucose.	• Treat hypoglycaemia if present (e.g., with glucose/glucagon). • Reduced GCS may be a sign of shock/exhaustion.	
E	• Temperature. • Brief abdominal exam – e.g., ascites, hepatomegaly. • Review of notes, etc.	• Will vary dependent on clinical picture and any additional pathology/causes of heart failure/ co-existing conditions that are identified.		

Continued

NEXT STEPS	Speak to senior doctor (e.g., medical registrar/cardiology registrar/high dependency/intensive care registrar) as appropriate. May need: • Echocardiogram – Can be done at the bedside to investigate for/exclude mechanical causes (e.g., acquired ventricular septal defect, mitral regurgitation, left ventricular aneurysm, cardiac tamponade). • Higher level care for continuous positive airway pressure (CPAP)/ventilation, insertion of arterial line, central venous line, or use of vasoactive drugs, e.g., inotropes for cardiogenic shock. Patients may sometimes need intraaortic balloon counterpulsation or haemofiltration. Return to the beginning and carry out in-depth history and examination *when appropriate*.
NOTES	Do not routinely offer: • *Morphine – increased risk of respiratory suppression, ICU admission, prolonged hospital stay, death.* • *Glyceryl trinitrate (GTN) – unless under cardiology advice or if there is co-existing evidence of ischaemia e.g., heart failure in context of ongoing myocardial infarction.*

Questions

1. Why might a patient with previously stable heart failure present with decompensated heart failure?
   - Decompensation of a previously stable heart failure patient may occur for many reasons – as well as treating the heart failure itself, it is equally important to identify and treat any underlying cause of decompensation, e.g., infection, arrhythmia, acute coronary syndrome, valvular disease, non-adherence with medications, etc.

2. What are the main ways in which diuretic medication might be prescribed in the patient with heart failure?
   - Diuretic medication is generally prescribed initially as an intravenous medication in the patient presenting with acute heart failure. Intravenous diuretics may be given as bolus doses (repeated if necessary) or sometimes as an infusion that is delivered at a constant rate over 24-hours.
   - Oral medications may not be absorbed well in the acute setting (due to gastrointestinal oedema) and are generally slower to act. When the patient is stable, intravenous medications should be switched to oral medications prior to discharge.

3. With a new diagnosis of heart failure, what medications might be started prior to discharge?
   - Patients with new diagnoses of heart failure should be started on a number of new medications prior to discharge, including:
     - All patients should be started on an angiotensin-converting enzyme (ACE) inhibitor or angiotensin II receptor antagonist – these act to reduce preload, reduce the ventricular remodelling seen in heart failure, reduce afterload on the heart and reduce salt and water retention. This improves the symptoms and prognosis in the patient with heart failure.
     - All patients should be started on a β-blocker – these act to reduce heart rate and as a result increase coronary blood flow. They also decrease the metabolic demand of the myocardium. In combination with ACE inhibitors, β-blockers improve survival and reverse ventricular remodelling.
     - Some patients may be started on an aldosterone antagonist (also known as mineralocorticoid receptor antagonist), such as spironolactone. These medications improve prognosis; they act to reduce preload by blocking aldosterone receptors in the distal convoluted tubule. Aldosterone promotes sodium retention and potassium excretion; it also has a number of unfavourable extra-renal effects, including promoting fibrosis and adverse remodelling of the heart, sympathetic stimulation, parasympathetic inhibition, vascular damage, and impairment of arterial compliance, all of which adversely affect cardiac function.
     - Most patients will be started on diuretic medications – these provide a symptomatic (but not prognostic) benefit by offloading oedema.
     - There are a number of other medications that may be used in certain situations, for example if other medications are insufficient or not tolerated. These include digoxin, nitrates, hydralazine, ivabradine, and combination sacubitril/valsartan.
     - Additional medications dependent on underlying cause of heart failure – e.g., patients may be started on aspirin and a statin if there is evidence of ischaemic heart disease, or warfarin if heart failure is due to atrial fibrillation.

4. What are the common adverse effects that a patient started on β-blockers may experience?
   - Some patients started on β-blockers may experience adverse effects, including bradycardia and resultant pre-syncope/syncope, cold hands/feet, fatigue, impotence, and sleep disturbance. β-blockers tend to be avoided in individuals with asthma as their use may provoke bronchospasm.

5. What information is it important to communicate to patients when starting them on ACE inhibitors?
    *   It is important to stress to patients that they will require regular monitoring of blood tests (particularly of electrolytes and renal function) as there is the potential for acute kidney injury and electrolyte abnormalities (especially hyperkalaemia) with ACE inhibitor treatment.
    *   It is especially important to advise patients to temporarily withhold ACE inhibitors when they are unwell (especially with conditions that are prone to causing dehydration, such as diarrhoea or vomiting) and to restart when they are well again – this reduces the risk of acute kidney injury.

OSCE 10 Acute care scenario – collapse

A 72-year-old patient on the acute medical unit has a collapse. A nurse has phoned for immediate review and is carrying out an ECG as she is concerned that the cardiac monitor shows an arrhythmia.

Example assessment template (Note: local guidelines may vary):

	Assessment	Investigations	Management	
A	• Patient position. • Is the patient talking? Are they confused? • Any audible added sounds?	• Nil.	• If breathless, sit the patient up. • If reduced consciousness, lie flat and consider airway manoeuvres/adjuncts.	
B	• Respiratory rate, oxygen saturations. • Cyanosis. • Chest sounds – e.g., bibasal crepitations.	• Arterial blood gas (ABG) if hypoxic. • Chest X-ray – look for evidence of heart failure.	• Oxygen 15L via non-rebreathe mask if hypoxic (this could be due to heart failure).	

C	• Heart rate and blood pressure (can be set to auto cycle).
	• Capillary refill time and peripheral perfusion.
	• Pulse rhythm and volume.
	• Jugular venous pressure.
	• Heart sounds – normal or additional sounds. Any murmurs?
	• Mucous membranes/peripheral oedema.
	• Urine output.
	History – Chest pain? Dizziness? Any precipitants – recent events, investigation results? History of heart disease? Allergies?
		• 12-lead ECG – crucial for diagnosis of arrhythmia.
		• Continuous cardiac monitoring– via defibrillator if very fast or unstable.
		• Bloods tests to consider:
		  o *Full blood count.*
		  o *Urea and electrolytes, magnesium and calcium* (electrolyte abnormalities may precipitate arrhythmia).
		  o *Troponin* (if concern arrhythmia is due to acute coronary syndrome).
		  o *Glucose.*
		  o *Venous blood gases* (if arterial sample not taken already).
			• Intravenous access.
			• Treatment of arrhythmia depends on the particular arrhythmia and whether the patient is stable with this arrhythmia – see **Chapter 15: Arrhythmias** for tachycardia and bradycardia algorithms.
			• Remember patient is peri-arrest if adverse features are present:
			- Shock
			- Syncope
			- Myocardial ischaemia
			- Heart Failure
			See below for more details.
				CALL FOR HELP early (or as soon as you identify an issue you may not be able to deal with yourself).
				
				REASSESS after interventions made.

D	• 'AVPU' (Alert/Responsive to pain/Responsive to Voice/Unresponsive) or GCS (Glasgow Coma Scale).	• Capillary blood glucose.	• Treat hypoglycaemia if present (glucose/glucagon). • Reduced GCS/confusion may be a sign of brain hypoperfusion.	
E	• Temperature. • Brief abdominal exam – e.g., ascites, hepatomegaly. • Review notes, etc.	• Will vary dependent on clinical picture and any additional precipitants or coexisting conditions that are identified.		

Continued

NEXT STEPS	Speak to senior colleague – e.g., medical registrar/cardiology registrar/high dependency unit (HDU) registrar/ intensive care unit (ICU) registrar as appropriate. May require:

- Higher level care (HDU/ICU/coronary care) for additional monitoring (e.g., continuous cardiac monitoring, central line and arterial line) or organ support (e.g., with inotropes).
- Treatment of any reversible conditions contributing to initiation and maintenance of arrhythmia. Treat ischaemia, hypotension, hypokalaemia and heart failure.
- Additional investigations – e.g., echocardiogram, coronary angiogram, or electrophysiological (EP) study to evaluate cause of arrhythmia.
- Medication may be given to prevent arrhythmia or reduce the risk or recurrence if treating the underlying cause is insufficient (e.g., use of amiodarone in ventricular tachycardia).

Patient may go on to require additional procedures, such as insertion of permanent pacemaker/implantable cardioverter defibrillator, catheter ablation, etc.

- Return to the beginning and carry out in-depth history and examination *when appropriate*.

Questions

1. What are the 'adverse features' of arrhythmia and how might these present clinically?
   - Shock – hypotension (generally a systolic blood pressure of <90 mmHg); the patient may also be pale, sweaty, clammy, confused, or have impaired consciousness.
   - Syncope – the patient may transiently lose consciousness due to a global reduction in cerebral blood flow.
   - Myocardial ischaemia – may present as typical ischaemic chest pain and/or evidence of ischaemia on the electrocardiogram.
   - Heart failure – may present with raised jugular venous pressure or pulmonary oedema (breathlessness, hypoxia, crepitations, and chest X-ray signs).

2. The patient is awake and responding but found to have a broad complex tachycardia on the ECG. If adverse features were present, then what should the next course of action be?
   - The patient fits the criteria for synchronized DC cardioversion. The patient is also conscious and should be anaesthetized or sedated before this is attempted. Therefore, call early for staff with these skills (e.g., anaesthetist, intensivist, A&E consultant). Another important concern is that some wards may have only automated external defibrillators (AEDs) which do not always have the capacity to deliver a synchronized shock; it is worth becoming familiar with local equipment.

3. What is the significance of cardioversion in this situation being 'synchronized'? What would happen if a shock was delivered without synchronization?

- If a patient has an arrhythmia but still has a pulse, and a shock is delivered during the ventricular repolarization (during the T wave), this can precipitate ventricular fibrillation and cardiac arrest – the 'R on T' phenomenon. In a synchronized shock the defibrillator monitors the heart's electrical activity and delivers a shock during the R wave, avoiding this risk.

4. Sometimes supraventricular tachycardia (SVT) with aberrant conduction can mimic ventricular tachycardia (VT). How can these be differentiated?
   - This can be difficult. A number of features are pathognomonic of VT:
     1. AV dissociation (P waves and QRS complexes at different rates).
     2. Capture beats – occur when the sinoatrial node transiently 'captures' the ventricles, in the midst of AV dissociation, to produce a QRS complex of normal duration.
     3. Fusion beats – occur when a sinus and ventricular beat coincide to produce a hybrid complex of intermediate morphology.

   Other features that suggest VT are:
   - Extreme left axis deviation – indeterminate or 'northwest' axis.
   - Very broad QRS complexes (>140 ms).
   - Tachycardia beats identical to ventricular ectopics during sinus rhythm.
   - Positive or negative concordance throughout the chest leads, i.e., leads V1–6 show entirely positive (R) or entirely negative (QS) complexes, with no RS complexes seen.
   - No response to carotid sinus massage or intravenous adenosine.

- o No known typical bundle branch block morphology or evidence of accessory pathway prior to onset of broad complex tachycardia.
- o History of myocardial infarction.

5. There is diagnostic uncertainty as to whether a patient is in VT or SVT with aberrant conduction. What is the safest course of action?
   - If in doubt in this situation, always treat as VT. VT is a life-threatening arrhythmia, whereas SVT generally is not.

OSCE 11 Acute care scenario – chest pain

A 64-year-old man comes into the Emergency Department with crushing central chest pain for the past hour. The ambulance ECG shows no ST segment elevation. Please assess him appropriately.

Example assessment template (Note: local guidelines may vary):

	Assessment	Investigations	Management	
A	• Patient position. • Is the patient talking? In full/short sentences? • Any added sounds?		• Sit the patient up if poorly positioned. • Oxygen – aim for 94%–98% in the patient without COPD.	
B	• Respiratory rate and oxygen saturations. • Work of breathing. • Cyanosis. • Trachea – is it central? • Chest expansion – equal and symmetrical? • Percussion. • Chest sounds – any added sounds?	• Chest X-ray – look for evidence of heart failure – ABCDE (**A**lveolar oedema, Kerley **B** lines, **C**ardiomegaly, upper lobe venous **D**iversion, **E**ffusions). • Arterial blood gases if patient hypoxic.	• Oxygen – aim for 94%–98% in the patient without COPD. • Consider nebulizers if wheezy (especially if patient has known history of COPD).	

C	• Heart rate and blood pressure (can be set to auto cycle).
	• Capillary refill and peripheral perfusion.
	• Pulse rhythm and volume.
	• Jugular venous pressure.
	• Heart sounds – normal or additional sounds. Any murmurs?
	• Mucous membranes/peripheral oedema.
	• Urine output.
	History – Ask about chest pain and heart disease. Any anticoagulation or recent bleeding?
		• 12-lead ECG - vital!
		• Continuous cardiac monitoring.
		• Blood tests:
		  o *Troponin* – vital!
		  o *Full Blood Count* (patients with anaemia, infection more prone to myocardial infarction).
		  o *Urea and electrolytes* (dehydration may increase risk of thrombotic events).
		  o *LFTs* (as baseline).
		  o *Lipid profile*.
		  o *Clotting screen*.
		  o *Glucose*.
			• Intravenous access.
			• If not contraindicated, give antiplatelet and anticoagulant therapy – local guidelines may vary but typical regime is:
			  o *Aspirin* 300 mg oral.
			  o *Ticagrelor* 180 mg oral or *clopidogrel* 300 mg oral.
			  o *Fondaparinux* 2.5 mg subcutaneous.
			• Give vasodilators and analgesia unless contraindicated, e.g., by hypotension:
			  o *Glyceryl trinitrate* 2 sprays sublingually.
			  o *Morphine* 1–10 mg titrated to response with prophylactic anti-emetic.
			• Consider urinary catheter to monitor urine output.
				CALL FOR HELP early (or as soon as you identify an issue you may not be able to deal with yourself).
				
				REASSESS after interventions made.

D	• 'AVPU' (Alert/Responsive to pain/Responsive to Voice/Unresponsive) or GCS (Glasgow Coma Scale). • Pupils/brief neurological exam if indicated.	• Capillary blood glucose.	• Treat any derangements in blood glucose appropriately. • Reduced GCS may be a sign of cerebral hypoperfusion.	
E	• Temperature. • Brief abdominal exam – e.g., ascites, hepatomegaly. • Review notes, etc.	Will vary dependent on clinical picture and any additional precipitants or coexisting conditions that are identified.		

Continued

NEXT STEPS	• Speak to senior colleague – e.g., medical registrar/cardiology registrar/high dependency unit (HDU) registrar/ intensive care unit (ICU) registrar as appropriate.

• Repeat troponin to confirm a rise indicative of myocardial damage. The timing of this repeat test will vary dependent on local guidelines, but with high-sensitivity troponins can be done as early as 3 hours.

• Most patients will require inpatient coronary angiography after non-ST elevation myocardial infarction. If moderate to high risk, discuss with cardiologist for consideration of *early* coronary angiography with view to percutaneous coronary intervention (PCI) or coronary artery bypass grafting (CABG). Some low risk patients or patients with multiple comorbidities may be managed medically in the first instance.

• Patients may require:
  o Higher level care (HDU/ICU/coronary care unit) for additional monitoring (e.g., continuous cardiac monitoring, central line and arterial line) or organ support (e.g., with inotropes).
  o Additional treatment of any complications of myocardial infarction (pacing, treatment of other arrhythmias or of heart failure, etc.).

Return to the beginning and carry out in-depth history and examination *when appropriate*. Remember to repeat the 12-lead ECG to detect evolving changes that may occur in myocardial infarction.

Questions

1. What would be the most important thing to do immediately if the patient was stable, but initial ECG showed ST elevation in the anterior leads?
   • Phone the catheterization laboratory ('cath lab') and cardiologist on call to make them aware of ST elevation myocardial infarction (STEMI) requiring primary percutaneous coronary intervention (PCI). These patients are often identified by the ambulance crew and taken directly for PCI if available.

2. What is the significance of new left bundle branch block in association with ischaemic sounding chest pain?
   • This should be treated as a STEMI until proven otherwise – the cardiologist on call should be contacted immediately.

3. If you saw ST elevation in leads II, III and aVF which region of the heart is affected? Occlusion of which coronary artery generally causes this picture?
   • This is an inferior STEMI and in the vast majority of cases the result of occlusion of the right coronary artery. Infrequently, inferior STEMIs can be due to occlusion of a dominant left circumflex artery

or rarely due to occlusion of a wraparound left anterior descending artery.

4. What is the significant difference between complete heart block in the context of inferior myocardial infarction and complete heart block in the context of anterior myocardial infarction?
   • When complete heart block occurs in inferior myocardial infarction, it is usually transient; temporary pacing may be required in some instances. Complete heart block in anterior myocardial infarction is generally permanent due to septal infarction and necrosis of the bundle branches; this will require permanent pacing.

5. If a patient came in with sharp chest pain and widespread ST segment elevation across multiple coronary artery territories, what is the most likely diagnosis?
   • This is most likely pericarditis. Patients develop widespread concave ST segment elevation (sometimes with PR segment depression) across multiple leads, rather than one coronary artery territory. They often describe pleuritic central chest pain that is worse on lying flat and relieved by sitting forward.

Abscess a collection of pus within a cavity.

Accessory pathway an abnormal connection between atrium and ventricle that is capable of propagating a cardiac impulse.

Acute coronary syndrome (ACS) a range of clinical presentations that includes myocardial infarction and unstable angina.

Afterload the pressure that the left ventricle must produce to eject blood out of the heart.

Ambulatory blood pressure monitoring (ABPM) monitoring of blood pressure during the day and night as the patient goes about their normal activities.

Anticoagulation treatment intended to prevent blood clotting.

Angina pectoris commonly known as angina, it is chest pain due to ischaemia (a lack of blood and hence oxygen supply) of the heart muscle, generally due to obstruction of one or more coronary artery/arteries.

Angiogram a technique where blood-filled structures, including arteries, veins and the heart chambers, are imaged, usually following the injection of a contrast medium.

Angioplasty see **Percutaneous coronary intervention**.

Apex beat the most inferior and lateral position on the chest wall where the cardiac impulse is palpable.

Arrhythmia a disturbance of cardiac rhythm.

Asystole absence of contraction. Asystole is when the heart has stopped beating. It is different from ventricular fibrillation where the heart is still contracting but not in a co-ordinated manner.

Atheroma an accumulation and swelling in artery walls consisting of cells (or cell debris) containing lipids (cholesterol and fatty acids), calcium and a variable amount of fibrous connective tissue.

Atrial fibrillation (AF) irregular uncoordinated contraction of the atria resulting from disorganized electrical activity, typically resulting in an irregularly irregular pulse.

Atrioventricular (AV) node region of specialized conducting tissue between the atria and ventricles that functions to regulate electrical conduction.

Atrium one of the two (upper) collecting chambers of the heart.

Bradycardia a heart rate <60 beats per minute.

Brain natriuretic peptide (BNP) a peptide released by ventricular cardiomyocytes in response to stretching; a clinical marker that can be used in the diagnosis of heart failure.

Bundle branch block failure of either the left (LBBB) or right (RBBB) bundle branches.

Cardiac catheterization an invasive procedure to access the coronary and pulmonary circulation and chambers of the heart using a catheter. It can be used for both diagnosis and treatment.

Cardiac failure also called **heart failure**, this is a reduction in cardiac pump function such that there is inadequate perfusion to metabolizing tissues. Patients may have left ventricular failure (**LVF**), right ventricular failure (**RVF**) or, more frequently, a combination of both.

Cardiac output (CO) the amount of blood pumped out by the heart every minute; the product of stroke volume (SV) and heart rate (HR), i.e., CO = SV × HR.

Cardiac tamponade compression of the heart as a result of accumulation of fluid in the pericardial space. This results in reduced cardiac output and can be fatal if untreated.

Cardiomyopathy disease of the myocardium (heart muscle).

Cardioversion reverting the heart to a normal rhythm, either electrically (with a DC shock) or using drugs (pharmacological or chemical cardioversion).

Central venous pressure (CVP) the pressure of blood in the great veins as they enter the right atrium.

Coarctation of the aorta a congenital defect characterized by an abnormal narrowing of part of the aorta.

Contractility the strength with which the myocardium contracts.

Cyanosis bluish discolouration of the skin due to the presence of deoxygenated haemoglobin.

Defibrillation the definitive treatment for the life-threatening cardiac arrhythmia of ventricular fibrillation. Defibrillation consists of delivering a therapeutic dose of electrical energy to the heart with a device called a defibrillator.

Defibrillator can be external, transvenous or implanted, depending on the type of device used.

Dehiscence reopening at the site of a surgical closure of apposition.

Diastole part of the cardiac cycle where the ventricles are relaxed and filling.

Echocardiogram an ultrasound scan of the heart, used to image two-dimensional slices of the heart.

Ectopic an event occurring at a place other than its normal location. For example, ventricular ectopic beats originate from the ventricles, not the sinoatrial node.

Electrocardiogram (ECG) a graphical representation of the electrical activity of the heart over time.

Electrophysiological (EP) study an invasive test used for accurate diagnosis (and potentially treatment) of arrhythmia and assessment of the heart's electrical pathways.

End-diastolic pressure (EDP) the amount of pressure in the ventricle at the end of diastole.

End-diastolic volume (EDV) the amount of blood in the ventricle at the end of diastole; the greatest amount found in the ventricle throughout the whole cardiac cycle.

Ejection fraction the proportion of the EDV which is ejected by contraction.

Glyceryl trinitrate (GTN) a vasodilator often used in patients with angina.

Heart block also called atrioventricular block; this is abnormal slowing or failure of conduction from the atria to the ventricles.

Holter monitor ambulatory ECG, usually attached to the patient for 24–48 hours.

Home blood pressure monitoring (HBPM) the patient monitors their own blood pressure in their own home.

Hypertension high blood pressure.

Hypertrophy increase in the size of a tissue or organ resulting from an increase in cell size.

Hypertrophic cardiomyopathy (HCM) an inherited disease of the heart muscle where the myocardium is hypertrophied (enlarged). HCM used to be called HOCM (hypertrophic obstructive cardiomyopathy) but has been renamed as obstruction occurs in a minority of cases.

Hypotension low blood pressure.

Hypoxia low oxygen levels.

Implantable cardioverter defibrillator (ICD) a device set up to detect an arrhythmia, delivering a shock to the patient as necessary.

Infective endocarditis infection of the endothelial surface of the heart or the heart valves by a microorganism.

Ischaemia lack of blood supply to a tissue.

Infarction tissue death caused by inadequate perfusion.

Jugular venous pressure (JVP) the visible pulsation of the internal jugular vein, seen in the neck.

Mean arterial pressure (MAP) the average pressure in the arterial system at any point in time, approximated as the diastolic pressure + (1/3 × pulse pressure).

Myocardial infarction death of heart muscle due to interruption of the blood supply, most commonly due to thrombosis of a ruptured atheromatous plaque in a coronary artery.

Myocarditis inflammation of the heart muscle.

Non-ST elevation myocardial infarction (NSTEMI) myocardial infarction without elevation of the ST segment on the ECG.

Pacemaker an area or device that generates cardiac electrical activity; this may be natural (such as the sinoatrial node) or artificial (such as a permanent pacemaker).

Percutaneous coronary intervention (PCI) commonly known as coronary angioplasty (or simply angioplasty); a therapeutic procedure to treat the stenotic (narrowed) coronary arteries of the heart found in coronary heart disease.

Perfusion movement of blood through an organ or tissue.

Pericarditis inflammation of the pericardium (the fibrous sac surrounding the heart).

Permanent pacemaker (PPM) an implantable device used to control the electrical activity of the heart.

Precordium the surface of the lower anterior chest wall.

Preload the degree of ventricular myocyte stretch before contraction; it is determined by the end-diastolic volume.

Pulse pressure the difference between systolic and diastolic blood pressure readings.

Radiofrequency ablation (RFA) the use of radiofrequency energy to create a therapeutic burn, intended to treat cardiac arrhythmia.

Septal defect a hole in the wall dividing the chambers of the heart; this may be between the ventricles (a VSD, or ventricular septal defect) or between the atria (an ASD, or atrial septal defect).

Shunt flow of blood through an abnormal communication between cardiac chambers or blood vessels (e.g., due to a septal defect). This may allow blood to flow between the pulmonary and systemic circulations.

Shock a situation where insufficient blood flow is reaching the body's tissues; causes commonly described as hypovolaemic, cardiogenic, distributive (e.g., anaphylactic, septic, etc.) or obstructive (e.g., due to tamponade, pulmonary embolism).

Sinoatrial (SA) node the impulse-generating (pacemaker) tissue located in the roof of the right atrium.

Sinus rhythm the 'normal' heart rhythm under direct control from the sinoatrial node.

Sphygmomanometer a device used for measuring blood pressure.

Starling's Law a phenomenon whereby the heart increases its output by increasing its strength of contraction when the fibres of the myocardium are stretched.

ST elevation myocardial infarction (STEMI) myocardial infarction with elevation of the ST segment on the ECG.

Stenosis an abnormal narrowing in a blood vessel or other tubular organ/structure.

Stent a tubular metal cage that is inserted to counteract a localized obstruction to flow. Often used in the coronary arteries during percutaneous coronary intervention (PCI).

Stroke volume (SV) the amount of blood ejected from the left ventricle with each beat.

Stroke work (SW) the amount of external energy expended in one ventricular contraction. Stroke work is the arterial pressure multiplied by stroke volume.

Supraventricular literally above the ventricle, i.e., originating from the atria or AV node.

Syncope temporary loss of consciousness as the result of reduced blood flow to the brain.

Systemic vascular resistance (SVR) the resistance to blood flow offered by all of the systemic vasculature (not including the pulmonary vasculature). It is calculated as (Mean Arterial Pressure – Right Atrial Pressure) / Cardiac Output.

Systole the part of the cardiac cycle where the ventricles are contracting.

Tachycardia a heart rate >100 beats per minute.

Tetralogy of Fallot a congenital heart condition characterized by four defects: ventricular septal defect, pulmonary stenosis, right ventricular hypertrophy and an overriding aorta (the aorta is positioned over the septal defect).

Torsades de pointes literally means 'twisting of the points', a polymorphic ventricular tachycardia (i.e., ventricular complexes have variable shapes).

Total peripheral resistance (TPR) the resistance to the flow of blood in the whole system. It is calculated as arterial pressure / cardiac output.

Transposition of the great arteries (TGA) a congenital heart defect where the aorta and the pulmonary artery are switched, i.e., the aorta arises from the anatomical right ventricle and the pulmonary artery arises from the anatomical left ventricle.

Troponin a complex of proteins that is integral to muscle contraction in skeletal and cardiac muscle (but not smooth muscle). Damage to cardiomyocytes leads to an elevation in cardiac specific troponin levels in the plasma.

Unstable angina angina with at least one of the following: occurring at rest or minimal exertion and usually lasting >20 minutes; being severe and of new onset; occurring in a crescendo pattern. May have ECG changes indicative of ischaemia but not elevation in troponin; if troponin is elevated, this is myocardial infarction.

Vasodilatation increase in the calibre of a blood vessel.

Vegetation a mass (generally consisting of fibrin, platelets and microorganisms) seen in infective endocarditis; they are generally associated with the valves of the heart.

Ventricular relating to the heart's ventricles.

Ventricular fibrillation (VF) irregular uncoordinated contraction of the ventricles, fatal if untreated.

Note: Page numbers followed by *f* indicate figures, *t* indicate tables and *b* indicate boxes.

Index